Cerebrovascular Surgery
Volume IV

Cerebrovascular Surgery

Volume IV

Edited by
Jack M. Fein and Eugene S. Flamm

With 194 Illustrations in 242 Parts

Springer-Verlag
New York Berlin Heidelberg Tokyo

JACK M. FEIN, M.D.
Department of Neurological Surgery, Albert Einstein College of Medicine, 1300 Morris Park Avenue, Bronx, NY 10461 USA

EUGENE S. FLAMM, M.D.
Department of Neurosurgery, New York University, 550 First Avenue, New York, NY 10016 USA

Library of Congress Catalog in Publication Data
Main entry under title:
Cerebrovascular surgery.
Includes bibliographies and index.
1. Cerebrovascular disease--Surgery. I. Fein, Jack M.
II. Flamm, Eugene S. [DNLM: 1. Cerebrovascular Disorders --surgery. WL 355 C4138]
RD594.2.C49. 1984. 617'.481. 84-13869

Typeset by Bi-Comp, Inc., York, Pennsylvania.
Printed and bound by Halliday Lithograph, West Hanover, Massachusetts.
Printed in the United States of America.

9 8 7 6 5 4 3 2 1

ISBN 0-387-96026-0 Springer-Verlag New York Berlin Heidelberg Tokyo
ISBN 3-540-96026-0 Springer-Verlag Berlin Heidelberg New York Tokyo

Dedicated to our children
Shari Fein
Andrew and Douglas Flamm

Foreword

Considerable impetus was given to the study and understanding of cerebrovascular anatomy by Thomas Willis and his contemporaries in the seventeenth century, yet almost two hundred years were to pass before further significant advances were made in this field. Then, from the mid-nineteenth century onwards, the dark ages of cerebrovascular research gradually lifted through the efforts of such workers as Luschka, Heubner, and Windle, whose pioneering anatomical studies formed the basis of the present-day understanding of the morphology of the cerebral circulation. The turn of the century saw an increasing influence of the early neurologists in describing anatomy of cerebral vessels in relation to their areas of distribution and to the production of focal deficits through specific vascular lesions and anomalies. Later still, Padget and others made important observations concerning phylogenetic and developmental aspects of the cerebral circulation.

These anatomical and clinical studies were remarkable enough but the real breakthrough in investigating cerebral pathophysiology and in devising appropriate corrective neurosurgical procedures had to await the remarkable advances in technology of the past fifty years. These began with the advent of cerebral angiography with all its subsequent refinements and progress has been accelerated through establishing noninvasive Doppler and high resolution ultrasound imaging techniques, methods for the accurate measurement of cerebral blood flow, CT scanning, PET scanning, and, most recently, imaging and metabolic NMR scanning. Also the electron microscope has facilitated investigation into the structural changes in brain blood vessels in various pathological conditions such as hemorrhagic stroke, cerebral infarction, and hypertension. In line with these numerous technical advances the number of investigations into CNS function carried out by neurosurgeons, neurologists, neuropathologists, physiologists, biochemists, and cell biologists has blossomed.

In contrast, cerebrovascular surgery might be considered still to be in its infancy. Early successes and advances in operative technique owed much to the individual brilliance and surgical expertise of surgeons such as Cushing and Dandy. Although cerebral arterial aneurysms have been operated upon directly for almost fifty years, and carotid occlusive disease since the 1950s, it is only in the past fifteen years that the introduction of the operating microscope, microtechniques, bipolar coagulation, and improved neuroanesthesia has brought about generally acceptable results for most surgeons in these fields.

In spite of the overall development of neuroscience on such a massive scale, we have to ask ourselves just how big are the steps we have taken in the understanding of cerebrovascular disease? Are we really that much nearer to knowing the true relationships of hypertension and cerebral arteriosclerosis, the development of aneurysms and AVMs, carotid occlusive disease, and the etiology and proper treatment of stroke and cerebral vasospasm? We are forced to admit that our therapeutic successes are still severely limited.

The present-day worker in almost every discipline of neuroscience is constantly assailed by steadily increasing numbers of scientific papers, journals, and monographs on his own and allied subjects. Their relevance and relative merits become increasingly difficult to discern in the context of what has gone before and what is currently acceptable theory.

These four volumes form a truly encyclopedic review of all aspects of cerebrovascular disease and its treatment yet remain uncluttered by irrelevant detail and yield so much more than simple lists of facts for reference. They present not only a remarkable perspective and clear review of what has been achieved so far in investigation and treatment of each subject considered, but each section reflects also a sensible and balanced opinion of current thinking in the field with some indication as to which direction we should next take.

I feel that the authors have achieved their aim in presenting these books not simply as reference volumes but in affording the discerning reader with an opportunity to open his mind to new perspectives which may thus stimulate further improvements in the understanding and treatment of cerebrovascular disease.

M. G. Yaşargil

Preface

In the last decade, cerebrovascular surgery has emerged as a distinct subspecialty within neurological surgery. Given the variety of diseases which involve the cerebral circulation and the large number of patients affected, cerebrovascular disorders are an important public health problem. A number of neurosurgeons now devote a major portion of their time to the study and treatment of these problems. Several centers of excellence have developed worldwide and a variety of innovative surgical approaches to these problems have been proposed. Clinical and basic research has widened the cerebrovascular horizon. There have been major advances in our understanding of the pathophysiology of ischemia, subarachnoid hemorrhage, vasospasm, and the hypertensive vasculopathies. Noninvasive imaging techniques such as digital subtraction angiography and quantitative metabolic and hemodynamic studies are becoming more important clinically. Intraoperative monitoring techniques have been refined and microvascular surgery is now a way of life for many surgeons. Many of these advances are described in journal publications, topical monographs, and symposium proceedings. With the growth of interest and concentration in this surgical subspecialty, however, there is a need for a more comprehensive treatment of cerebrovascular surgery.

Cerebrovascular operations require precise surgical skills. These skills are an amalgam of technical facility, knowledge, judgment, experience, and discipline. All four volumes of *Cerebrovascular Surgery* describe technical innovations which have been found useful through trial and error. They provide the fundamental concepts and facts which should form the basis for surgical judgments.

The experience required to formulate a logical surgical plan and the discipline required to carry it through to completion is difficult to describe. Given the variety of approaches to the various cerebrovascular disorders, we felt that this should be a multiauthored work. By pooling such a fund of knowledge the reader is given the opportunity for a broad education in cerebrovascular surgery.

Cerebrovascular surgery cannot be carried out in a vacuum. A sophisticated appreciation of the heart as a pump and the brain as a functional organ are requisite ingredients. Volume I was therefore designed to address these issues and to provide the reader with the insights into the anatomy and physiology of the cerebral circulation. Since microsurgery has become an important component in the treatment of all cerebrovascular disorders, the concluding chapters in Volume I describe the fundamental principles, instrumentation, and techniques utilized in microvascular surgery. Volume II describes the specific management of patients with cerebrovascular occlusive disease. Volume III describes the surgery of arterial aneurysm. This volume completes the series with a description of the surgical treatment of arteriovenous malformations, spontaneous hematomas, and surgery of the sagittal sinus.

The editors would like to acknowledge the efforts of the senior surgeons and their staff who participated in this effort. These individuals will undoubtedly continue to provide the creative leadership needed to reduce the morbidity and mortality due to cerebrovascular disease.

JACK M. FEIN
EUGENE S. FLAMM

Contents of Volume IV

Foreword by *M. G. Yaşargil* vii
Preface.. ix
Contents of Volume I...................................... xiii
Contents of Volume II..................................... xv
Contents of Volume III.................................... xvii
Contributors to Volume IV................................. xix
Contributors to Volumes I–IV.............................. xxi

1 The Pathology of Angiomas 1073
William F. McCormick

2 Supratentorial Arteriovenous Malformations 1097
Bennett M. Stein

3 Infratentorial Arteriovenous Malformations 1117
Francis W. Gamache, Jr. and Russel Patterson, Jr.

4 Venous Angiomas of the Brain 1139
Hajime Handa and Kouzo Moritake

5 Embolization of Cerebral Arteriovenous Malformations...... 1151
W. Jost Michelsen and Sadek K. Hilal

6 Radiosurgery in Cerebral Arteriovenous Malformations...... 1161
Ladislau Steiner

7 Spinal Cord Arteriovenous Malformations 1217
Ayub Khan Ommaya

8 Treatment of Carotid Cavernous and Vertebral Fistulas 1229
Gerard Debrun

9 Surgical Treatment of Hypertensive Intracerebral Hemorrhage
Masahiro Mizukami 1259

10 Posterior Fossa Hematomas 1283
George W. Sypert

11 Cerebellar Infarction....................................... 1299
George W. Sypert

12 Surgery of the Dural Sinuses 1311
R. M. Peardon Donaghy

Index to Volumes I–IV I–1

Contents of Volume I

1 Historical Introduction
Jack M. Fein

2 The Vascular Anatomy of the Cerebral Hemispheres
Georges Salamon, Andre Gouaze, Sharon E. Byrd, and Jean-Marie Corbaz

3 Vascular Anatomy of the Posterior Fossa
Ajax E. George and In-Sup Choi

4 Cerebrovascular Physiology
Niels A. Lassen and Jens Astrup

5 Hematologic Considerations in Cerebrovascular Surgery
Charles A. Owen, Jr. and E. J. Walter Bowie

6 Cardiovascular Considerations in Cerebrovascular Surgery
William H. Frishman, Jack M. Fein, and Marc Kirschner

7 Neurological Evaluation in Cerebrovascular Disease
O. M. Reinmuth and P. N. Karanjia

8 Clinical Evaluation of Cerebral Hemodynamics
Robert H. Ackerman

9 Anesthesia for Neurovascular Surgery
James E. Cottrell and Philippa Newfield

10 The Operating Microscope in Microvascular Surgery
Jack M. Fein

11 Instrumentation for Microvascular Neurosurgery
Leonard I. Malis

12 Photodocumentation in Microvascular Neurosurgery
Ronald I. Apfelbaum

13 The Microsurgical Laboratory
Norman Chater, Z. Szabo, and H. J. Buncke

14 Acquisition of Technical Skills in Microvascular Neurosurgery
Jack M. Fein and Rodney Olinger

Index

Contents of Volume II

1 Neuroradiology of Cerebrovascular Disease
Norman E. Leeds and Robert D. Zimmerman

2 Digital Subtraction Angiography in the Evaluation of Patients with Cerebrovascular Disease
Robert D. Zimmerman, Norman E. Leeds, and Mark J. Goldman

3 Antithrombotic Therapy in Ischemic Cerebrovascular Disease
Robert Coté, C. W. McCormick, and Henry J. M. Barnett

4 Principles of Vascular Surgery
Charles G. Rob

5 Carotid Endarterectomy
Jack M. Fein

6 Occlusive Disease of the Aortic Arch and the Innominate, Carotid, Subclavian, and Vertebral Arteries
Michael E. DeBakey and George P. Noon

7 Subclavian Steal Syndrome
Jim L. Story, Willis E. Brown, Jr., George L. Bohmfalk, and Moustapha Abou-Samra

8 Extracranial-Intracranial Bypass Surgery
Jack M. Fein

9 Intracranial Bypass Grafts for Vertebrobasilar Ischemia
Thoralf M. Sundt, Jr. and David G. Piepgras

10 The Use of Tissue Adhesives in Cerebrovascular Surgery
Hajime Handa, Sen Yamagata, and Waro Taki

11 Dissection of Internal Carotid, Vertebral, and Intracranial Arteries
Robert G. Ojemann

12 Vertebral Artery Insufficiency and Cervical Spondylosis
Chikao Nagashima

13 "Moyamoya" Disease: Clinical Review and Surgical Treatment
Yasuhiro Yonekawa, Takehiko Okuno, and Hajime Handa

14 Cerebral Arteritis
Bennett M. Derby and Humberto M. Cravioto

Index

Contents of Volume III

1 Microsurgical Anatomy of Intracranial Aneurysms
Albert L. Rhoton, Jr., Kiyotaka Fujii, Naokatsu Saeki, David Perlmutter, and Arnold Zeal

2 The Natural History of Intracranial Aneurysms
H. Richard Winn, Alan E. Richardson, and John A. Jane

3 Neuroradiology of Intracranial Aneurysms
Joseph P. Lin and Irvin I. Kricheff

4 The Management of Aneurysmal Subarachnoid Hemorrhage
Eugene S. Flamm

5 Cerebral Vasospasm: Diagnosis and Treatment
Jack M. Fein

6 Graded Carotid Litigation for Aneurysms of the Anterior Circulation
George T. Tindall, Miguel A. Faria, and Alan S. Fleischer

7 Carotid-Ophthalmic Aneurysms
Beniamino Guidetti and Sandro Nicole

8 Internal Carotid Posterior Communicating Artery Aneurysms
Jack M. Fein

9 Middle Cerebral Artery Aneurysms
Eugene S. Flamm and Jack M. Fein

10 Anterior Cerebral Artery Aneurysms
Eugene S. Flamm

11 Stereotactic Thrombosis of Intracranial Aneurysms
John F. Alksne

12 Posterior Circulation Aneurysms
Donald L. Erickson and Shelley N. Chou

13 The Frontotemporal Approach to Basilar Aneurysms
Duke Samson

14 Subarachnoid Hemorrhage in Children
Kenneth Shapiro

15 Electrothrombosis
Hajime Handa, Masatsune Ishikawa, and Shunichi Yoneda

16 Management of Multiple and Asymptomatic Aneurysms
Ronald Brisman

17 Vascular Clips: An Historical and Biomechanical Perspective
Manuel Dujovny, Nir Kossovsky, Ram Kossowsky, Debra Nelson, Norman Wackenhut, Alfred Perlin, and Ranjit K. Laha

18 Infectious Intracranial Aneurysms
Robert G. Ojemann

19 Special Problems Associated with Subarachnoid Hemorrhage
Paul O'Boynick and Charles E. Brackett

Index

Contributors to Volume IV

Gerard Debrun, M.D.
Visiting Professor of Radiology, Harvard Medical School, Director of Interventional Neuroradiology, Massachusetts General Hospital, Boston, Massachusetts 02114 USA

Francis W. Gamache, Jr., M.D.
Assistant Professor of Neurosurgery, Cornell University Medical College, Attending Surgeon, Neurosurgery, New York Hospital, Cornell Medical Center, New York, New York 10021 USA

Hajime Handa, M.D.
Professor and Director of Neurosurgery, Kyoto University Medical School, Sakyo-ku, Kyoto 606, Japan

Sadek K. Hilal, M.D., Ph.D.
Professor of Radiology, Director of Neuroradiology, Columbia University, New York, New York 10032 USA

William F. McCormick, M.S., M.D.
Professor of Neurology, Neurosurgery and Pathology, University of Texas Medical Branch, Galveston, Texas 77550 USA

W. Jost Michelsen, M.D.
Associate Attending Neurosurgeon, Department of Neurosurgery, Columbia Presbyterian Medical Center, New York, New York 10032 USA

Masahiro Mizukami, M.D.
Director, Department of Neurosurgery, Mihara Memorial Hospital, Isesaki, Gunma 372, Japan

Kouzo Moritake, M.D.
Department of Neurosurgery, Kyoto University Medical School, Sakyo-ku, Kyoto 606, Japan

Ayub Khan Ommaya, M.D., M.A., F.R.C.S.
5530 Wisconsin Avenue, Chevychase, Maryland 20815 USA

Russel Patterson, Jr., M.D.
Professor of Surgery, Cornell University Medical College, New York Hospital, New York, New York 10021 USA

Raymond M. Peardon Donaghy, M.D.
Professor Emeritus Neurosurgery, Department of Surgery, University of Vermont, Director, Neurosurgical Research Laboratory, Burlington, Vermont 05405 USA

Bennett M. Stein, M.D.
The Byron Stookey Professor and Chairman, Department of Neurological Surgery, Columbia University, College of Physicians and Surgeons, Director of Neurosurgery, The Neurological Institute of the Presbyterian Hospital of New York, New York, New York 10032 USA

Ladislau Steiner, M.D., Ph.D.
Associate Professor of Neurosurgery, Department of Neurosurgery, Karolinska Institute, Neurosurgeon in Chief, Karolinska Hospital, Stockholm 10401, Sweden

George W. Sypert, M.D., C.M., K.E.
Overstreet Professor of Neurological Surgery and Neuroscience, University of Florida College of Medicine, Gainsville, Florida 32610 USA

Contributors to Volumes I–IV

Abou-Samra, M. *Vol. II, Ch. 7*
Ackerman, R. H. *Vol. I, Ch. 8*
Alksne, J. F. *Vol. III, Ch. 11*
Apfelbaum, R. I. *Vol. I, Ch. 12*
Astrup, J. *Vol. I, Ch. 4*
Barnett, H. J. M. *Vol. II, Ch. 3*
Bohmfalk, G. L. *Vol. II, Ch. 7*
Bowie, E. J. W. *Vol. I, Ch. 5*
Brackett, C. E. *Vol. III, Ch. 19*
Brisman, R. *Vol. III, Ch. 16*
Brown, W. E., Jr. *Vol. II, Ch. 7*
Buncke, H. J. *Vol. I, Ch. 13*
Byrd, S. E. *Vol. I, Ch. 2*
Chater, N. *Vol. I, Ch. 13*
Choi, I-S. *Vol. I, Ch. 3*
Chou, S. N. *Vol. III, Ch. 12*
Corbaz, J-M. *Vol. I, Ch. 2*
Coté, R. *Vol. II, Ch. 3*
Cottrell, J. E. *Vol. I, Ch. 9*
Cravioto, H. M. *Vol. II, Ch. 14*
DeBakey, M. E. *Vol. II, Ch. 6*
Debrun, G. *Vol. IV, Ch. 8*
Derby, B. M. *Vol. II, Ch. 14*
Dujovny, M. *Vol. III, Ch. 17*
Erickson, D. L. *Vol. III, Ch. 12*
Faria, M. A. *Vol. III, Ch. 6*
Fein, J. M. *Vol. I, Ch. 1, 6, 10, 14; Vol. II, Ch. 5, 8; Vol. III, Ch. 5, 8, 9*
Flamm, E. S. *Vol. III, Ch. 4, 9, 10*
Fleischer, A. S. *Vol. III, Ch. 6*
Frishman, W. H. *Vol. I, Ch. 6*
Fujii, K. *Vol. III, Ch. 1*
Gamache, F. W. *Vol. IV, Ch. 3*
George, A. E. *Vol. I, Ch. 3*
Goldman, M. J. *Vol. II, Ch. 2*
Gouaze, A. *Vol. I, Ch. 2*
Guidetti, B. *Vol. III, Ch. 7*
Handa, H. *Vol. II, Ch. 10, 13; Vol. III, Ch. 15; Vol. IV, Ch. 4*
Hilal, S. K. *Vol. IV, Ch. 5*
Ishikawa, M. *Vol. III, Ch. 15*
Jane, J. A. *Vol. III, Ch. 2*
Karanjia, P. N. *Vol. I, Ch. 7*
Kirschner, M. *Vol. I, Ch. 6*
Kossovsky, N. *Vol. III, Ch. 17*
Kossowsky, R. *Vol. III, Ch. 17*
Kricheff, I. I. *Vol. III, Ch. 3*
Laha, R. K. *Vol. III, Ch. 17*
Lassen, N. A. *Vol. I, Ch. 4*
Leeds, N. E. *Vol. II, Ch. 1, 2*
Lin, J. P. *Vol. III, Ch. 3*
Malis, L. I. *Vol. I, Ch. 11*
McCormick, C. W. *Vol. II, Ch. 3*
McCormick, W. F. *Vol. IV, Ch. 1*
Michelsen, W. J. *Vol. IV, Ch. 5*
Mizukami, M. *Vol. IV, Ch. 9*
Moritake, K. *Vol. IV, Ch. 4*
Nagashima, C. *Vol. II, Ch. 12*

Nelson, D. *Vol. III, Ch. 17*
Newfield, P. *Vol. I, Ch. 9*
Nicole, S. *Vol. III, Ch. 7*
Noon, G. P. *Vol. II, Ch. 6*
O'Boynick, P. *Vol. III, Ch. 19*
Ojemann, R. G. *Vol. II, Ch. 11; Vol. III, Ch. 18*
Okuno, T. *Vol. II, Ch. 13*
Olinger, R. *Vol. I, Ch. 14*
Ommaya, A. K. *Vol. IV, Ch. 7*
Owen, C. A. *Vol. I, Ch. 5*
Patterson, R. *Vol. IV, Ch. 3*
Peardon Donaghy, R. M. *Vol. IV, Ch. 12*
Perlin, A. *Vol. III, Ch. 17*
Perlmutter, D. *Vol. III, Ch. 1*
Piepgras, D. G. *Vol. II, Ch. 9*
Reinmuth, O. M. *Vol. I, Ch. 7*
Rhoton, A. L., Jr. *Vol. III, Ch. 1*
Richardson, A. E. *Vol. III, Ch. 2*
Rob, C. G. *Vol. II, Ch. 4*
Saeki, N. *Vol. III, Ch. 1*
Salamon, G. *Vol. I, Ch. 2*
Samson, D. *Vol. III, Ch. 13*
Shapiro, K. *Vol. III, Ch. 14*
Stein, B. M. *Vol. IV, Ch. 2*
Steiner, L. *Vol. IV, Ch. 6*
Story, J. L. *Vol. II, Ch. 7*
Sundt, T. M., Jr. *Vol. II, Ch. 9*
Sypert, G. W. *Vol. IV, Ch. 10, 11*
Szabo, Z. *Vol. I, Ch. 13*
Taki, W. *Vol. II, Ch. 10*
Tindall, G. T. *Vol. III, Ch. 6*
Wackenhut, N. *Vol. III, Ch. 17*
Winn, H. R. *Vol. III, Ch. 2*
Yamagata, S. *Vol. II, Ch. 10*
Yaşargil, M. G. *Foreword*
Yoneda, S. *Vol. III, Ch. 15*
Yonekawa, Y. *Vol. II, Ch. 13*
Zeal, A. *Vol. III, Ch. 1*
Zimmerman, R. D. *Vol. II, Ch. 1, 2,*

1

The Pathology of Angiomas

William F. McCormick

Introduction

Angiomas are vascular malformations that derive from the failure of normal maturation ("resolution") of embryonic vascular networks. Despite the name "angioma," they are not neoplastic. Their histologic classification is based on the morphologic type of the component vessels. The following classification is both simple and practical; it also allows for considerable prognostication of behavior.

The literature on angiomas is now so voluminous that a truly comprehensive review is impractical if not impossible. Many of the more important references prior to 1970 can be found in the bibliography of several earlier papers.[37–43,45]

A brief statement detailing how my opinions on classification and natural history were derived is necessary. Over the past quarter of a century, I have had the opportunity to examine more than 1,000 angiomas in the central nervous system; about half of them were derived from my own direct autopsy and surgical services and the others from the Armed Forces Institute of Pathology and from consultations and gifts from many kind colleagues. The very large total number of cases has allowed me to feel secure in making what would otherwise be very presumptious and overly dogmatic statements. Prevalence figures are derived from my consecutive autopsy material of the last 19 years.

Classification and Descriptions

The chief justification for any classification of angiomas is its ability to distinguish biologic differences between the various types. It is now abundantly clear that there are such differences, and that each major type has its own natural history as well as morphologic appearance. Many of these differences will be discussed in later sections of this chapter.

I have been able to divide the angiomas I have studied into four major types based on their component vessels and intervascular neural parenchyma. Forms transitional between the major types do occur, and these are also discussed. Diagnosis of the angioma type is based on both gross and microscopic patterns. Elastic tissue stains are often needed to rule out arterial components. Multiple sections, often encompassing the entire specimen, are frequently employed in my laboratory. Brief formal definitions and descriptions are given below.

Arteriovenous Malformations (AVM)

These angiomas are masses of arteries, "arteriolized veins," and veins (Figs. 1.1 and 1.2).

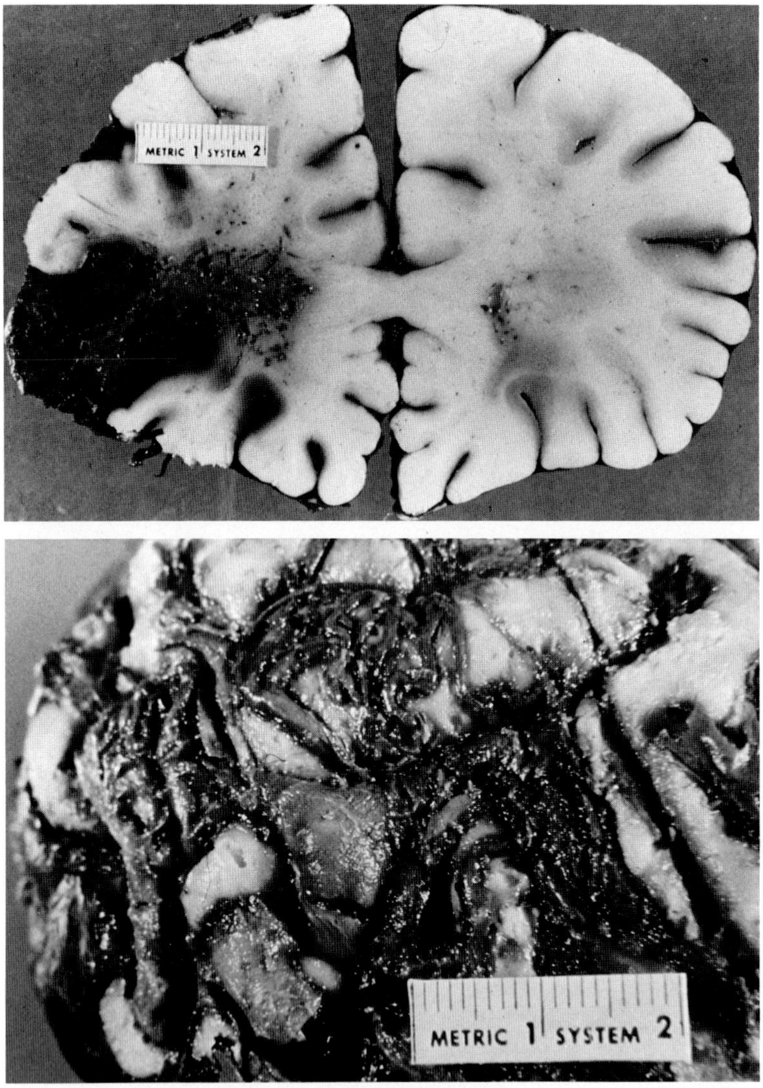

A

B

Fig. 1.1. **A.** Coronal section of a typical large lobar AVM with its conical configuration and deep penetration of the brain parenchyma. **B.** Frontal lobe with leptomeninges removed to show surface vessels of the large AVM seen in Fig. 1a. The larger vessels are arteriolized veins.

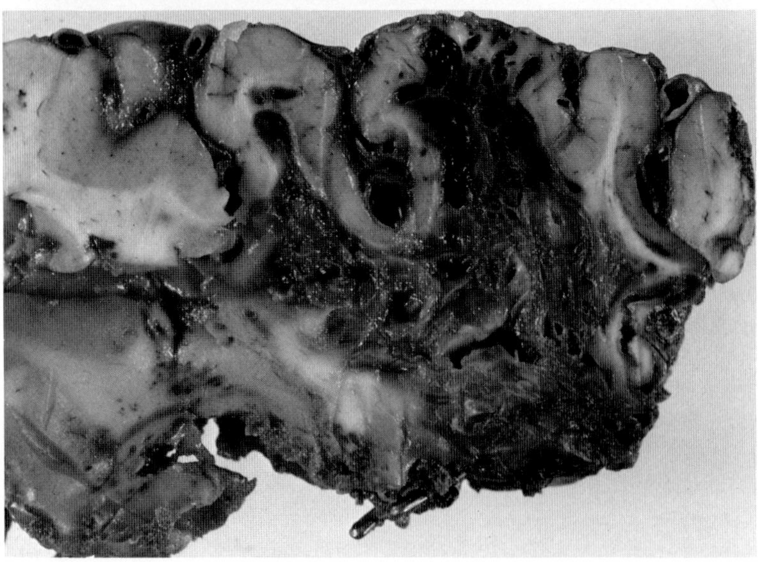

Fig. 1.2. Cross-section of a large, surgically resected AVM. Both cortex and white matter are involved. The neural parenchyma within the angioma is abnormal.

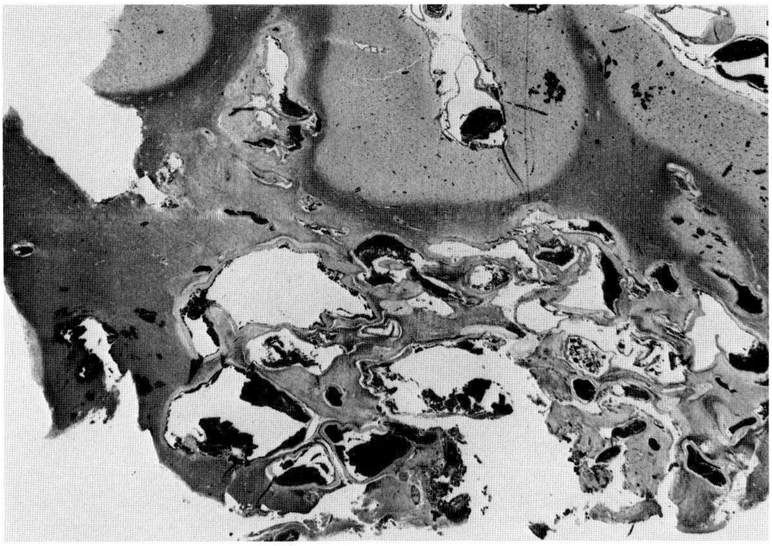

Fig. 1.3. Photomacrograph of typical cerebral AVM with variable-sized vessels and severely damaged and malformed parenchyma between the component vessels. The larger vessels are veins. (Trichromc; ×3)

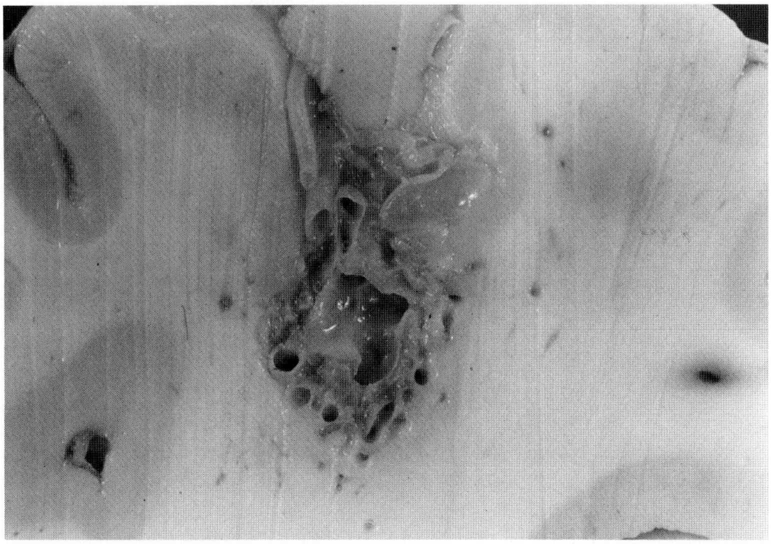

Fig. 1.4. Cryptic AVM in the frontal lobe. Note the very large arteriolized central vein.

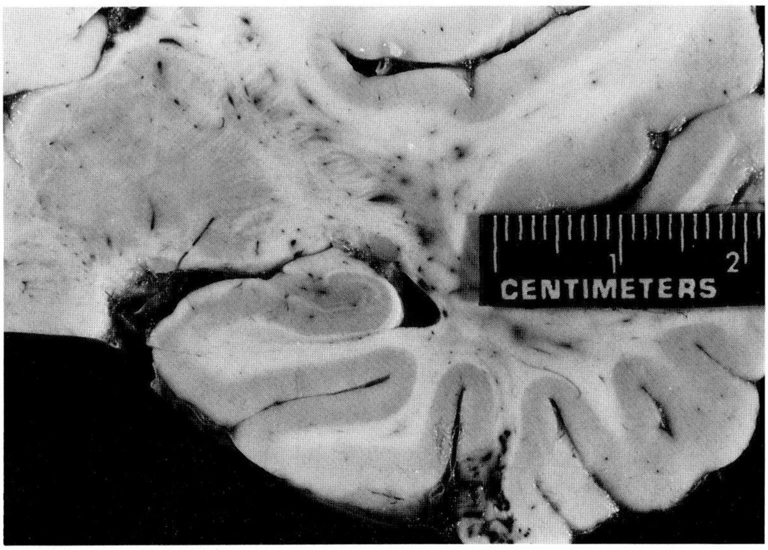

Fig. 1.5. Cryptic AVM in fusiform gyrus. There has been a mild acute hemorrhage from this very small angioma.

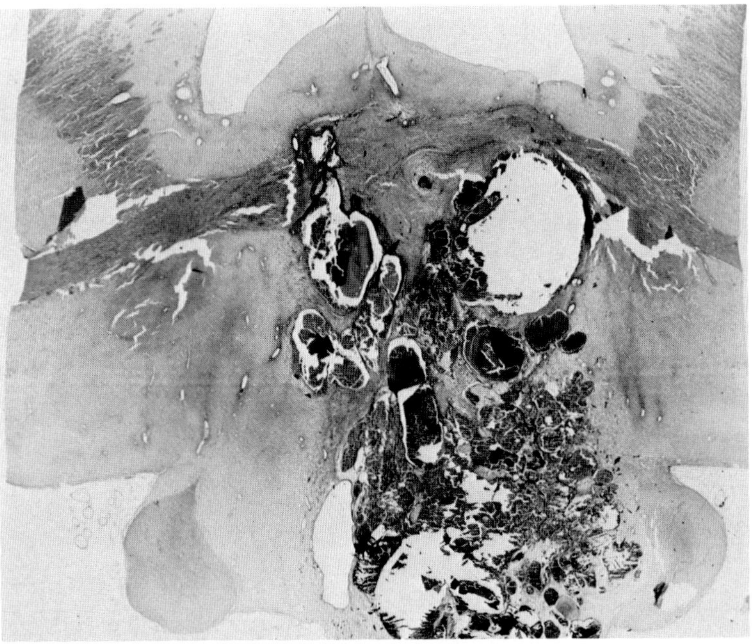

Fig. 1.6. Cryptic AVM in hypothalamus with compact vessels grossly closely resembling a cavernous angioma. (H&E; ×3)

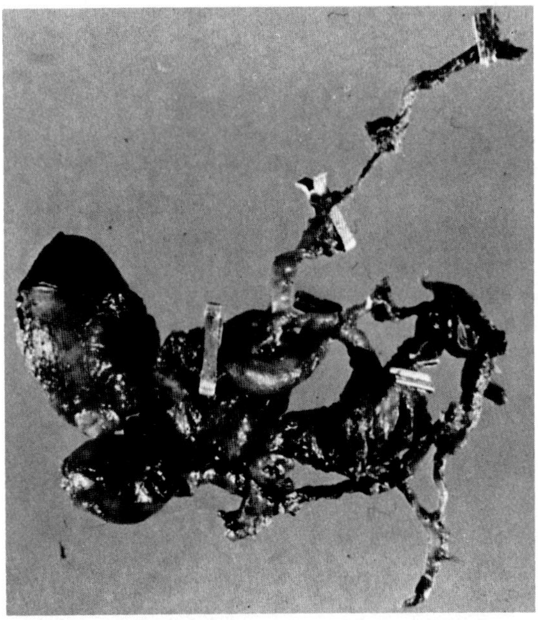

Fig. 1.7. Dissected AVM with neural parenchyma removed to illustrate the marked segmental venous sacculations that are typical of these angiomas.

The component vessels vary greatly in size with the larger vessels always of the venous type (Figs. 1.2 and 1.3). In many instances, especially the smaller "cryptic" forms (Figs. 1.4 and 1.5), the arterial supply is small and difficult to demonstrate. The compactness of the component vessels varies considerably from specimen to specimen; some are so compact as to resemble cavernous angiomas in many ways (Fig. 1.6). Segmental dilatation, even to the point of discrete sacculations of component vessels, is common (Figs. 1.4 and 1.7). The majority of these greatly dilated vessels are clearly venous in origin (Fig. 1.8), and true arterial sacculations (i.e., arterial aneurysms) do not appear to be a component of the AVM. Varying sized nodules of smooth muscle and intima often project into the lumena of the component veins (Fig. 1.9) and amyloid-like material is sometimes encountered in the vessel walls. Abnormal, gliotic parenchyma occurs between many of the component vessels (Fig. 1.10), and foci of hemosiderin-laden macrophages are commonly encountered (Fig. 1.11). No recognizable normal capillary bed is found in any of these angiomas.[40,63] Mineralization of some of the component vessels and/or the intermeshed and adjacent gliotic neural parenchyma is found in about 10% of cases.* Bone formation is far

* References 8, 16, 21, 37, 38, 39, 40, 42, 62.

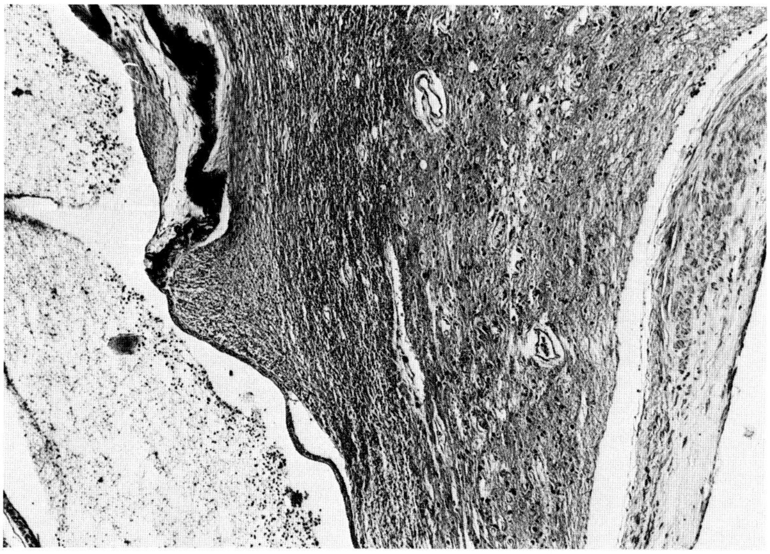

Fig. 1.8. Photomicrograph of an AVM showing parts of the walls of two large arteriolized venous sacculations. There is considerable variation in wall thickness and smooth muscle content in these veins. (Trichrome; ×80)

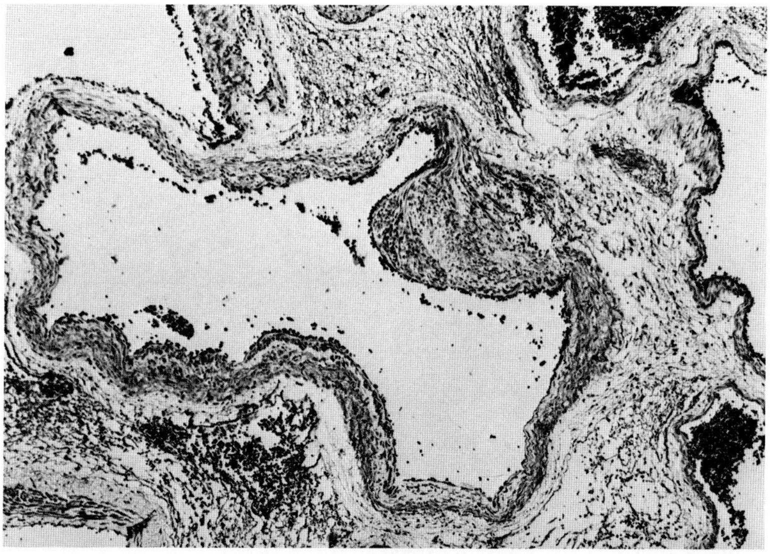

Fig. 1.9. Photomicrograph of AVM with dysplastic smooth muscle nodule projecting into an arteriolized vein. (Trichrome; ×200)

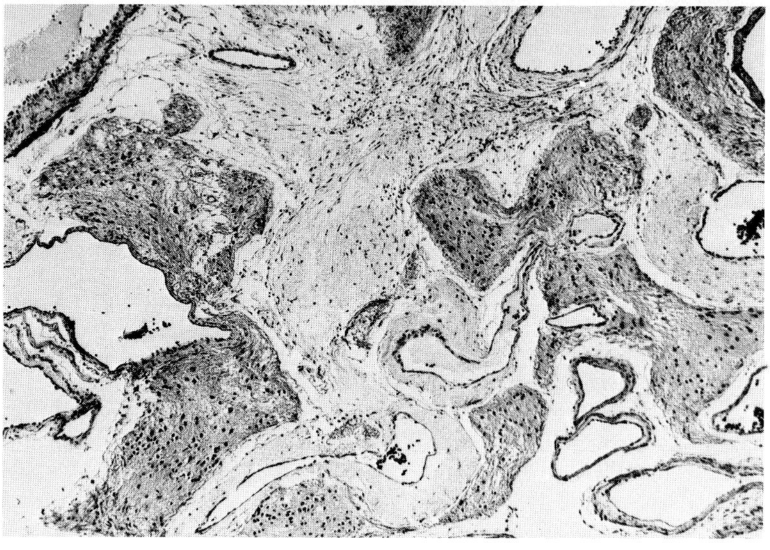

Fig. 1.10. Photomicrograph illustrating tongues of gliotic neural parenchyma projecting between the component vessels of the AVM. (H&E; ×80)

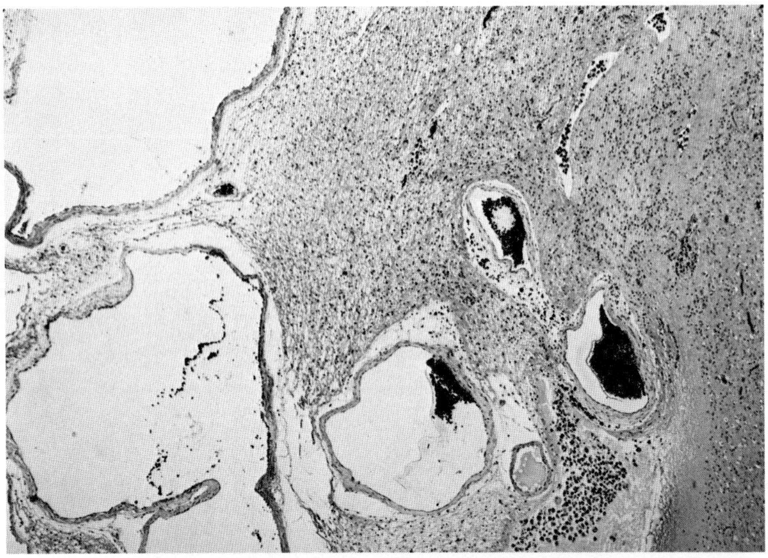

Fig. 1.11. Hemosiderin deposited in abnormal parenchyma about an AVM (Trichrome; ×50)

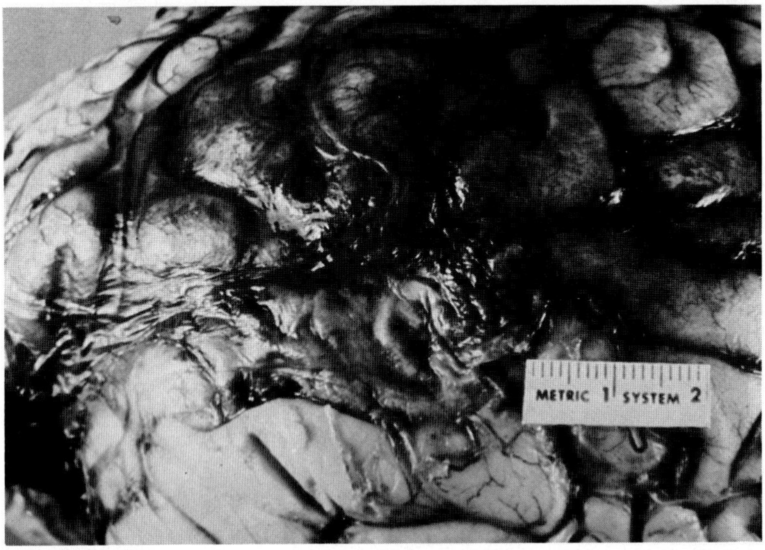

Fig. 1.12. Gross appearance of thickened leptomeninges overlying an AVM in the Sylvian fissure.

less often encountered in these angiomas than in the cavernous variety.[37,38,40,42,45] Varying degrees of spontaneous thrombosis of component vessels are common in these angiomas and may be so complete as to cause them to spontaneously disappear on angiography.** Inflammation associated with thrombosis may be so marked that it simulates infection both clinically and pathologically. Progressive thrombosis with and without significant inflammation is occasionally particularly prominent in the spinal angiomas in the so-called Foix-Alajouanine syndrome, a condition historically misdiagnosed as a phlebitis. The leptomeninges overlying superficial AVMs are often quite thickened and opacified a milky-white (Fig. 1.12).[37,40,45]

Symptoms due to "steal"* are most common in this type of angioma, which is by far the best known type of angioma and the one that is most often clinically symptomatic. Angiography will usually demonstrate a shunt from arterial to venous circulation, unlike the general failure of

** References 1, 7, 8, 13, 14, 15, 20, 21, 32, 34–36, 39, 40, 42, 45, 48, 50, 55, 62, 69, 72.

* References 14, 17, 25, 28, 33, 39, 40, 42, 48, 57, 63.

such demonstrable shunting in the other angioma types.

Venous Angiomas

These angiomas are composed of a group of anomalous veins and are by far the most frequently recognized type found at autopsy (Table 1.1) (Fig. 1.13).[11,39,40,45,58,60] The component

Table 1.1. Histologic type of angiomas in 274 patients (from consecutive autopsy series of 5,850 patients).

Age		Types	Patients[a]
Youngest:	new born	Venous (+ varix)	175 (+4)
Oldest:	89 years	Telangiectasis	52
		Arteriovenous	30
		Cavernous	19
Sex[b]			
Male:	172		
Female:	102		

[a] Of these 274 patients, 16 had multiple angiomas. One patient had Sturge-Weber disease and two had massive bilateral arteriovenous angiomas with Galen's vein aneurysms. Sixteen patients also had saccular aneurysms. Some of these patients had two different types of angiomas (such as a venous angioma in the cerebellum and a cavernous angioma in the cerebrum) and would be listed here under both venous and cavernous headings. The total number of angiomas found is therefore different from the total number of patients.

[b] Our autopsy population is approximately M : F = 1.7 : 1.

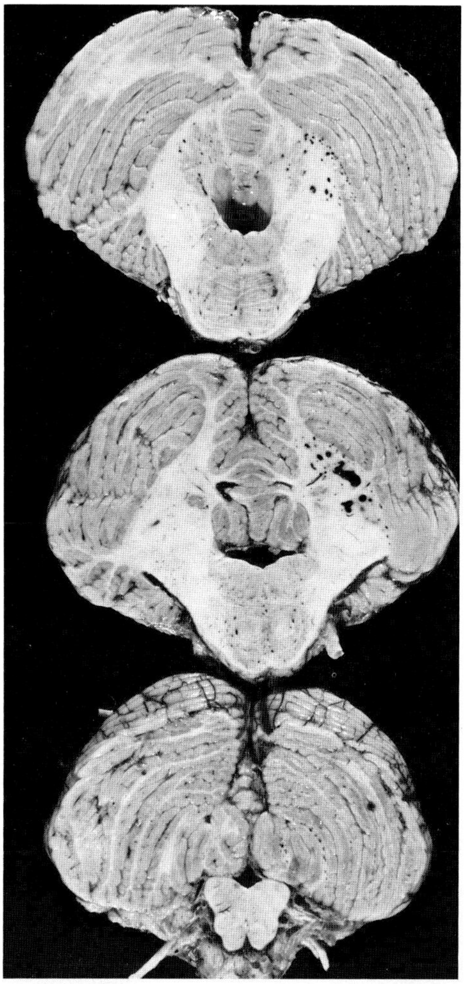

Fig. 1.13. Cryptic venous angioma in right cerebellar hemisphere. Large central draining vein is seen in middle section.

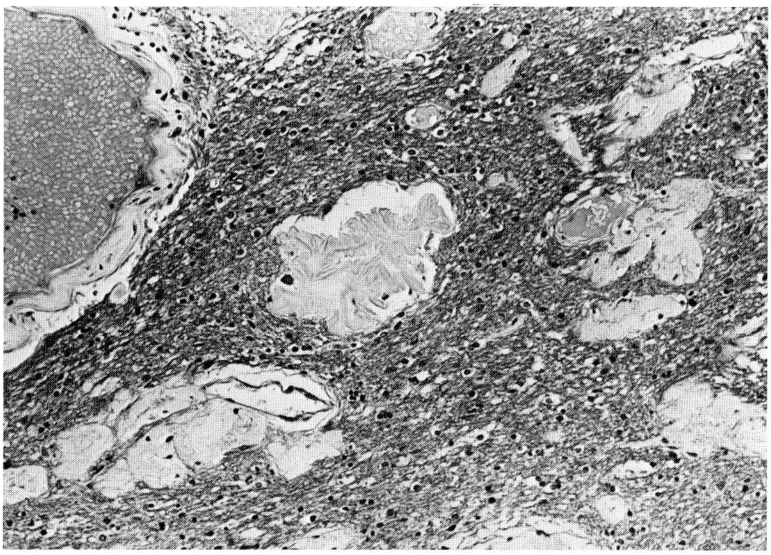

Fig. 1.14. Photomicrograph of venous angioma showing the essentially normal neural parenchyma between the component vessels of the angioma. Many of the veins are quite sclerotic and hyalinized. (H&E; ×80)

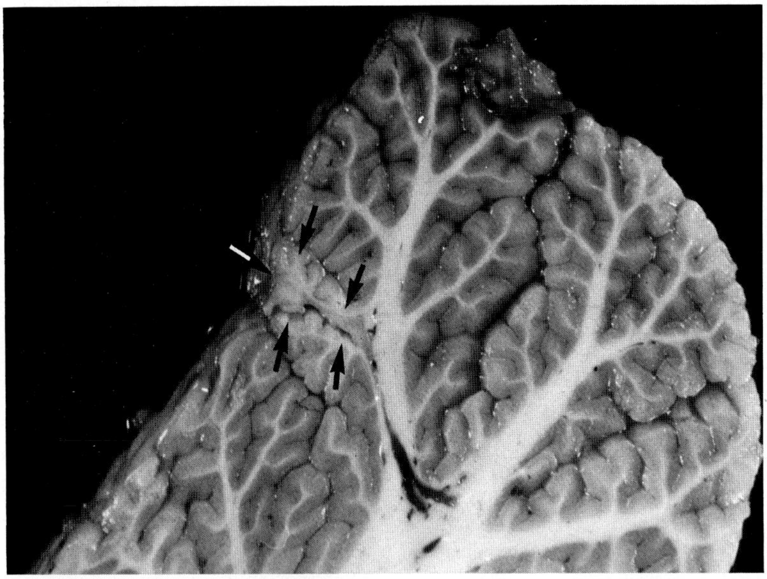

Fig. 1.15. Venous angioma in cerebellum with focal folial sclerosis due to "steal."

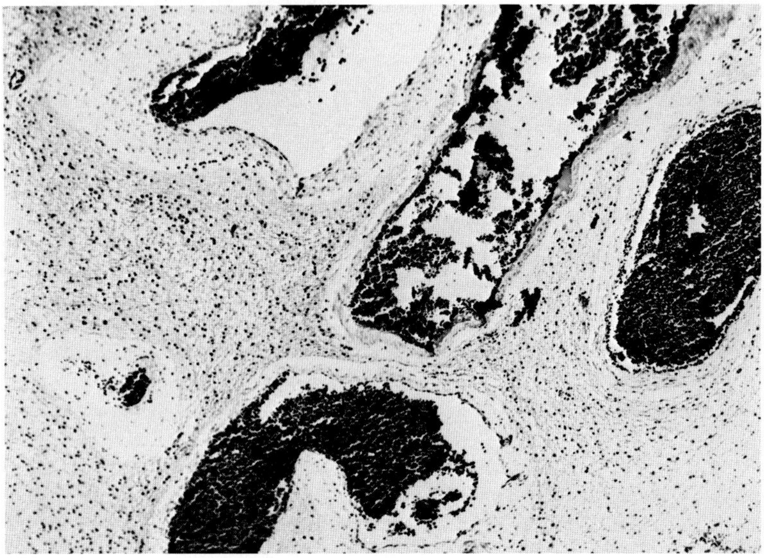

Fig. 1.16. Thickened walls in a venous angioma, best seen in vein at top. (H&E; Box)

veins are separated by neural parenchyma, which is usually morphologically normal (Fig. 1.14). One or more central draining veins are generally conspicuous (Fig. 1.13) and may be very large and varicose. Gliosis and evidence of neural ischemia ("steal") can occur, but are not frequent; it may be quite focal (Fig. 1.15).[39,40,45] Mineralization in or about these angiomas is distinctly rare. The walls of the veins in these angiomas may become quite thick and hyalinized (Figs. 1.14 and 1.16). Composed as they are only of veins and with no direct arterial input, these angiomas will not opacify during the arterial phases of angiography.[11,40,58,60]

The "varix" is a single dilated vein, often with a thickened and fibrotic hyalinized wall. In the past, I have classified these anomalies as a separate type of angioma,[37–39,41–43,45] but the fact that they are composed of only one vein prompts me to reconsider them as a variant of the venous angioma.[40] These congenital malformations appear to be uncommon, but their apparent infrequency may reflect only an inability to recognize a single anomalous vein unless large. They can reach a size sufficient to produce symptoms from compression of adjacent structures. Occasionally, venous-phase angiography clearly demonstrates these anomalies.

Cavernous Angiomas

These angiomas are composed of a relatively compact mass of sinusoidal-type vessels immediately in apposition to each other with no intervening parenchyma (Figs. 1.17 and 1.18). They appear as a compact purplish mass and, when small, may resemble a parenchymal hemorrhage (Figs. 1.19 and 1.20). There is often gross and usually microscopic evidence of blood leakage, with numerous hemosiderin-laden macrophages in the adjacent, often gliotic neural parenchyma (Figs. 1.21 and 1.22). Marked hyalinization and thickening of component vascular channels especially the more peripheral ones, are common (Fig. 1.23). Mineralization or even ossification[19,37,42,45] occurs in some of the larger cavernous angiomas. These angiomas, especially when superficial and large, may become virtually encapsulated.

Cavernous angiomas can be found in all parts of the CNS, including the spinal cord (Figs. 1.22 and 1.24). These angiomas do not visualize well if at all on angiography owing to the absence of a direct arterial input.[40,68]

Capillary Angiomas (Telangiectasis)

These angiomas are composed of small, capillary type vessels. Typically of very limited size (0.3–1.0 cm) (Fig. 1.25), they appear as a pinkish, discolored, sometimes finely spongy area (Fig. 1.26). They are apparently most common in but by no means confined to the pons (Table 1.2) (Fig. 1.27). The component vessels may reach a diameter larger than normal for a capillary, but their walls are morphologically capil-

Table 1.2. Location of 173 angiomas in 164 consecutive angioma autopsies.[a]

Type of angioma	No. of specific type	Location of angioma
Venous	112 (2 with extensive hemorrhage)	81 cerebral lobar 26 cerebellar 3 basal ganglia 2 brainstem
Capillary (telangiectases)	41 (none with extensive hemorrhage)	21 striate (basis) pons 2 medulla 4 basal ganglia 13 cerebral lobar 1 cerebellar
AVM	11 (3 with extensive hemorrhage)	6 cerebral lobar 2 basal ganglia 1 massive and bilateral cerebral with vein of Galen aneurysm 1 spinal cord (lumbar) 1 medulla and upper cervical cord
Cavernous	5 (none with extensive hemorrhage)	4 cerebral lobar 1 spinal cord (thoracic)
Transitional	4 (none with extensive hemorrhage) (1 venous-cavernous; 2 venous-telangiectasis; 1 cavernous-telangiectasis)	3 cerebral lobar 1 pons (tegmentum)

[a] 9 cadavers contained multiple CNS angiomas; 7 cadavers contained angiomas and saccular aneurysms.

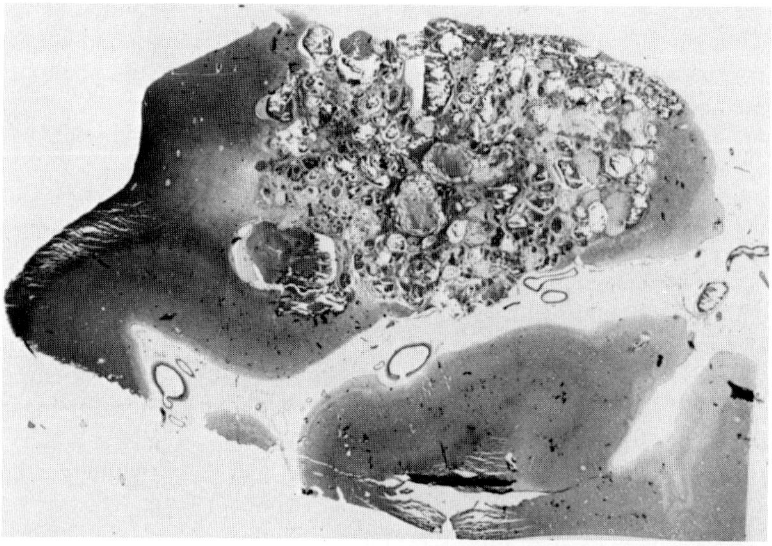

Fig. 1.17. Photomacrograph of small cavernous angioma with compact, sinusoidal vessels. (Trichrome; ×3)

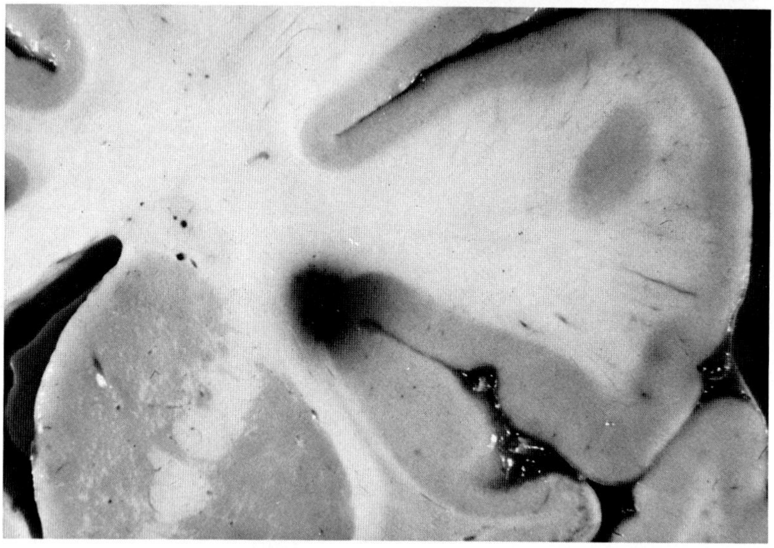

Fig. 1.18. Cavernous angioma with sinusoidal vessels adjacent to each other without intervening neural parenchyma. (H&E; ×80)

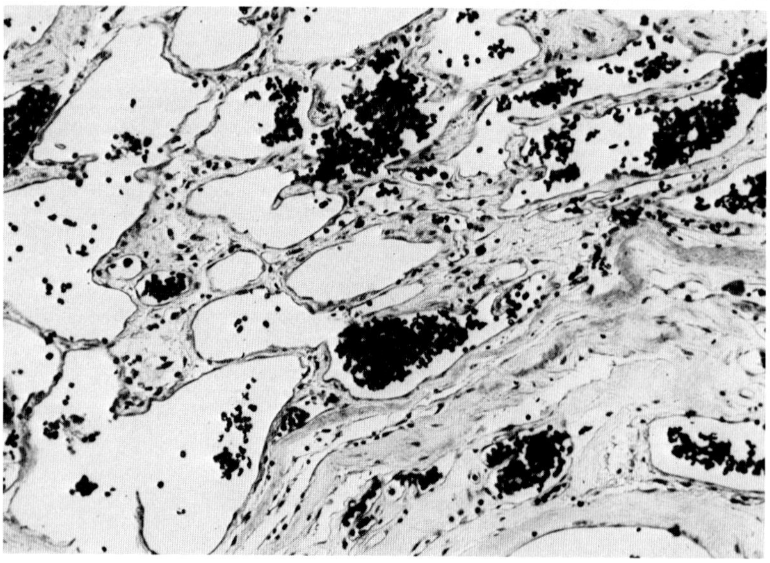

Fig. 1.19. Small cavernous angioma at cortical-white matter junction resembling a small fresh hemorrhage.

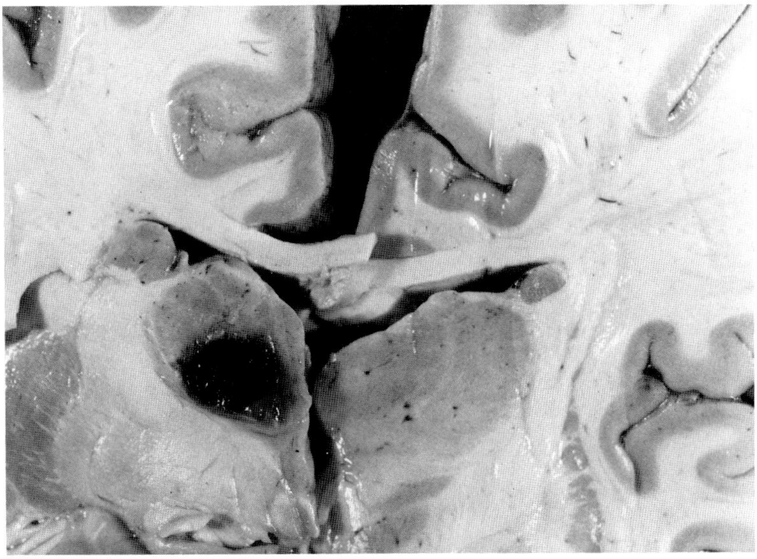

Fig. 1.20. Cavernous angioma in thalamus.

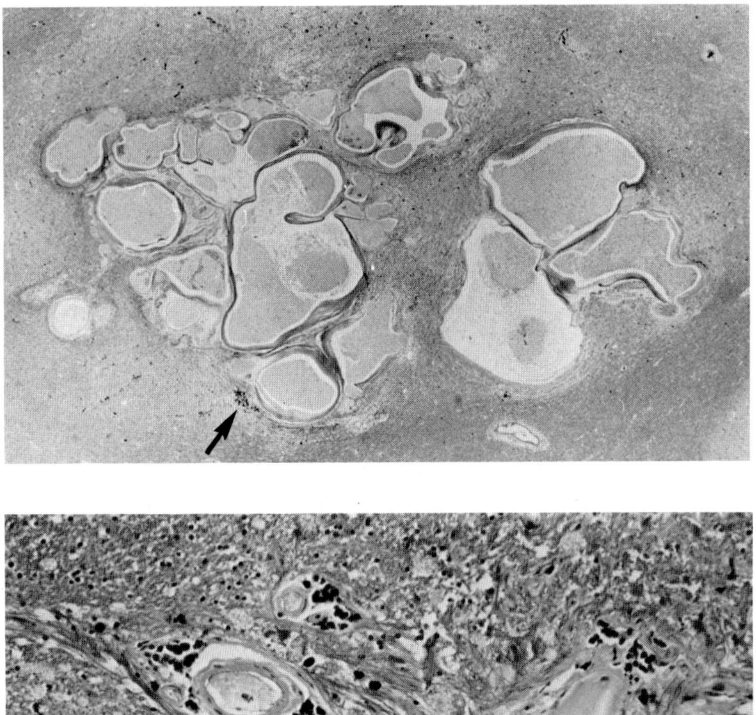

Fig. 1.21. Photomacrograph of small cavernous angioma with deposits of hemosiderin-laden macrophages in adjacent neural parenchyma (*arrow*). (H&E; ×3)

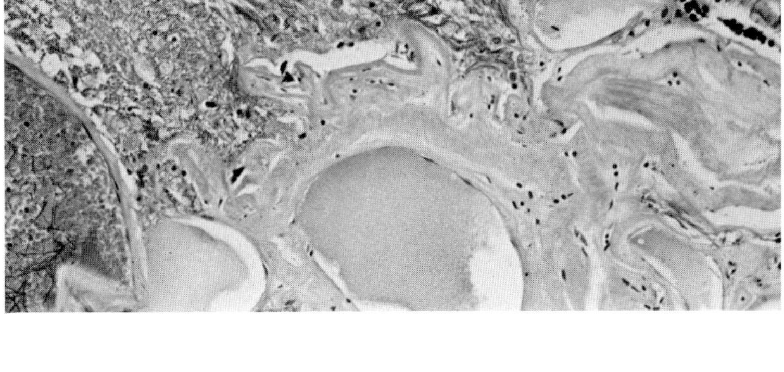

Fig. 1.22. There is evidence of remote bleeding from this spinal cord cavernous angioma. Hemosiderin and reactive gliosis may be quite abundant about cavernous angioma. (H&E; ×200)

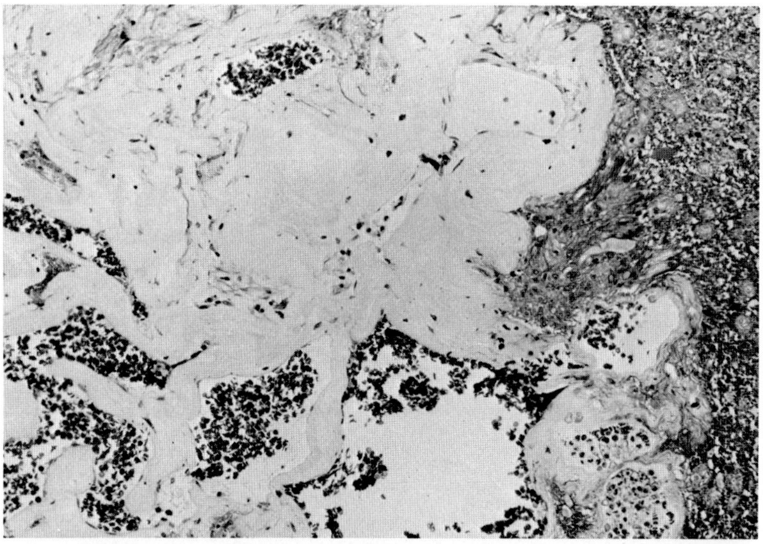

Fig. 1.23. The sinusoidal vessels of a cavernous angioma often become thickened and hyalinized. (Trichrome; ×80)

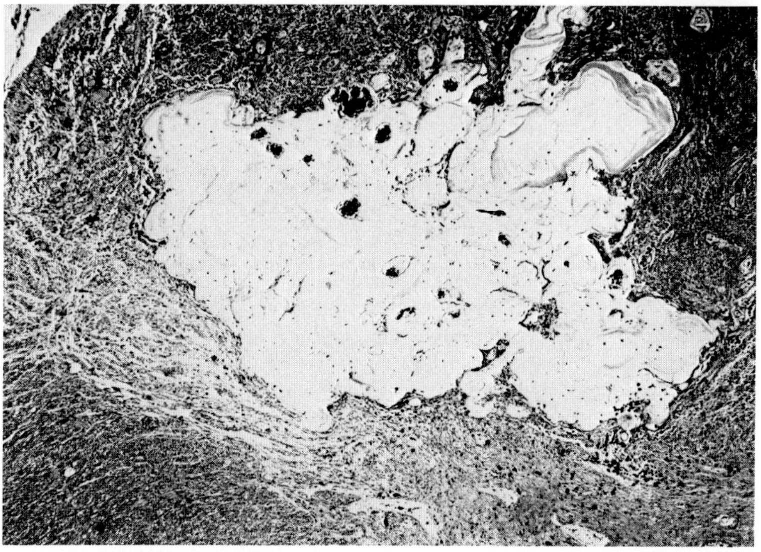

Fig. 1.24. Cavernous angioma in the spinal cord. These angiomas can occur in any part of CNS. (Trichrome; ×3)

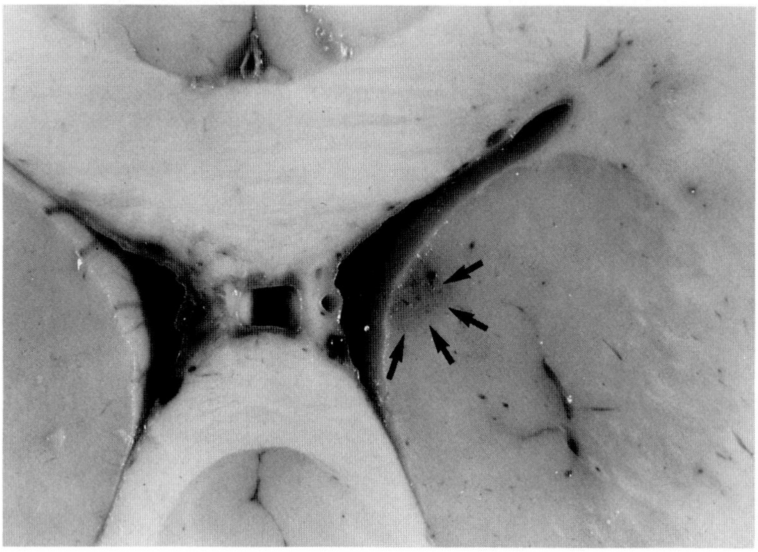

Fig. 1.25. Capillary angioma (telangiectasis) in caudate nucleus. These angiomas generally appear as a pinkish area and are typically small.

lary-like (Figs. 1.28 and 1.29). The component vessels are separated from each other by more or less normal neural parenchyma (Fig. 1.30). Gliosis, mineralization, and significant hemorrhage are very uncommon but can occur (Table 1.3). Transitional forms between these malformations and either the cavernous and venous types are sometimes encountered.[39,40]

These angiomas are not visualized at angiography.

Transitional Forms

Transitional types of angiomas that do not fit cleanly into one of the four types described are encountered. The great majority of these angiomas have discrete areas that are grossly and histologically of one type and adjacent areas of another (Figs. 1.31 to 33). I tend to classify these angiomas according to the most abundant (extensive) vessel type (in much the same way we classify gliomas according to their predominant cell type) unless the two component types are about equally voluminous. Angiomas reported as cavernous but with angiographically demonstrated arterial inflow[49,55] are almost certainly of this transitional type. This method of

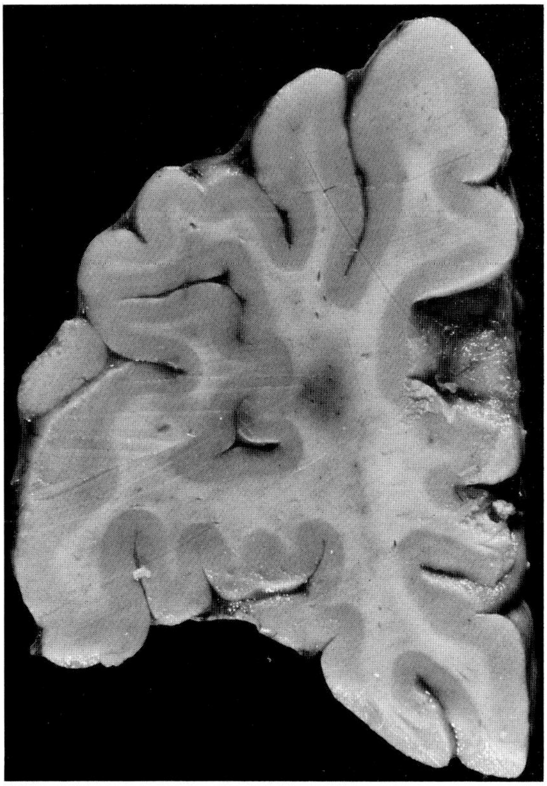

Fig. 1.26. Capillary angioma (telangiectasis) in left frontal white matter. These angiomas often appear as a pink, fine spongy area.

Table 1.3. Angiomas causing massive brain hemorrhage.[a]

Age/sex	Hypertension	Location	Type
17 M	−	Thalamus and hypothalamus	Telangiectasis
15 M	−	L striate	Arteriovenous
29 F	−	Thalamus and hypothalamus	Arteriovenous
12 F	−	Cerebellar vermis and L hemisphere	Arteriovenous
55 M	+	L striatum	Arteriovenous
48 F	−	L striatum	Arteriovenous
61 M	+	L cerebellar hemisphere	Arteriovenous
64 M	+	L temporal	Arteriovenous
15 M	−	L frontal	Arteriovenous
1-Day M	−	L cerebellar hemisphere	Arteriovenous
37 M	−	L cerebellar hemisphere	Arteriovenous
31 F	−	L cerebellar hemisphere	Arteriovenous
48 F	+	R temporal	Arteriovenous
65 F	−	Pons and medulla	Arteriovenous
61 M	−	L parietal	Arteriovenous
25 F	−	R parietal lobar	Venous
52 M	−	R temporal lobar	Arteriovenous
26 M	−	L parietal and thalamic	Arteriovenous

[a] From an autopsy series of 274 consecutive angioma autopsies.

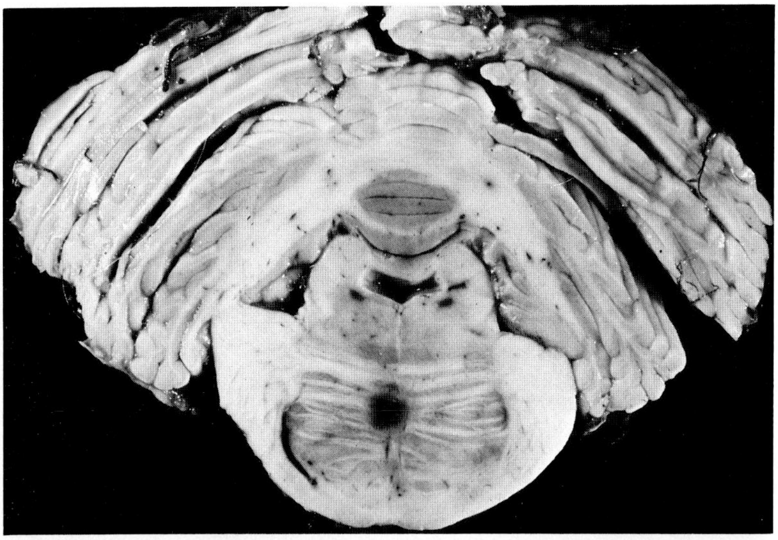

Fig. 1.27. Capillary angioma (telangiectasis) in striate pons. This is the most common location for these angiomas.

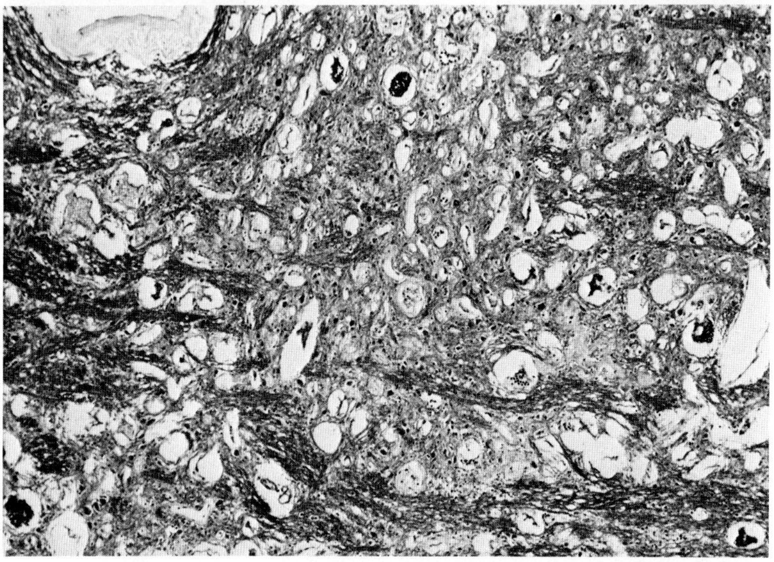

Fig. 1.28. Capillary angioma in striate pons. (H&E; ×50)

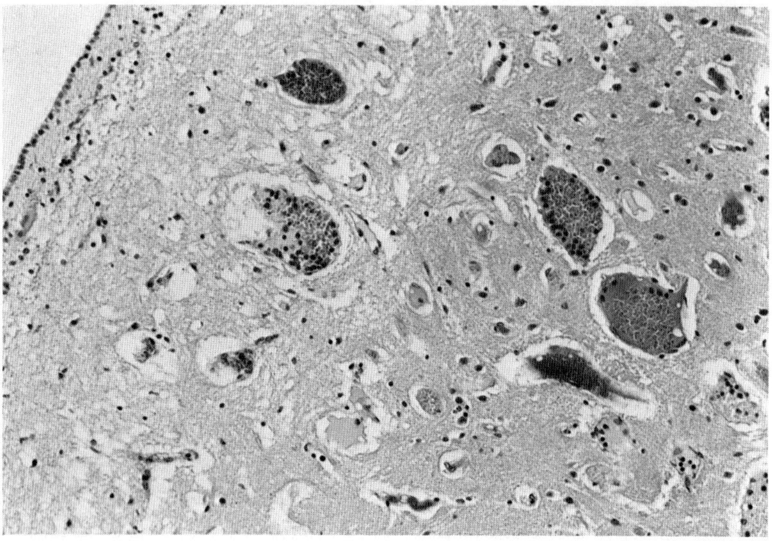

Fig. 1.29. Capillary angioma (from caudate; Fig. 1.25) showing variable vessel diameter but capillary-type wall. (H&E; ×80)

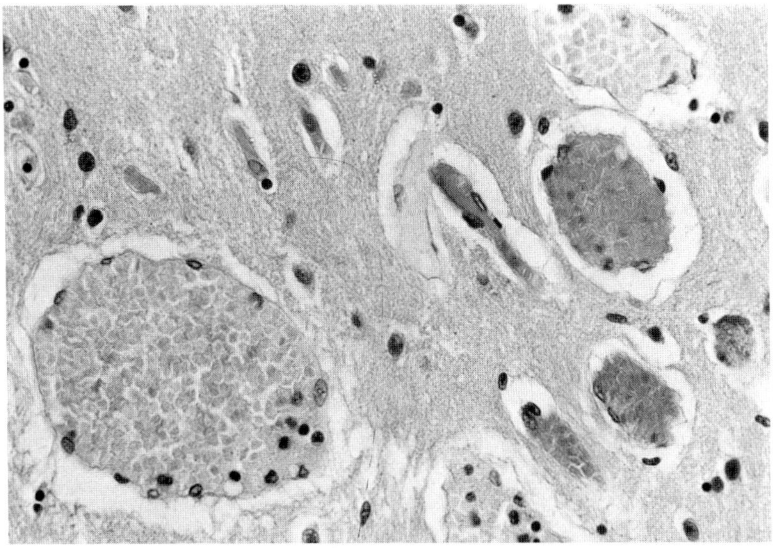

Fig. 1.30. Photomicrograph of a capillary angioma illustrating normal neural parenchyma between component capillaries of the angioma. (H&E; ×200)

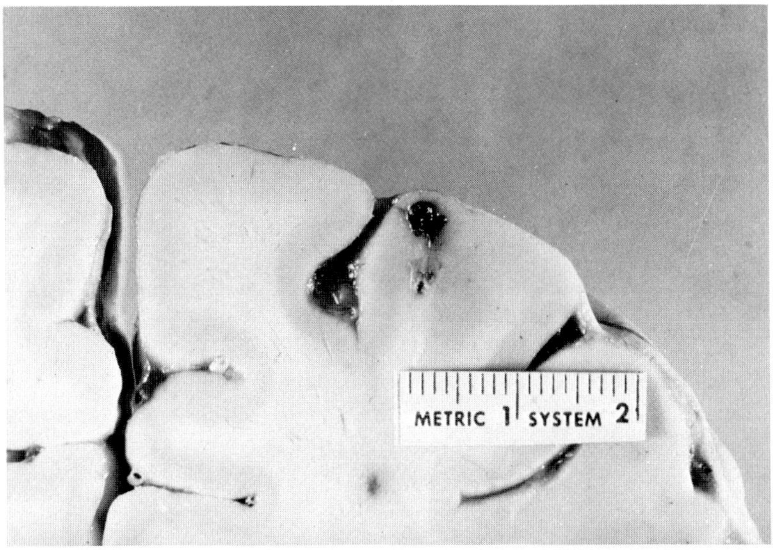

Fig. 1.31. Cryptic angioma transitional in form between cavernous and venous. The compact mass in the cortex is the cavernous component.

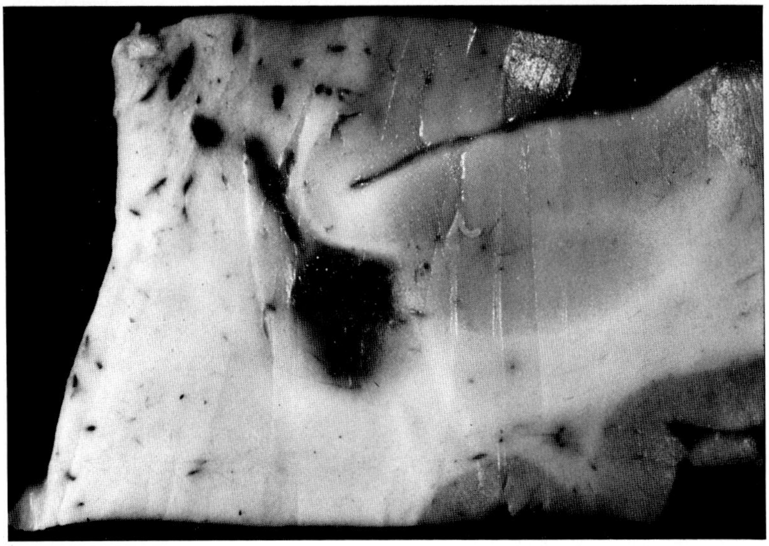

Fig. 1.32. Transitional cavernous and venous angioma in the cerebrum. The venous component appears above the compact cavernous area.

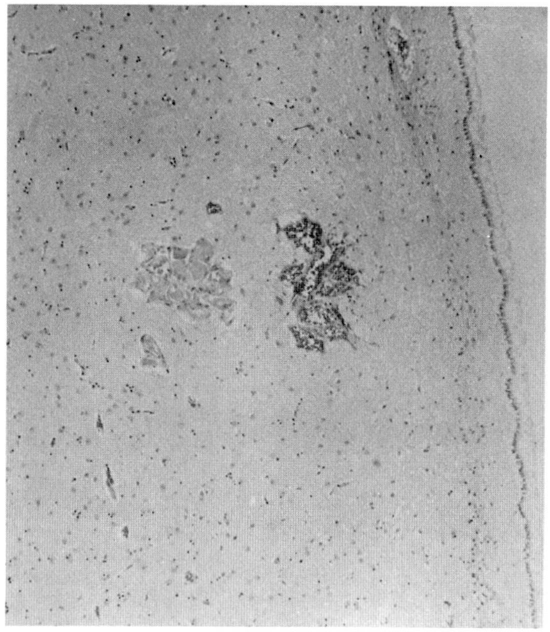

Fig. 1.33. Two minute cavernous angiomas in the subependymal region of the caudate nucleus. These angiomas appeared grossly as petechiae. (H&E; ×30)

classification seems to be consistent with biological behavior.

The histologic types of angiomas in a personal consecutive autopsy series is shown in Table 1.1.

"Cryptic" Angiomas

The term "cryptic" is applied to small (Figs. 1.3–1.5), at times virtually microscopic (Figs. 1.34 and 1.35), clinically silent angiomas popularized in 1954 by Dorothy Russell. This group of angiomas have in common only their hidden (i.e., cryptic quality) and can be of any histologic type and occur at any location.[43] At one time considered uncommon medical "curiosities," it is now clear that small, clinically silent angiomas are the rule and not the exception.* Indeed, in my consecutive autopsy material, it is obvious that completely asymptomatic angiomas are ten times as common as symptomatic ones due principally to the overwhelming predominance of venous and capillary (telangiectasis) forms. Many believe these small angiomas pose a greater risk of rupture than do their larger counterparts,[1,6,8,21,22,39] but this has not been substantiated in several large studies of mine[40,42] in which the larger malformations more often bled. As small, "cryptic" angiomas are far more common than larger angiomas, more frequent bleeding from cryptic angiomas would not be unexpected and may not actually reflect a different biology. Many of the cryptic angiomas can not be demonstrated by angiogra-

* References 6–9, 20, 21, 27, 40, 51, 54, 56, 64, 65.

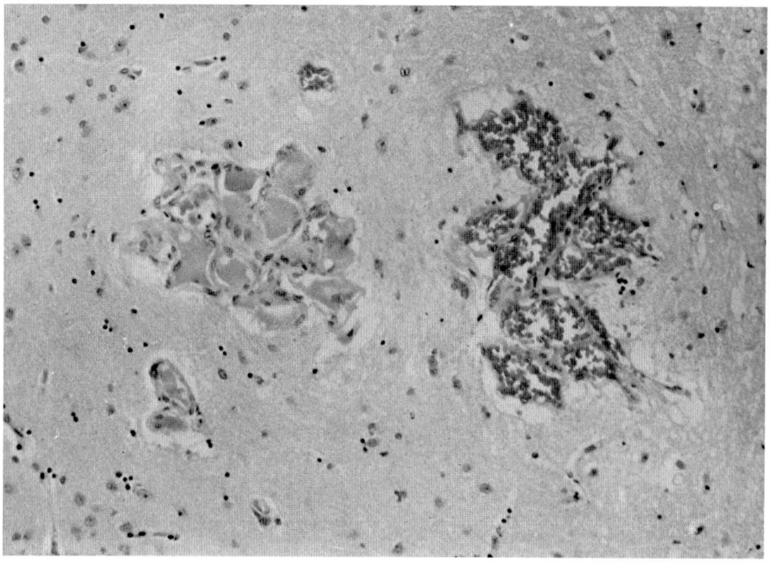

Fig. 1.34. Same cavernous angiomas as seen in Fig. 1.33 illustrating their true cavernous nature. (H&E; ×80)

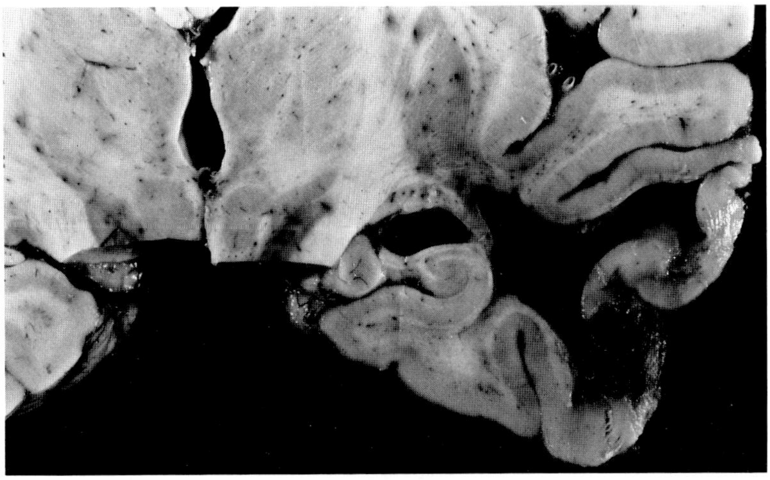

Fig. 1.35. Cryptic AVM in right inferior temporal gyrus with massive hematoma cavity medial to it. This patient survived the hemorrhage and died of unrelated causes five months later.

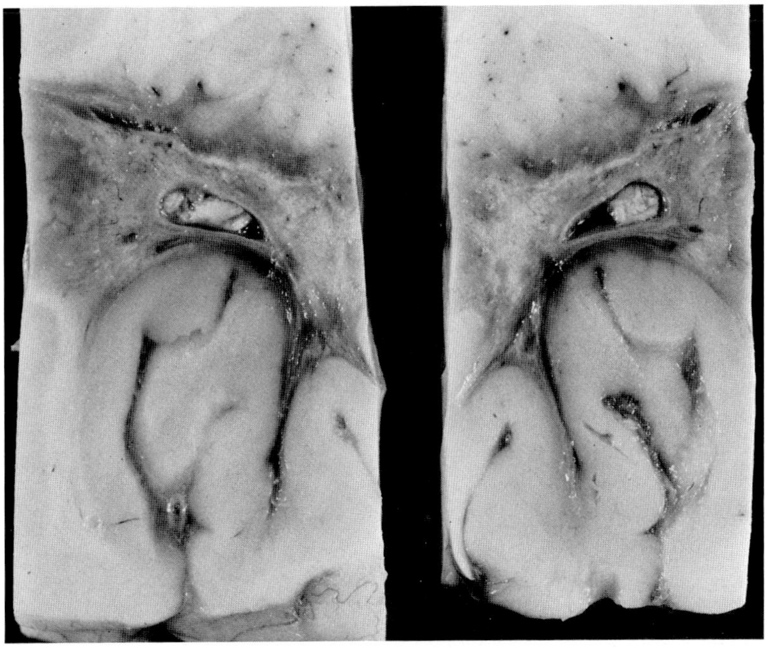

Fig. 1.36. Close-up of almost totally, spontaneously obliterated venous angioma. A phlebolith is seen in the central chaining vein.

phy, even with careful searching.* Computed tomography often indicates their location usually by demonstrating periangioma parenchymal changes (hemorrhage, necrosis) (Fig. 1.36).

Prevalence of Angiomas

The vast majority of the literature deals with clinically derived material and thus unavoidably reflects biases toward symptomatic cases or cases of unusual (and thus "reportable") presentations or appearances. Such publications collectively may give the reader a view that does not reflect what I believe to be the natural history of these malformations. For example, anyone familiar only with the older literature would quite naturally believe that the arteriovenous type of angioma was the most common, that angiomas were at least moderately dangerous (prone to bleed, produce hydrocephalus, etc.), and that an angiogram will invariably diagnose them. I hope to show that most esti-

* References 1, 6, 8, 9, 15, 16, 21, 22, 38, 40, 43, 54, 56, 63, 73.

mates of the prevalence of angiomas derived from clinical material are little more than crude guesses.

I have already mentioned the heavy clinical bias toward AVMs. Cryptic angiomas of all types are typically grossly underestimated owing to their very inconspicuousness. The commonly held belief that venous angiomas are rare illustrates the unreliability of most published estimates of prevalence. As Tables 1.1 and 1.2 summarize, angiomas of all types are relatively common (approximately that of intracranial saccular aneurysms) and the venous type greatly dominates. These two points (prevalence of 4%–5% and venous type predominance) have been stressed before.[39,40,60] If symptomatic (often lethal) clinically derived cases are used, as in my largely Armed Forces Institute of Pathology-derived material,[42] the relative frequency of the different histologic angioma types changes, with AVMs appearing most commonly.

Table 1.4 Location of angiomas in 274 patients.

Location of angiomas	Patients
Cerebrum (nonstriate)	166
Corpus striatum and thalamus	22
Cerebellum	54
Brainstem	36
Spinal cord	6
Location of ruptured angiomas	
Cerebrum (nonstriate)	11
Corpus striatum	4
Cerebellum	5
Brainstem	1
Spinal cord	1

Multiple Angiomas

Angiomas are often multiple.* Nearly 6% of patients with an angioma had one or more additional angiomas in my autopsy series (Table 1.1).[40] All histologic types of angiomas can occur multiply,** and different morphologic types can occur in the same individual. In my consecutive autopsy material from Texas (Table 1.2), 9 of 170 cadavers with angiomas had two or more. One patient had 6, one 3, and the others 2 each. The histologic types in these 9 decedents were venous and telangiectasis in two, all venous in 6, and both telangiectasis in one. I have also had several cases with multiple cavernous angiomas in my cumulative material, one with more than 20. None of these multiple cases were in recognized phakomatosis patients.

Location of Angiomas

Table 1.4 lists the general anatomic location of angiomas found in 274 patients in my prospective autopsy series of 5,850 total cadavers from Iowa and Texas. In general, there appears to be a rough correlation between the volume of tissue in an anatomic site (e.g., cerebral "lobar") and the prevalence of angiomas in that site. Figures comparing relative frequency of angiomas by area (for example, posterior fossa, spinal cord, choroid plexus)* and size[22,43] are available, but most are generally unreliable due to strong biases related to method of diagnosis and ascertainment. Some types, such as AVMs with vein of Galen aneurysms,** tend to be vastly overreported (i.e., reported more often because of their spectacular nature) whereas others are clearly underreported. Table 1.2 identified the specific angioma type by location in the last 170 cadavers with angiomas in my Texas series. A cerebral location has been most often observed and reported. In Table 1.4, 187 of 274 patients had a cerebral (either lobar or ganglionic) location for their angioma. (Several of these patients also had another angioma elsewhere in the CNS.) This cerebral "lobar" location appears to be true of all types of angiomas (Table 1.2). Among cases of cryptic angiomas reported prior to 1966,[43] 161 of 308 were located in the cerebrum. Of these 161, 136 were "lobar" and 25 were confined to the basal ganglia. In a review of angiomas with emphasis on those occurring in the posterior fossa,[42] 346 cerebral angiomas were found in a study population also

* References 20, 22, 39, 40, 45, 60, 65, 73.

** References 20, 22, 39, 40, 60, 65, 73.

* References 1, 5, 6, 8, 10, 11, 16, 22–24, 28, 35, 42, 56, 59, 61, 66.

** References 2, 12, 14, 25, 45, 48, 62, 70, 71.

containing 164 posterior fossa angiomas. Choroid plexus angiomas occur overwhelmingly most often in the glomi of the lateral ventricles,[9,23,38,66] but may occur in other areas.[56]

Although uncommonly reported, they are certainly more common than the literature would indicate. A subependymal location of angiomas has been suggested as a common site.[1] Although angiomas certainly occur in such locations (Figs. 1.26 and 1.33),[54] no real predilection is obvious (Table 1.2). Dural or combined meningeal (dural and leptomeninges) and cerebral angiomas are well known* and were found in from 3% to 27% of patients with supratentorial AVMs.[46,52]

Spinal cord angiomas are uncommon compared with those occurring in the brain, but are well known clinically and pathologically,[5,24,28,35,43] Most are AVMs, but I have studied several cavernous examples (Fig. 1.24).

Angiomas and Saccular Aneurysms

There have been a number of reports of the concurrence of angiomas and saccular arterial intracranial aneurysms.* Several authors[24,28] have noted the relationship of spinal AVMs with arterial aneurysms. In my own material, this association seems to be due largely to the relatively high prevalence of both angiomas (approx. 5%) and aneurysms (approx. 7%) in the population. The expected concurrence based on these prevalences is what I have observed—16 patients with both angiomas and arterial saccular aneurysms in approximately 4,400 patients over 1 year of age. Table 1.5 summarizes the cases with both angiomas and aneurysms.

There does appear to be a somewhat greater than expected concurrence of saccular aneurysms and AVMs. If abnormal vascular dynamics can give rise to saccular aneurysms, it is indeed the arteriovenous angioma that would be expected to be the offending type of angioma. More critical data are needed to prove or disprove a cause and effect relationship between angiomas and aneurysms.

* References 3, 4, 26, 30, 31, 44, 46, 47.

* References 22, 33, 39, 40, 42, 45, 52, 63, 70.

Vascular Malformations and Gliomas

Fischer, et al[18] have recently discussed the possibility that angiomas, particularly the cavernous type, may be associated with gliomas and that coincidence is not fortuitous. I have recently described a small, clinically unsuspected cavernous malformation at the margin of an oligodendroglioma among cases seen on our surgical service,[40] and I have had the opportunity to examine several similar cases from the AFIP material.[42] The occurrence of cavernous malformation-like areas in both central and peripheral neurinomas suggests—but clearly does not prove—an association between at least the Schwannian/oligodendroglial neoplasms and cavernous malformations. The relative prevalence of both gliomas and vascular malformations in the population and the probabilities of their being coincident are important considerations. Their coincidence in the same patient in the same location is at least intriguing.

Natural History

Our knowledge of the true natural history of angiomas has slowly advanced over the past generation, but we are not yet to the point where we can predict which ones will become clinically symptomatic. It is now clear that most angiomas, perhaps 90%, will remain silent. It is also clear that the arteriovenous type is the most agressive in its behavior. We are aware that most angiomas are small, less than 2 or 3 cm in maximal size, and appear to remain so.

Growth

Arteriovenous and cavernous angiomas occasionally grow (i.e., increase in volume of brain occupied),[34,38–40,52,63] although clearly not all angiomas grow appreciably over time. The increase in size appears to be due both to enlargement of the component vessels of the angioma and to "recruitment" of vessels from the adjacent, initially uninvolved tissues. With growth, an increase in (or initiation of) clinical symptoms and signs often occurs owing to the increase in mass of the angioma per se and an increase in the area of ischemia associated with the angioma ("steal"). This "growth," with its

Table 1.5. Angiomas and arterial saccular aneurysms.

	Angiomas			Aneurysm(s)
Age, race, sex	Type	Location	No.	Location(s)
81 WM	Telangiectasis	Pons	2	Right MCA and anterior communicating-median artery of corpus callosum (unruptured)
75 WF	Venous	R frontal lobar	1	Right IC-anterior choroidal (unruptured)
49 WF	Venous	L frontal lobar	1	Left IC-ophthalamic (unruptured)
35 BM	AVM	R Sylvian	3	Basilar tip (ruptured); Right AC-anterior communicating-Right MCA (unruptured)
62 WM	Venous	L frontal lobar	1	Left IC-anterior choroidal (unruptured)
37 WM	AVM with hemorrhage	Cerebellum	2	Left basilar-anterior inferior cerebellar; L PICA (unruptured)
61 WM	Venous	R parietal lobar	1	Left AC-anterior communicating-(unruptured)
71 WF	Telangiectasis	Pons	2	Right MCA and Right IC posterior communicating (unruptured)
65 WM	Venous	Pons	1	Right MCA (unruptured)
69 WF	Venous	Cerebellum	1	Right AC-anterior communicating-(remote rupture)
62 BF	Telangiectasis	R frontal lobal	1	Anterior Communicating (unruptured)
31 WM	Venous	Cerebellum	1	Left MCA (ruptured)
65 WF	Venous	L Occipital	1	Left IC-anterior choroidal (unruptured)
69 WM	Telangiectasis	R frontal	1	Right MCA (unruptured)
71 WM	Venous	R frontal	1	Left IC-anterior choroidal (unruptured)
50 BF	Venous	L frontal	1	Left MCA (unruptured)

MCA, middle cerebral arteries; IC, internal carotid artery; PICA, posterior inferior cerebellar artery; AC, anterior cerebral artery.

increasingly obvious clinical presentation, was the reason that some physicians years ago considered angiomas to be neoplasms.

Rupture

Many, perhaps most, angiomas show at least microscopic evidence of bleeding (Figs. 1.11, 1.21 and 1.22). Only occasionally is this bleeding massive, most often in the AVM. Table 1.3 summarizes the angiomas that have bled massively. In these 18 autopsies, all but two were AVMs. Grossly evident but submassive hemorrhage (Fig. 1.4) is considerably more common in all angiomas than is massive hemorrhage (Fig. 1.35), but less common than microscopic bleeding.

No cause for angioma rupture has been established to my satisfaction. Activity, even strenuous, plays no demonstrable role,[39,40,53,63] nor does hypertension.[39,40,44] Several authors have noted posttraumatic rupture of AVMs,[66,67] but a close association between head trauma and rupture is difficult or impossible to prove in most patients. I have seen numerous patients with angiomas who died from severe closed head injury without rupture of the angioma. Considering the frequency of head trauma in contemporary civilization and the prevalence of angiomas in the population, a close association between trauma and rupture should be easy to prove—it has not been.

"Steal"

Deprivation of the adjacent neural tissues of normal blood supply by an angioma produces "steal."* It is seen most often with large AVMs

* References 14, 17, 25, 28, 30, 38–40, 42, 45, 48, 57, 63.

but has been observed in other types of angiomas as well. Morphologic examples of steal from venous angiomas have been published[39,40,45] and an example is shown in Fig. 1.15.

Increasing neurologic dysfunction and epilepsy presumably are clinical manifestations of steal in many patients.

Spontaneous Thrombosis

Once considered rare, it is now apparent that many angiomas of all types undergo varying degrees of spontaneous thrombosis of their component vessels.**

This thrombosis may result in virtually complete obliteration of the angioma (Fig. 1.36) with complete disappearance on angiography.* It is probably the cause of the decrease in size of radiographically demonstrated angiomas in many patients and is most often due to subclinical bleeding.

Summary

Angiomas are congenital malformations of vessels and are of four major histologic types. The venous type is by far the most common. Small, silent (cryptic) angiomas occur far more frequently than large ones and appear in all parts of the CNS. The arteriovenous type is clinically the most agressive, most prone to massive hemorrhage, steal and mass effect, but is one of the less common types. The cause of rupture of angiomas of any type is unknown but does not seem to be related to preictal physical activity; it is probably multifactorial. Multiplicity is relatively frequent, and several different histologic types may be found in the same patient. None of my cases have been familial, but several families with angiomas have been reported. Angiomas as a group are biologically quite benign, but individual patients with angiomas, especially large AVMs, may develop devastating disorders.

** References 2, 7, 8, 12, 13, 16, 17, 26, 28–30, 39, 40, 42, 45, 48, 50, 55, 62, 68, 72.

* References 13, 15, 29, 34, 36, 50, 56, 69, 72.

References

1. Abroms IF, L Yessayan, J Shillito, Barlow CF: Spontaneous intracerebral haemorrhage in patients suspected of multiple sclerosis. J Neurol Neurosurg Psychiatry 34:157–162, 1971
2. Agee OF, Musella R, Tweed CG: Aneurysm of the great vein of Galen. Report of two cases. J Neurosurg 31:346–351, 1969
3. Aminoff MJ: Vascular anomalies in the intracranial dura mater. Brain 96:601–612, 1973
4. Aminoff MJ, Kendall BE: Asymptomatic dural vascular anomalies. Br J Radiol 46:662–667, 1973
5. Bailey WL, Sperl MP: Angiomas of the cervical spinal cord. J Neurosurg 30:560–568, 1969
6. Becker DH, Townsend JJ, Kramer RA, Newton TH: Occult cerebrovascular malformations. A series of 18 histologically verified cases with negative angiography. Brain 102:249–287, 1979
7. Bell BA, Kendall BE, Symon L: Angiographically occult arteriovenous malformations of the brain. J Neurol Neurosurg Psychiatry 41:1057–1064, 1978
8. Bicknell JM, Carlow TJ, Kornfeld M, Stovring J, Turner P: Familial cavernous angiomas. Arch Neurol 35:746–749, 1978
9. Britt RH, Connor WS, Enzmann DR: Occult arteriovenous malformations of the brainstem simulating multiple sclerosis. Neurology 31:901–904, 1981
10. Britt RH, Silverberg GD, Enzmann DR, Hanbery JW: Third ventricular choroid plexus arteriovenous malformation simulating a colloid cyst. Case report. J Neurosurg 52:246–250, 1980
11. Cabanes J, Blasco R, Garcia M, Tamarit L: Cerebral venous angiomas. Surg Neurol 11:385–389, 1979
12. Carroll CPH, Jakoby RK: Neonatal congestive heart failure as the presenting symptom of cerebral arteriovenous malformation. J Neurosurg 25:159–163, 1966
13. Conforti, P: Spontaneous disappearance of cerebral arteriovenous angioma. J Neurosurg 34:432–434, 1971
14. Diebler C, Dulac O, et al: Aneurysms of the vein of Galen in infants aged 2 to 15 months. Diagnosis and natural history.
15. Eisenman JI, Alekoumbides A, Priebram H: Spontaneous thrombosis of vascular malformations of the brain. Acta radiol 13:77–85, 1972
16. Erenberg G, Rubin R, Shulman K: Cerebellar haematomas caused by angiomas in children. J Neurol Neurosurg Psychiatry 35:304–310, 1972
17. Feindel W Yamamoto YL, Hodge CP: Red cerebral veins and the cerebral steal syndrome. Evidence from fluorescein angiography and mi-

croregional blood flow by radioisotopes during excision of an angioma. J Neurosurg 35:167–179, 1971
18. Fischer EG, Sotrel A, Welch K: Cerebral hemangioma with glial neoplasia (angioglioma ?). J Neurosurg 56:430–434, 1982
19. Galzio RJ, Zenobii M, et al: Hemangioma calcificans. Surg Neurol 14:331–335, 1980
20. Giombini S, Morello G: Cavernous angiomas of the brain. Account of 14 personal cases and review of the literature. Acta Neurochir 40:61–82, 1978
21. Golden JB, Kramer RA: The angiographically occult cerebrovascular malformation. Report of three cases. J Neurosurg 48:292–296, 1978
22. Graf CJ, Perret GE, Torner JC: Bleeding from cerebral arteriovenous malformations as part of their natural history. J Neurosurg 58:331–337, 1983
23. Hamer J: Small angioma of the choroid plexus as a cause of primary intraventricular haemorrhage. Acta Neurochir 47:83–89, 1979
24. Herdt JR, Di Chiro G, Doppman JL: Combined arterial and arteriovenous aneurysms of the spinal cord. Radiology 99:589–593, 1971
25. Hoffman HJ, Chuang S, et al: Aneurysms of the vein of Galen. J Neurosurg 57:316–322, 1982
26. Houser OW Jr, Baker HL Jr, Rhoton AL Jr, Okazaki H: Intracranial dural arteriovenous malformations. Radiology 105:55–64, 1972
27. Jonutis AJ, Sondheimer FK, Klein HZ, Wise BL: Intracerebral cavernous hemangioma with angiographically demonstrated pathologic vasculature. Neuroradiology 3:57–63, 1971
28. Kaufman HH, Ommaya AK, Di Chiro G, Doppman JL: Compression vs "Steal." The pathogenesis of symptoms in arteriovenous malformations of the spinal cord. Arch Neurol 23:173–178, 1970
29. Kim YH, Gildenberg PL, Duchesneau PM: Angiographic evidence of spontaneous closure of nontraumatic arteriovenous fistula of the vertebral artery. Case report. J Neurosurg 38:658–661, 1973
30. Kosnik EJ, Hunt WE, Miller CA: Dural arteriovenous malformations. J Neurosurg 40:322–329, 1974
31. Kühner A, Krastel A, Stoll W: Arteriovenous malformations of the transverse dural sinus. J Neurosurg 45:12–19, 1976
32. Kushner J, Alexander E Jr: Partial spontaneous regressive arteriovenous malformation. Case report with angiographic evidence. J Neurosurg 32:360–366, 1970
33. Kusske JA, Kelly WA: Embolization and reduction of the "steal" syndrome in cerebral arteriovenous malformations. J Neurosurg 40:313–321, 1974
34. Lakke JPWF: Regression of an arteriovenous malformation of the brain. J Neurol Sci 11:489–496, 1970
35. Logue V: Angiomas of the spinal cord: Review of the pathogenesis, clinical features, and results of surgery. J Neurol Neurosurg Psychiatry 42:1–11, 1979
36. Mabe H, Furuse M: Spontaneous disappearance of a cerebral arteriovenous malformation in infancy. Case report. J Neurosurg 46:811–815, 1976
37. McCormick WF: The pathology of vascular ("arteriovenous") malformations. J Neurosurg 24:807–816, 1966
38. McCormick WF: Vascular disorders of nervous tissue: Anomalies, malformations and aneurysms. In Bourne GE (ed.): Structure and function of nervous tissue. Vol 3. Academic Press, New York, 1969, pp 537–596
39. McCormick WF: Classification, pathology, and natural history of angiomas of the central nervous system. Weekly Update: Neurology and Neurosurgery. Vol 1, No 14, Biomedia Inc, Princeton, 1978
40. McCormick WF: Pathology of vascular malformations of the brain. In Wilson CB, Stein BM (eds.): Intracranial Arteriovenous Malformation: Current Neurosurgical Practice. Williams and Wilkins, Baltimore, 1984
41. McCormick WF, Boulter TR: Vascular malformations ("angiomas") of the dura mater. Report of 2 cases. J Neurosurg 25:309–311, 1966
42. McCormick WF, Hardman JM, Boulter TR: Vascular malformations ("angiomas") of the brain, with special reference to those occurring in the posterior fossa. J Neurosurg 28:241–251, 1968
43. McCormick WF, Nofzinger J: "Cryptic" vascular malformations of the central nervous system. J Neurosurg 24:892–894, 1966
44. McCormick WF, Rosenfield DB: Massive brain hemorrhage: A review of 144 cases and an examination of their causes. Stroke 4:946–954, 1973
45. McCormick WF, Schochet SS Jr: Atlas of cerebrovascular disease. WB Saunders Co, Philadelphia, 1976, pp 72–105
46. Newton TH, Cronqvist S: Involvement of dural arteries in intracranial arteriovenous malformations. Radiology 93:1071–1078, 1969
47. Newton TH, Weidner W, Greitz T: Dural arteriovenous malformation in the posterior fossa. Radiology 90:27–35, 1968
48. Norman MG, Becker LE: Cerebral damage in neonates resulting from arteriovenous malforma-

tion of the vein of Galen. J Neurol Neurosurg Psychiatry 37:252–258, 1974

49. Numaguchi Y, Kishikawa T, et al: Prolonged injection angiography for diagnosing intracranial cavernous hemangiomas. Radiology 131:137–138, 1979
50. Omojola MF, Fox AJ, et al: Spontaneous regression of intracranial arteriovenous malformations. J Neurosurg 57:818–822, 1982
51. Pak H, Patel SC, Malik GM, Ausman JI: Successful evacuation of a pontine hematoma secondary to rupture of a venous angioma. Surg Neurol 15:164–167, 1981
52. Parkinson D, Bachers G: Arteriovenous malformations. Summary of 100 consecutive supratentorial cases. J Neurosurg 53:285–299, 1980
53. Peräsalo J, Waltimo O, Heiskanen T: Cardiovascular dimensions in patients with intracranial arteriovenous malformation. Stroke 4:787–794, 1973
54. Pozzati E, Gaist G, et al: Microsurgical removal of paraventricular cavernous angiomas. J Neurosurg 55:308–311, 1981
55. Prensky AL, Gado M: Angiographic resolution of a neonatal intracranial cavernous hemangioma coincident with steroid therapy. Case report. J Neurosurg 39:99–103, 1973
56. Roda JM, Moneo JH, et al: Cryptic arteriovenous malformation of the choroid plexus of the third ventricle. Surg Neurol 16:353–356, 1981
57. Rodda RA, Calvert GD: Postmortem arteriography of cerebral arteriovenous malformations. J Neurol Neurosurg Psychiatry 32:432–439, 1969
58. Saito Y, Kobayashi N: Cerebral venous angiomas. Radiology 139:87–94, 1981
59. Sansone ME, Liwnicz BH, Mandybur TI: Giant pituitary cavernous hemangioma. Case report. J Neurosurg 53:124–126, 1980
60. Sarwar M, McCormick WF: Intracerebral venous angioma. Case report and review. Arch Neurol 35:323–325, 1978
61. Stahl SM, Johnson KP, Malamud N: The clinical and pathological spectrum of brain stem vascular malformations. Arch Neurol 37:25–29, 1980
62. Stehbens WE, Sahgal KK, Nelson L, Shaher RM: Aneurysm of vein of Galen and diffuse meningeal angiectasia. Occurrence in a neonate with cardiac failure. Arch Pathol 95:333–335, 1973
63. Stein BM, Wolpert SM: Arteriovenous malformations of the brain. I: Current concepts and treatment. Arch Neurol 37:1–5, 1980
64. Terao H, Hori T, Matsutani M, Okeda R: Detection of cryptic vascular malformations by computerized tomography. Report of 2 cases. J Neurosurg 51:546–551, 1979
65. Tindall RSA, Kirkpatrick JB, Sklar F: Multiple small cavernous angiomas of the brain with increased intracranial pressure. Ann Neurol 4:376–378, 1978
66. Towfighi J, Bilaniuk LT, Zimmerman RA, Langfitt TW, Gonatas NK: Hemorrhage in bilateral choroid plexus hemangiomas demonstrated by computed tomography. Case report. J Neurosurg 45:218–222, 1976
67. Tyson GW, Jane JA, Strachan WE: Intracerebral hemorrhage due to ruptured venous aneurysm. Report of 2 cases. J Neurosurg 49:739–743, 1978
68. Vaquero J, Leunda G, et al: Cavernomas of the brain. Neurosurgery 12:208–210, 1983
69. Wakai S, Chen C-H, et al: Spontaneous regression of a cerebral arteriovenous malformation. Arch Neurol 40:377–380, 1983
70. Walter W: The influence of the type and location of the angioma on the clinical syndrome. In Pia HW et al (eds.): Cerebral Angiomas. Springer-Verlag, New York, 1975, p 27–37
71. Watson DG, Smith RR, Brann AW Jr: Arteriovenous malformation of the vein of Galen. Treatment in a neonate. Am J Dis Child 130:520–525, 1976
72. Wharen RE, Scheithaurer BW, Laws ER Jr: Thrombosed arteriovenous malformations of the brain. J Neurosurg 57:520–526, 1982
73. Wolf PA, Rosman NP, New PFJ: Multiple small cryptic venous angiomas of the brain mimicking cerebral metastases. A clinical, pathological, and angiographic study. Neurology 17:491–502, 1967

2

Supratentorial Arteriovenous Malformations

Bennett M. Stein

Introduction

Arteriovenous malformations (AVMs) are vascular lesions of the brain representing an abnormal shunt between arteries and veins.[3,24] Although congenital, they usually become symptomatic during the mid decades of life. Anatomically they are represented by an abnormal tangle of arteries, large sinusoids and veins involving the surface and deep portions of the brain. These malformations are uncommon, representing one-tenth the frequency of intracranial arterial aneurysms.[26,30,33,40,41] Approximately 2,500 new cases per year are identified in the United States. Despite their infrequency there has been an intensified interest in these lesions because of the development of techniques designed to obliterate AVMs—even those involving large or crucial areas of the brain. Parallel to the development of surgical techniques, neuroradiologic intravascular techniques aimed at thrombosis of intracranial vessels have been particularly applicable to these lesions. These intravascular techniques may be used primarily or as an adjuvant to surgical resection in the treatment of AVMs.

This chapter is confined to a discussion of those AVMs involving the supratentorial portion of the brain. In addition to the true AVMs, which range in size from extremely large to small "cryptic" lesions (Fig. 2.1) sometimes not visualized on angiography,[22] there are other rare vascular anomalies involving the cerebrum. They include pure venous malformations,[46] cavernous malformations, and capillary telangiectases associated with Weber-Osler disorder. Most of these latter lesions are anatomic curiosities and do not hold the same implications for surgical or intravascular therapy as do the AVMs.

Anatomic Considerations

Most anatomic data relevant to AVMs have been obtained from the gross and histologic evaluation of autopsy material or from surgical experience with these lesions. Lacking is an in-depth study of the three-dimensional anatomy of these malformations. This study is needed to correlate with angiographic data, which may be obtained in stereoscopic form, and with surgical anatomy. The few existing three-dimensional dissection studies show that AVMs are composed of attenuated arterial channels and cavernous vascular structures (probably abnormal veins).[8,12] The malformations are drained by a group of tortuous veins, often originating deep within the lesion, that reach the surface and gain either the cortical veins or the deep periventricular veins. I have recently been injecting resected specimens with an inert sub-

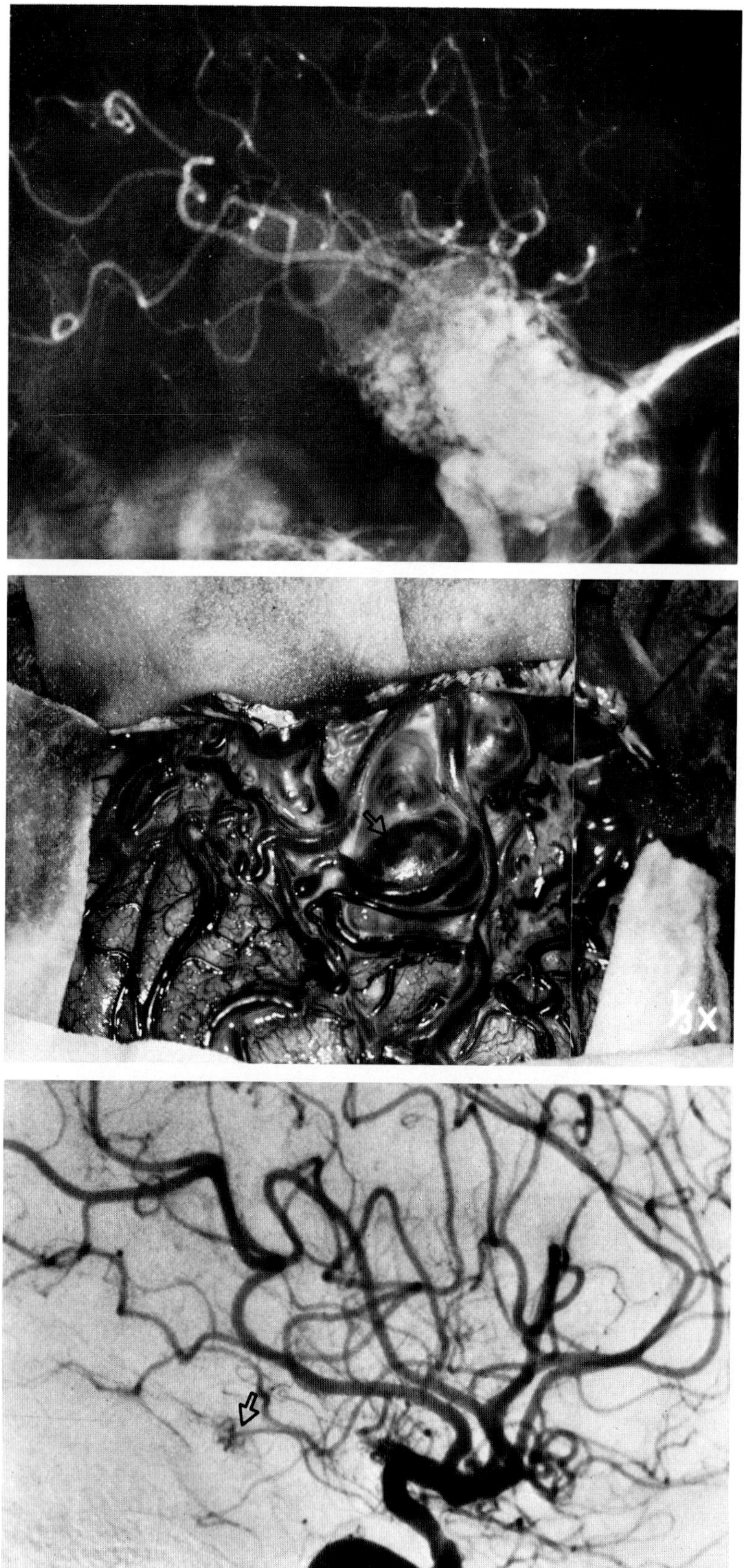

A

B

C

Fig. 2.1. **A.** Right lateral carotid angiogram demonstrating a large AVM involving branches of the middle cerebral artery. **B.** Operative photograph of large AVM involving the parietal lobe. *Arrow* denotes one of many large arterialized venous "aneurysms." **C.** Right lateral carotid angiogram demonstrating a small AVM (*arrow*) fed by branch of anterior choroidal artery.

stance, later dissolving the surrounding soft tissue so that a dissecting microscopic study of the vascular anatomy may be carried out (Fig. 2.2). Results of these studies confirm that very little within the malformation represents a capillary bed, inferring an absence of viable cerebral tissue within the confines of the AVM.

The entire extent of an AVM is rarely delineated on the cerebral cortex. The bulk rather lies subcortical with normal-appearing cortex over a varying portion of the lesion (Fig. 2.3). The deep extent of the lesion into the white matter may be in a wedge or globoid configuration. The arterial supply often enters the malformation deep in sulci and is not readily visible at the cortical margins of the malformation (Fig. 2.4).

Drawing a blood supply in parasitic fashion, AVMs often receive arterial feeders from many cerebral arteries, commonly from all three major cerebral circulations to include the anterior, middle, and posterior cerebral arteries (Fig. 2.5). The arteries supplying a malformation are often tortuous, ectatic, and thin walled. On the surface of the brain they may be indistinguishable, except for their anatomic location, from large arterialized veins draining the malformation. Presumably the structural changes in these arteries are the explanation for a 10% incidence of aneurysms involving the arterial supply to AVMs.[23,24,26,30,33] The venous drainage of these lesions gains the pial surface of the brain directly over or adjacent to the malformation and joins either the cortical veins or the venous sinuses. Deep-draining veins are buried in the white matter and extend to the periventricular venous plexus, often producing dilated clusters of veins lying free within the ventricular system, unprotected by a gliotic or ependymal membrane.

Histologic evaluation of AVMs demonstrates a gliotic core associated with the nidus and gliosis surrounding the AVM.[21] The former allows one to remove an AVM that otherwise would be situated in eloquent portions of the brain. Presumably the development of the AVM coincident with the brain results in a displacement of normal anatomic structures so that the only tissues lying within the malformation are blood vessels and nonfunctional brain. The gliotic wall around the malformation permits a precise surgical dissection in a relatively avascular plane, aiding in the total removal of these malformations.

Thrombosis has been histologically demonstrated within malformations.[4] Hemorrhages, both macroscopic and microscopic, without an antecedent clinical history have been observed both at surgery and at postmortem. In approximately 15% of our operations we have observed evidence of an old hemorrhage without clinical manifestations. The question of growth or involution of AVMs is pertinent to any treatment plan.[11,16,28,31,37] Our experience in a small number of cases followed by arteriography has shown that one-third of AVMs involute, one-third remain the same, and one-third enlarge. Most series, based on clinical and surgical experience, would indicate that AVMs generally grow at a rate no greater than the rate of cerebral growth and therefore remain static in proportion to brain size. However, dramatic exceptions have been reported.[37]

Natural History of Arteriovenous Malformations

Arteriovenous malformations are an affliction of the middle ages. As an initial manifestation, they most commonly become symptomatic with either hemorrhage or seizures.*

Hemorrhage from AVMs, generally parenchymal, occurs in approximately 75% of the patients. Once hemorrhage has occurred the statistical probability of another hemorrhage is much higher; however, these recidivous hemorrhages often occur at long intervals.[23] Many of these patients suffer repeated hemorrhages from AVMs and yet escape serious permanent neurologic deficits. Rupture of blood into the subarachnoid space gives rise to all the classic signs of subarachnoid hemorrhage. Therefore the rupture of an AVM may be clinically indistinguishable from that of an intracranial arterial aneurysm. However, the possibility of an intraparenchymal hematoma with focal neurologic deficits would naturally be higher in the AVM at the time of rupture. Perhaps because most hemorrhages occur from the dilated venous channels of an AVM, the initial mortality from the hemorrhage of an AVM is less than that from

* References 6, 20, 26, 27, 29–31, 33, 40, 41.

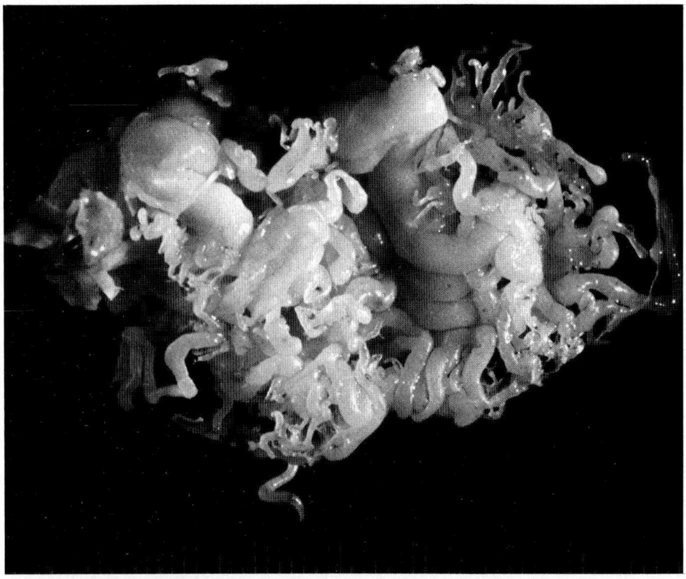

Fig. 2.2. Corrosion specimen of resected AVM. Demonstrated are the numerous large, tortuous vascular channels.

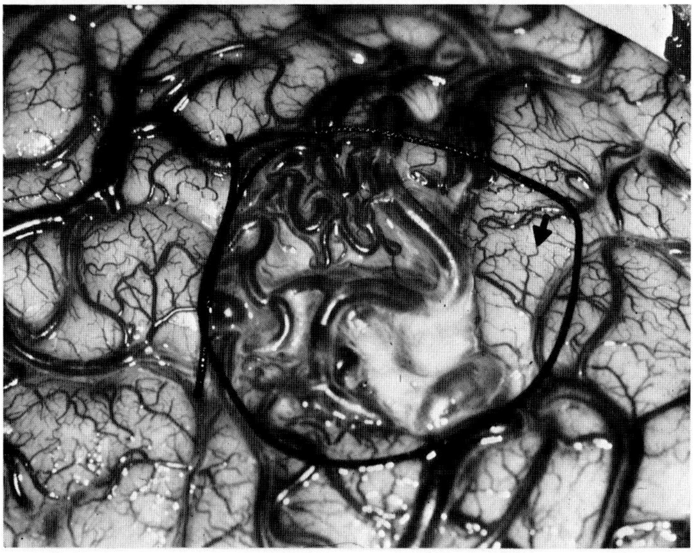

Fig. 2.3. Operative photograph showing obvious surface component of a frontoparietal AVM. Entire AVM encompasses area outlined by silk suture, indicating significant hidden portion under normal cortex (*arrow*).

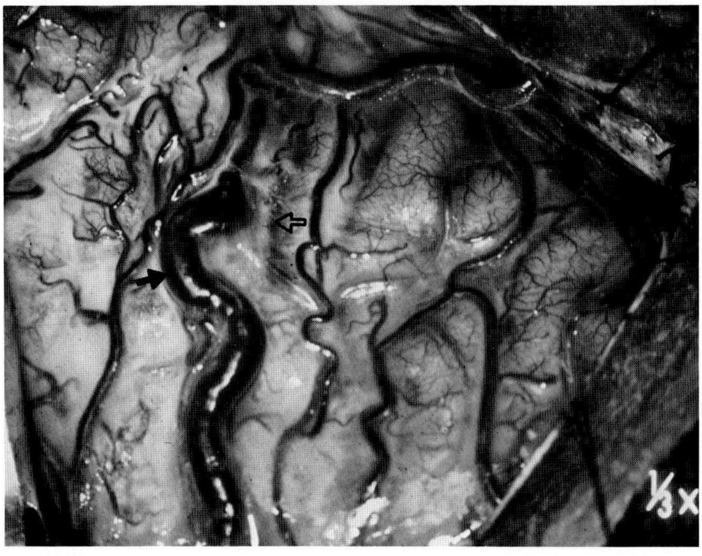

Fig. 2.4. Operative photograph of frontoparietal AVM. Large draining vein is obvious (*arrow*); feeding artery lies deep and hidden by thick arachnoid (*open arrow*).

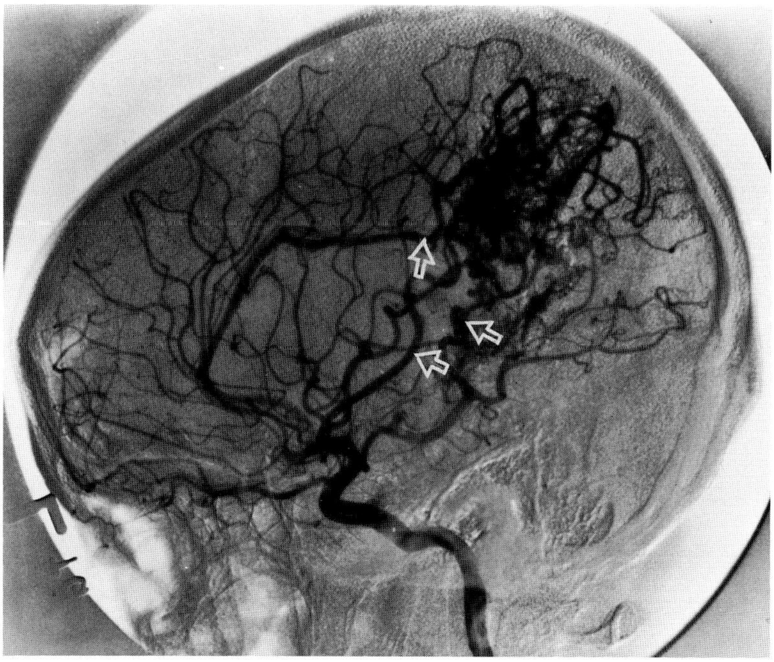

Fig. 2.5. Left lateral carotid angiogram demonstrating vascular supply to parietal lobe AVM from anterior, middle, and posterior cerebral arteries (*arrows*).

the rupture of an intracranial arterial aneurysm. Additionally, the possibility of an imminent repeat hemorrhage is much lower in an AVM than it is following rupture of an intracranial aneurysm. No correlation can be drawn between the size or configuration of an AVM and its propensity for hemorrhage.[45]

The second common presentation of an AVM is a seizure disorder either focal or generalized. The difficulty with which these seizures are controlled appears to be unrelated to the location or size of the AVM. With the increased use of computed tomographic (CT) scanning to evaluate single seizures, AVMs are being uncovered that heretofore might have gone unrecognized for many years during the development of a seizure disorder secondary to their presence.

Severe intractable headaches, even a classic migraine syndrome, have been associated with AVMs. Other more subtle symptomatology includes progressive mental deterioration and audible bruits.

Since hemorrhage, both parenchymal and subarachnoid, is the most serious complication of AVMs, it is a paramount factor in determining the risk associated with leaving these lesions to their natural course. Furthermore, since the initial hemorrhage is associated with low mortality—morbidity and repeated hemorrhages occur at long intervals—the overall risk in mortality and morbidity must be measured in decades. Obviously a younger patient is at greater risk over the extended time involved than is an older one. Evaluating the added risk factor of recurrent hemorrhage is further complicated by the fact that clinically silent hemorrhages have been discovered at autopsy and during surgery. Therefore, to base statistics solely on clinical information must be accepted with caution.

A significant body of literature is available on the role of hemorrhage and the risks in the natural history of these AVMs.** Much, unfortunately, is based on speculation, and a purely objective perspective is lacking. Available information indicates a 40% to 50% risk of severe morbidity or mortality over a long time frame in the life of a young person who has not been treated. One extensive review reported that 56% of nonsurgically treated patients were either dead or incapacitated as the result of the natural course of their AVMs.[33] In those patients whose only clinical symptom is seizures, a 12% mortality and 16% overall morbidity over a prolonged period of follow-up has been re-

** References 5, 10, 13, 23, 30–33, 35, 40–44.

ported.[13] It is plausible that the intracranial vascular steal associated with large AVMs leads to focal and general neurologic deficits, the latter being manifested by progressive dementia. The bulk of clinical evidence testifies to the dangerous nature of these lesions.[43]

The sparse data available indicates a balanced ledger between those AVMs that expand and those that involute. Whether or not these changes can be related to the intrinsic risk of the lesion is uncertain. Taking the distillate of the available clinical evidence, I explain to young patients that they have from a 40% to 50% risk factor of severe morbidity (hemiplegia, aphasia, or severe cortical sensory loss) or mortality from an untreated lesion.

Diagnosis

Rarely do the routine neurologic evaluations such as EEG, plain skull x-rays, and CSF evaluation lead to the positive diagnosis of an intracranial AVM. With the increasing use of CT scanning—especially for common neurologic complaints such as seizures, headaches, and intermittent symptomatology referrable to the cortical motor and sensory areas—AVMs are being discovered unexpectedly. The CT findings that are highly suggestive of an AVM consist of small areas of calcification and on a contrast-enhanced scan, the telltale tortuous or serpiginous channels representing the enlarged draining veins or feeding arteries of an AVM. It remains, however, for angiography to define the anatomy and flow characteristics of an AVM. We have found selective arteriography most useful in determining the arterial contributions to complex AVMs. Subtraction techniques are mandatory, and magnification angiography may be utilized to define the smaller AVMs or those lying in deep regions of the brain and being fed by numerous small arterial channels. Of great use to the surgeon in planning an operative approach to these lesions is stereoscopic angiography. This is performed during the lateral run of an internal carotid or vertebral arteriogram. Stereoscopic pairs may be utilized in the operating room during the resection of an AVM. Since important arteries may be intertwined or closely circumscribed AVMs, a stereoscopic representation of such anatomy is invaluable to the surgeon while dissecting these vessels. In some malformations the degree and rapidity of blood flow require that serial angiography be carried out rapidly with at least a rate of six or more films per second to precisely define the hemodynamics of the lesion.

The combined use of CT scan and angiography will define the relationship between a hematoma, which results from a rupture of an AVM, and the actual malformation. In those cases without hematoma the mass effect of an AVM is minimal. Therefore when mass plays a prominent role in a highly vascular lesion, one must also consider the possibilities of a vascular tumor, such as a hemangioblastoma, malignant glioma, or an angioblastic meningioma. In most instances the differential diagnosis should not be difficult.

Treatment

Small AVMs situated in polar regions of the brain, such as the frontal, temporal or occipital poles, which are easily accessible and supplied by relatively few small arteries, offer little challenge for resection (Fig. 2.1C). In such cases, with or without hemorrhage, a decision for surgical resection can be made without difficulty. The dilemma occurs in the majority of cases that are extensive or that involve crucial areas of the brain, such as the motor and speech regions (Figs. 2.1A, B). In such cases surgical resection with a risk of mortality and morbidity must be balanced against the inherent risk of the natural course of these lesions. Olivecrona's statement is germane in which he points out that the only reasonable therapeutic alternative to no treatment is surgical resection.[27] It would appear that any treatment short of total obliteration or removal of an AVM may be less than adequate.[27,30–33] Follow-up studies on cases of selective ligation of feeding arteries or in which embolization failed to totally obliterate the lesion would indicate the continued high incidence of recurrent hemorrhage.[19] A similar situation exists following the partial obliteration of an AVM by radiotherapy.[15] Recently, proton-beam therapy has been advocated in the treatment of AVMs.[15] The effects of this radiation, however, are slow to evolve and therefore long-term follow-up is mandatory

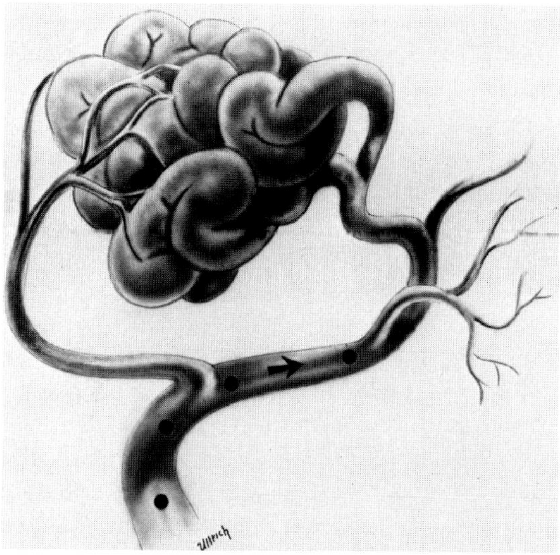

A

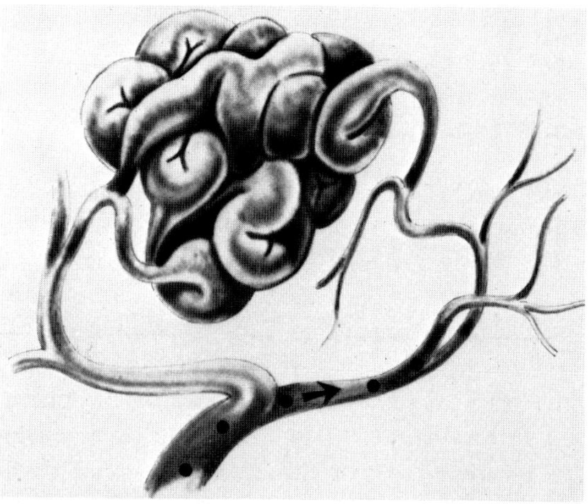

B

Fig. 2.6. A. Ideal situation for embolization in which a large middle cerebral artery branch is primary supply to an AVM and angulation of pertinent arterial system is appropriate. **B.** Situation not ideal for embolization, the middle cerebral branch to AVM being no larger than the normal branches permits emboli to travel to normal brain.

to gauge the result. One must also include a significant complication of radionecrosis and recurrent hemorrhage in those patients treated solely by radiation therapy by whatever means.

Ligation of the carotid or vertebral arteries in the neck has proved to be ineffectual and dangerous, as the ensuing overall reduction in blood flow to the brain is more deleterious to normal regions than to the malformation, which continues to act as a parasite to the blood flow.[9]

Contemporary therapy of AVMs relies on a multidisciplinary attack: by the neuroradiologist utilizing intravascular techniques to obliterate portions of the AVM and by the neurosurgeon performing a resection of the lesion.[2,18,36,39,48,49]

Intravascular thrombosis of portions of an AVM is most practically accomplished by the embolization technique developed by Luessenhop et al.[18] Emboli of various artificial substances, including metal and plastic, have been utilized. We currently use silastic emboli 1.5 to 3 mm in diameter and impregnated with barium.[48] Numerous emboli may be injected through a catheter that is positioned into either the internal carotid or the vertebral arteries on the side appropriate to the malformation. These catheters are fluoroscopically directed from an insertion site at the femoral artery. Catheters with a maximum internal diameter of 3 mm may be used in a lengthy procedure similar to angiography. When the size of the emboli and configuration of the arterial tree proximal to the malformation are appropriate, the emboli enter the malformation (Fig. 2.6). Best results are obtained when the emboli lodge within the malformation rather than occlude the feeding arteries proximal to the malformation.[39] In the former instance emboli within the interstices of a malformation reduce the potential of collateralization following embolization. Numerous factors must be taken into consideration in predicting the course of emboli. Most critical is the ratio of diameter of the major feeding arteries to an AVM and the diameter of arteries supplying the adjacent brain. Ideally this ratio should be 4 : 1 or greater.[49] The position of an AVM either peripheral or proximal to an arterial system and the character of the intervening arteries, either straight or tortuous, are also important. Paramount attention is given to the angulation between the arteries that feed the malformation and the parent artery from which it arises, whether they be the internal carotid or basilar arteries. A gradual curving angulation provides the most appropriate direction for blood flow and thereby the course of emboli, which are flow-directed (Fig. 2.7). Acute or right angles, such as the origin of the lenticulostriate arteries from the middle cerebral artery, preclude embolization (Fig. 2.8). Taking these factors into consideration, it has been difficult to embolize those malformations fed primarily by the anterior cerebral or lenticulostriate arteries,

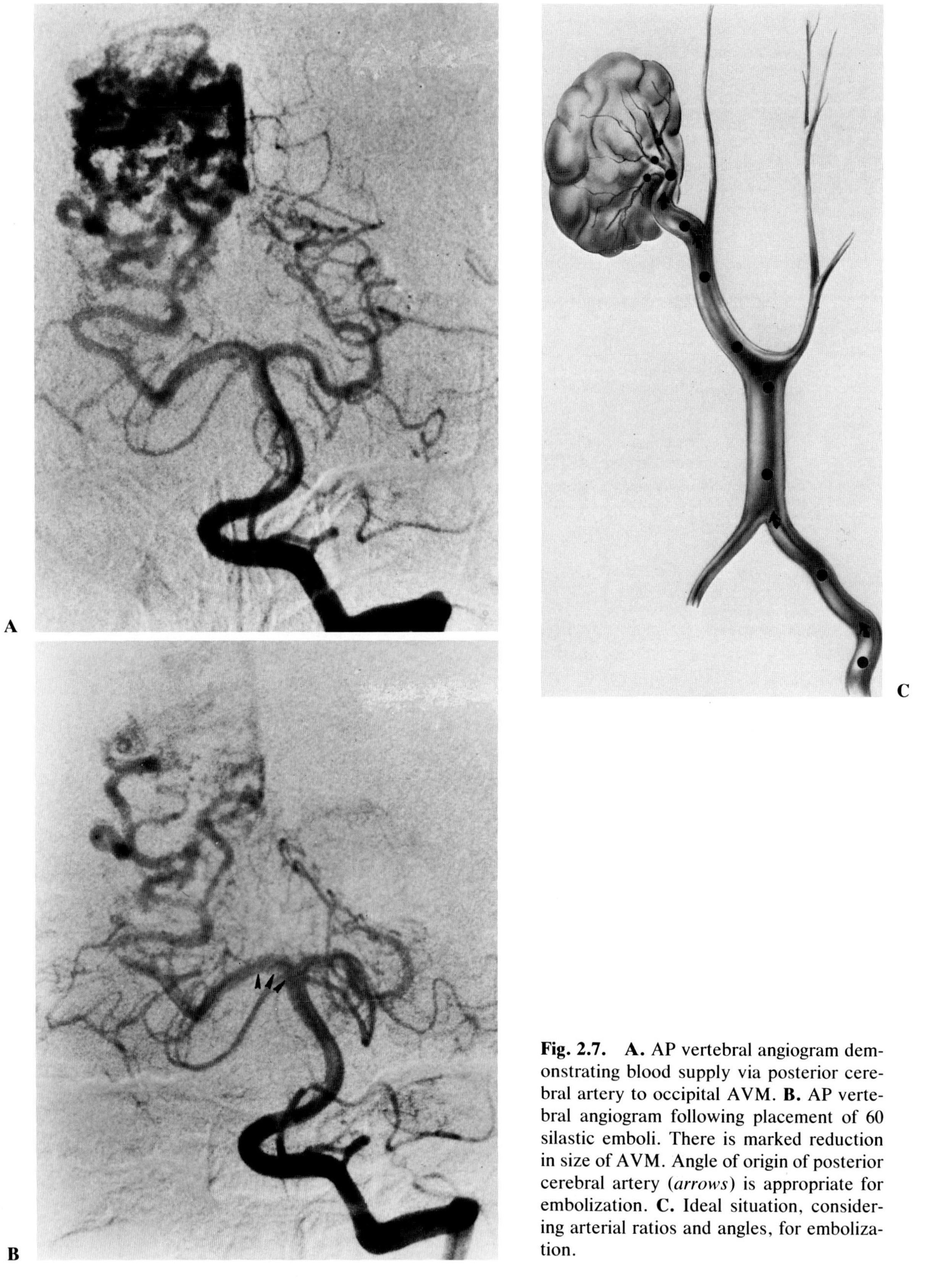

Fig. 2.7. **A.** AP vertebral angiogram demonstrating blood supply via posterior cerebral artery to occipital AVM. **B.** AP vertebral angiogram following placement of 60 silastic emboli. There is marked reduction in size of AVM. Angle of origin of posterior cerebral artery (*arrows*) is appropriate for embolization. **C.** Ideal situation, considering arterial ratios and angles, for embolization.

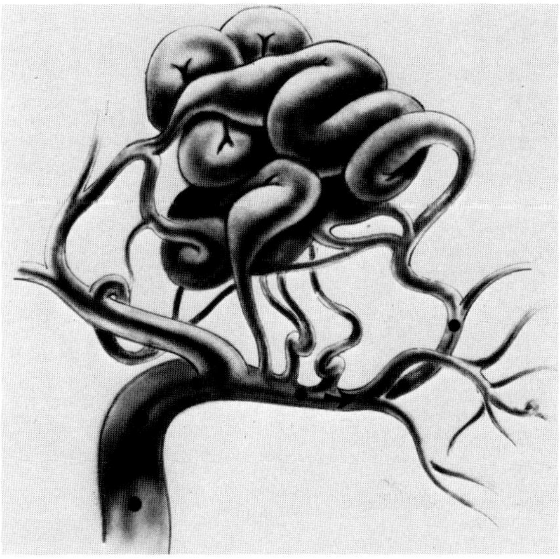

Fig. 2.8. Pattern of arterial supply to AVM in which emboli tend to avoid anterior cerebral and lenticulostriate arteries because of inappropriate angle of origin even though these arteries may be the dominant supply of the lesion.

even though these vessels may convey the dominant blood supply to the malformation. All other factors being equal, those malformations fed primarily by middle and posterior cerebral arteries are the easiest to embolize (Figs. 2.6, 2.9). In our experience, when embolization is carried out meticulously, with frequent checks on the position of emboli, the procedure has a wide margin of safety. In more than 70 instances of embolization, we have had only one serious complication.

The limitations and usefulness of embolization must be thoroughly considered in any treatment regimen. It is virtually impossible to eliminate a malformation by embolization. As additional emboli reduce blood flow to the malformation, there is less propensity for ensuing emboli to follow a course to the malformation. At a critical point when blood flow dynamically shifts away from the malformation to the brain, a high percentage of emboli will go astray into the normal circulation. Therefore, in the majority of cases we use embolization not as a primary mode of therapy but as a preliminary adjuvant to the surgical resection of these lesions. Besides generally reducing blood flow to and turgor within the malformation, embolization may be used specifically to reduce or obliterate deep inaccessible arterial feeders to a large malformation. Such an instance is the obliteration of the posterior cerebral arterial supply to a malformation which is additionally supplied by the middle and anterior cerebral arteries (Fig. 2.7). Obliteration of the posterior cerebral artery facilitates the resection of the lesion.

Experience indicates that the sudden removal or obliteration of a large malformation with massive arteriovenous shunting can displace an intolerable vascular load to adjacent normal brain, resulting in hemorrhage or uncontrolled edema in the normal brain. An analogous situation is the sudden strain placed on the cardiovascular system when a large systemic arteriovenous shunt is interrupted. In addition, experimental evidence indicates the loss or compromise of autoregulation in the normal vasculature surrounding an AVM.[38] This further compromises the ability of the normal circulation to compensate for the sudden elimination of the A-V shunt and a shift in circulatory dynamics. Embolization, by gradually eliminating the shunt, reduces these problems. We have frequently resorted to a number of embolizations before being satisfied that a maximum result has been achieved by such a procedure. In a select group of patients, in consideration of certain factors, embolization has been the sole form of treatment. In these cases surgery has not been recommended following embolization for the following reasons: (1) failure to significantly modify a large lesion by embolization, (2) the presence of large lesions in critical portions of the brain, or (3) patients over 55 years of age without a history of previous hemorrhage and normal neurologic evaluation. The angiographic follow-up in these patients has demonstrated the very gradual development of a collateral circulation to the AVM over many months. Our data are not of sufficient magnitude nor has enough time elapsed to indicate whether or not these patients have been protected against recidivous hemorrhages. Luessenhop and Presper indicate that in such cases recurrent hemorrhage is still a significant factor.[19]

When the arterial blood supply to the malformation is common to the brain surrounding the AVM, resection of the malformation would compromise this important vasculature and lead to infarction of crucial areas of the brain. By limited but repeated embolization, these ar-

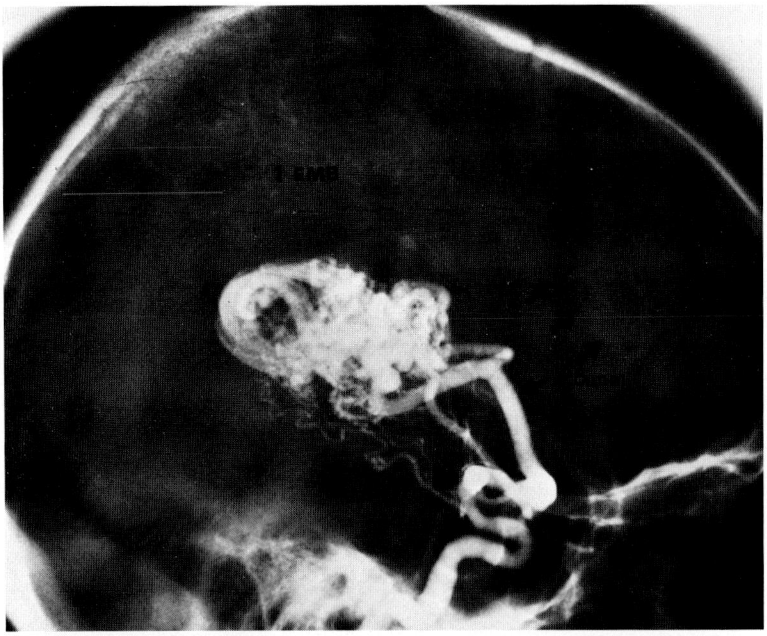

A

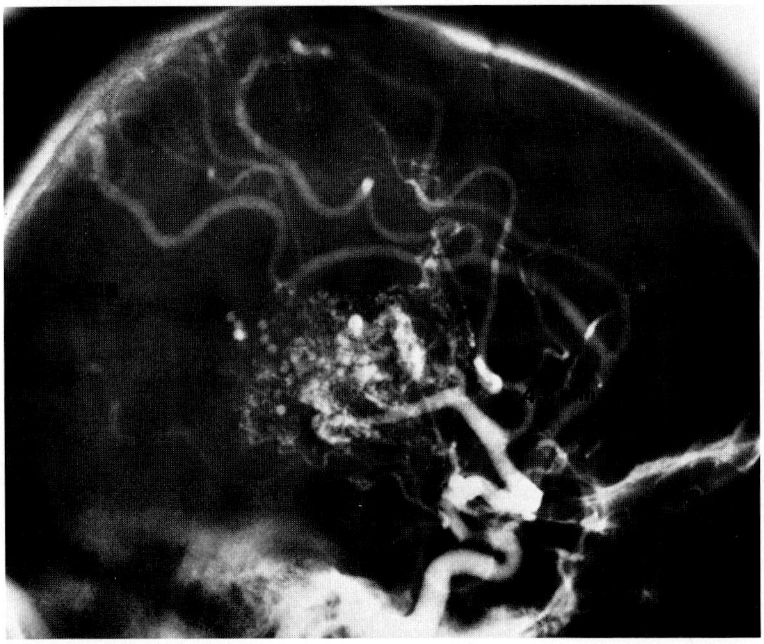

B

Fig. 2.9. **A.** Right lateral carotid angiogram after one embolization. Anterior cerebral artery is faintly visualized (*arrows*). **B.** Angiogram following second, effective embolization with 45 silastic emboli. AVM is reduced in size and circulation to normal regions is enhanced. Note that proximal middle cerebral artery temporarily enlarges (from 4.5 to 4.6 mm).

teries are compromised gradually resulting in temporary periods of ischemia to the brain which are rapidly compensated for by the development of collateral circulation through arteries not supplying the malformation. In addition to significantly reducing blood flow and turgor within the malformation, such a technique prepares the surrounding brain tissue for the eventual resection of the malformation. At the time of surgery, previously important middle cerebral arterial branches, which were intimate to the AVM, no longer hold significance for the normal brain and can be interrupted during the removal of the AVM without permanent neurologic deficit. Although we have used this modification of the embolization procedure in only a few cases, it appears to be useful, as when an AVM is in the territory of the middle

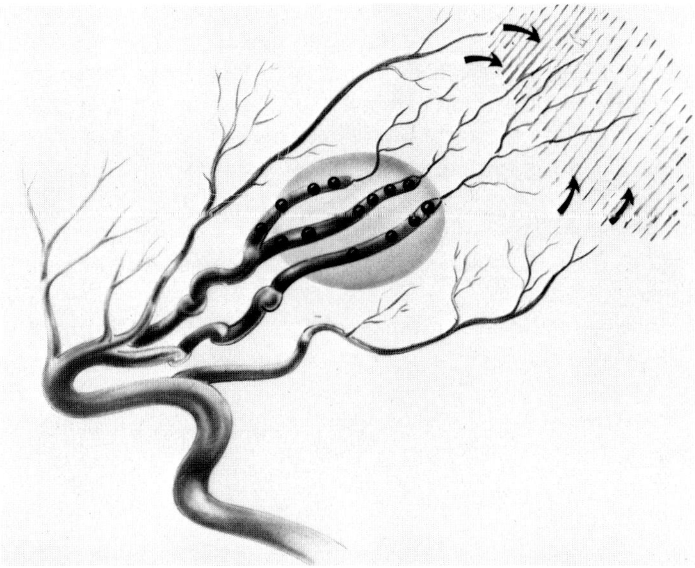

Fig. 2.10. Gradual intentional occlusion of middle cerebral artery branches common to normal brain and AVM. Area distal to AVM (*shaded area*) is rendered temporarily ischemic until collateral circulation is established (*arrows*).

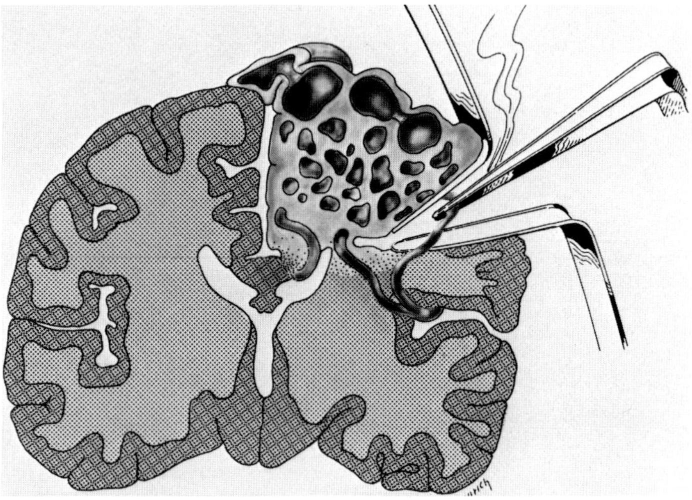

Fig. 2.11. Resection of AVM. Close adherence to margin of AVM and bipolar cautery with division of feeding arteries is essential.

cerebral artery involving the speech area (Fig. 2.10).

Techniques utilizing small balloon catheters that are placed in the arteries adjacent to an AVM and through which polymerizing agents may be injected directly into the AVM offer hope in the treatment of AVMs.[14]

Surgical removal of an AVM offers the only hope for total obliteration of the lesion and thereby a cure.* In the past, resection of large lesions situated in crucial areas of the brain frequently met with disastrous results. However, the mortality and morbidity from such procedures have been significantly reduced by a better understanding of the anatomy of these lesions, the use of embolization prior to surgery, and the use of sophisticated microneurosurgical techniques. Now lesions situated in crucial regions of the brain such as the motor and speech areas may be resected as well as some lesions involving deep portions of the brain.[7,17,39] It is recognized that in general the tissue within an AVM is composed of abnormal blood vessels and gliotic, nonfunctional brain tissue. Because of the congenital nature of these lesions, function is displaced from normal anatomic patterns. Therefore, working close to the margin of an AVM, one can remove the lesion without producing permanent neurologic deficit (Fig. 2.11). There is still concern, however, for the

* References 1, 3, 17, 25, 32, 34, 39, 47.

occurrence of disasters during the resection of such lesions, such as inadvertent violation of the confines of the malformation, with massive and often uncontrolled bleeding. Also one must be careful not to compromise vessels that are common to the normal brain and to the malformation. The exception to this situation is that previously mentioned where the vascular bed of the brain and the AVM is prepared by preoperative embolization.

In my experience with more than 200 AVMs, 170 of which have been resected, there has been under 2% mortality and less than 10% morbidity. Patients have been selected for surgery, and obviously not all AVMs are appropriate for resection. However, utilizing the principles previously outlined, we can remove not only small polar lesions but also large AVMs and those lying directly within or adjacent to eloquent areas of the brain. Factors militating against surgery include patients of advanced age; extensive, ill-defined malformations covering wide areas of the cortex or subcortex; and those lesions extensively involving the diencephalon or brain stem. In general, approximately two-thirds of patients evaluated will have resection of their AVM.

General anesthesia has been utilized in all cases, and although we consider intraoperative angiography useful, technical limitations have

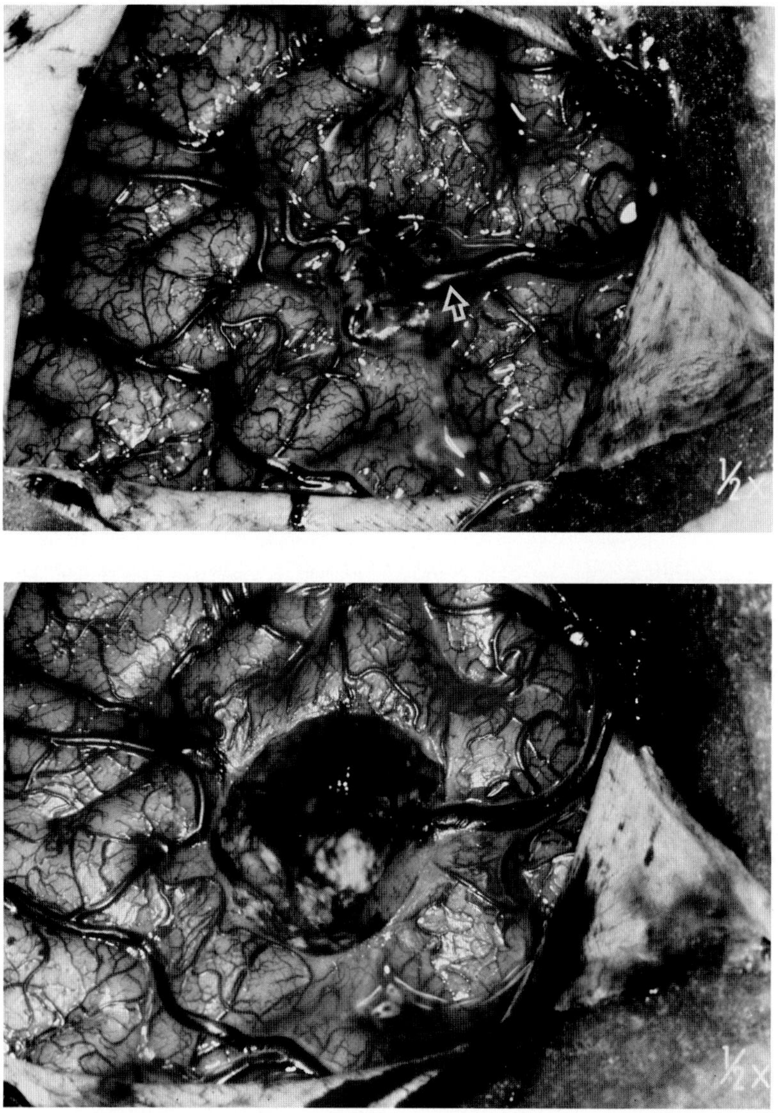

A

B

Fig. 2.12. A. Large draining vein (*arrow*) from a deep AVM involving motor region. Feeding arteries are not readily visible. **B.** After resection of AVM.

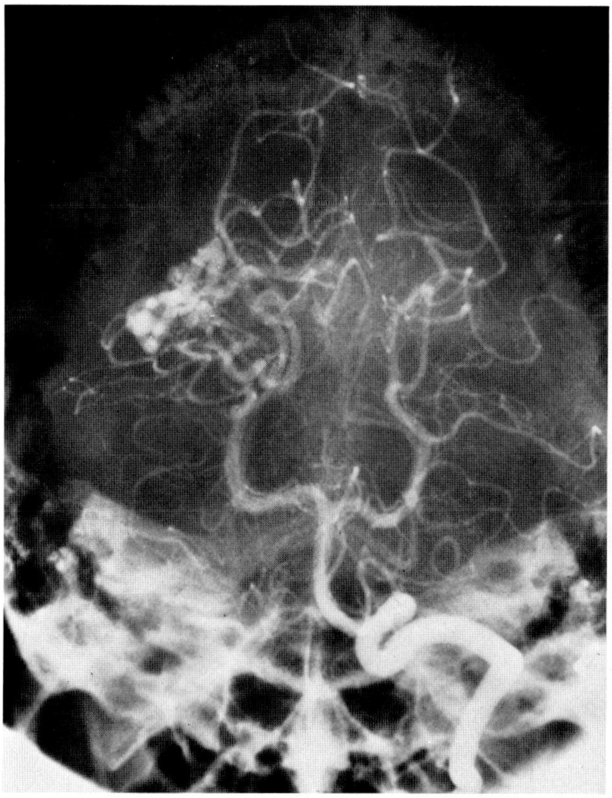

Fig. 2.13. AP vertebral angiogram demonstrating AVM involving medial temporal lobe adjacent to tectum of midbrain.

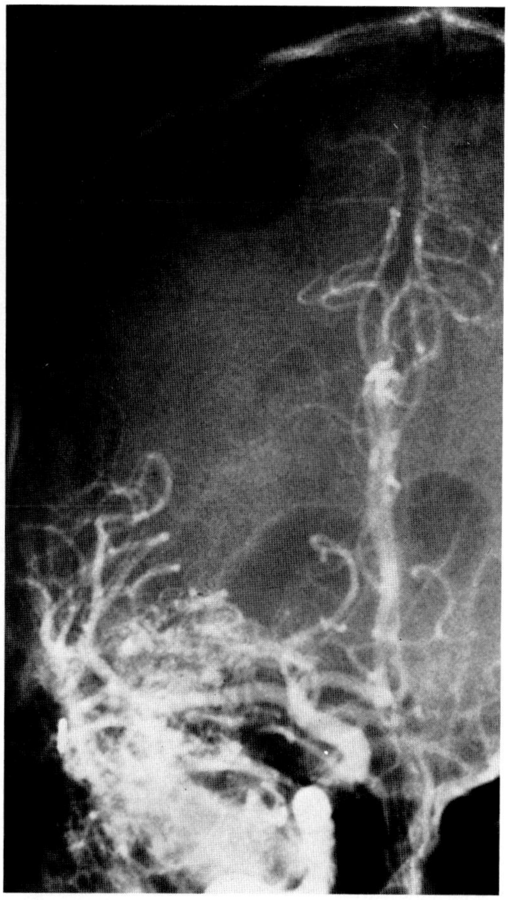

Fig. 2.14. AP right carotid angiogram demonstrating AVM partially involving lenticulostriate and anterior choroidal arteries. Stereolateral angiogram showed that the AVM could be separated from these important vessels.

precluded its routine use. Intra-arterial monitoring of blood pressure is essential for control, and spinal drainage is instituted for maximal relaxation of the brain. We have found that the most useful adjuvants are hypotension, often for a prolonged period, and liberal use of techniques to relax the brain.

The patient is positioned so that the surface of the lesion is horizontal and above cardiac level to ensure maximum venous drainage and reduction in turgor of the malformation. For midline lesions and those in the region of the vein of Galen, the patient is positioned in a semisitting posture. For lesions associated with the basal ganglion and lenticulostriate arteries, the head is well extended. A large craniotomy with wide exposure of the involved area is essential.

The margins of most malformations are not defined on the cortical surface. The most prominent landmarks are the veins draining the malformation; conversely the feeding arteries may lie buried in the sulci adjacent to the malformation and not be visible (Fig. 2.12). We have utilized templates of the arteriogram (drawings of both arterial and venous phases) to superimpose on the cortex. Measurements from routine angiography and the operating-room evaluation of stereoscopic angiograms are also important in deciphering the anatomy of these lesions.

The operation microscope is used throughout the resection of the malformation. A 275-mm objective with magnification of 10× or 16× is most satisfactory. I prefer the bipolar cautery with irrigation for occlusion of the feeding arteries rather than clips, except for large arteries.

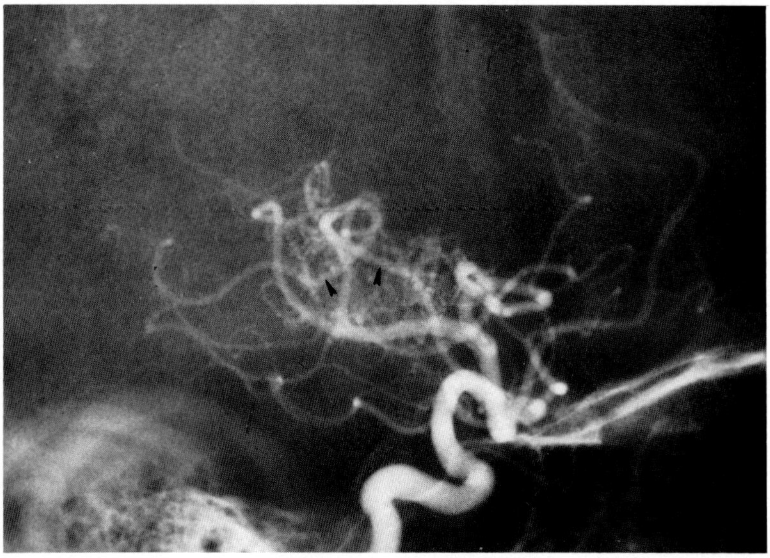

A

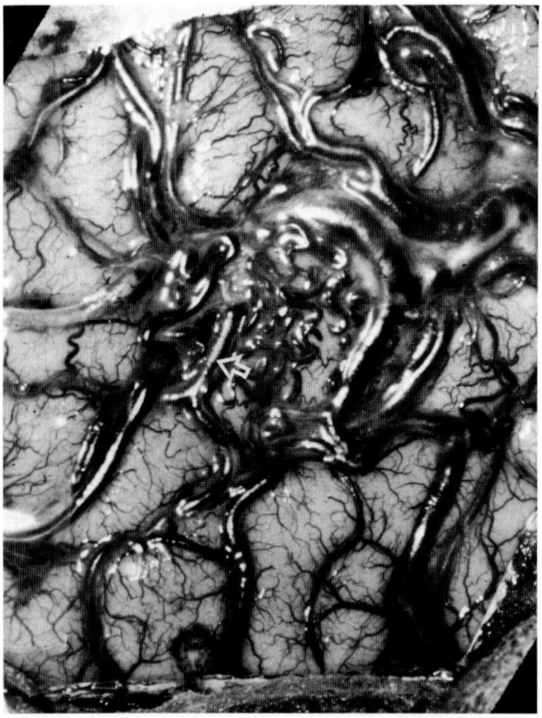

B

Fig. 2.15. **A.** Right lateral carotid angiogram demonstrating AVM fed by branches of middle cerebral. One important branch (*arrow*) is intimately involved by the AVM. This branch is partially visible (*open* (*arrow*) on the operative photograph **(B)** of the AVM. **C.** After resection of AVM showing preservation of middle cerebral branch intimate to the AVM (*open arrows*). This branch is seen (*arrows*) on the postoperative arteriogram **(D)**.

Metallic clips present a confusing picture on the postoperative CT scan. Furthermore, these clips do not satisfactorily occlude many of the thin-walled vessels associated with an AVM.

The major feeding arteries must be identified early in the resection. This step may require discrete transcortical incisions or the separation of gyri to visualize the arteries within their sulci. To mobilize the lesion and identify deep arterial feeders, it may be necessary to divide some of the arterialized draining veins. However, one large draining vein must be left intact until the very end of the surgical resection. Compromise of the dominant draining venous system may lead to premature rupture of the lesion and to a disastrous hemorrhage. Nevertheless, leaving cortical veins intact until the latter stage of the operation presents some problem, as feeding arteries often lie adjacent to the deep surface of these veins. As the arterial blood supply is gradually occluded, dissection is carried close to the AVM in the gliotic plane, which is invariably present around the margin of the lesion. Deep arterial feeders are the most difficult to identify and divide. This is doubly hazardous since it is impossible to debulk the lesion as one would a tumor. At this stage of the operation—often the most critical—mobile, gentle retraction on the AVM by an assistant and low-volume cautery of the surface of the lesion to toughen and shrink it are of consider-

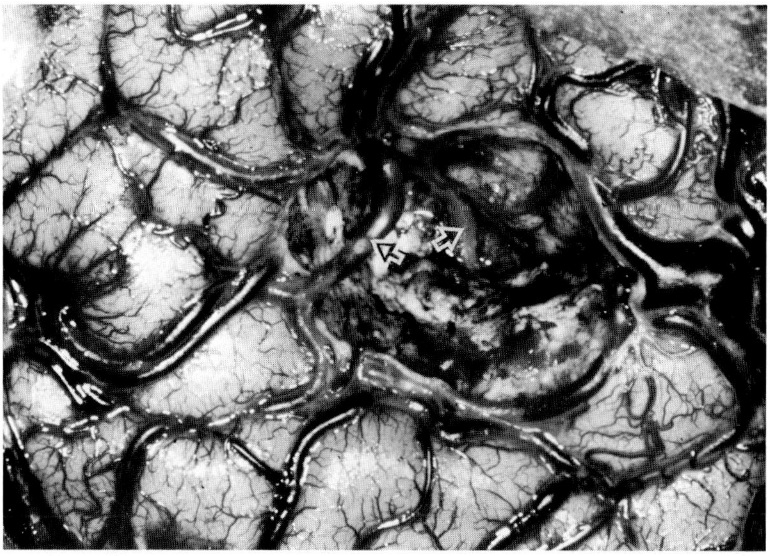

C

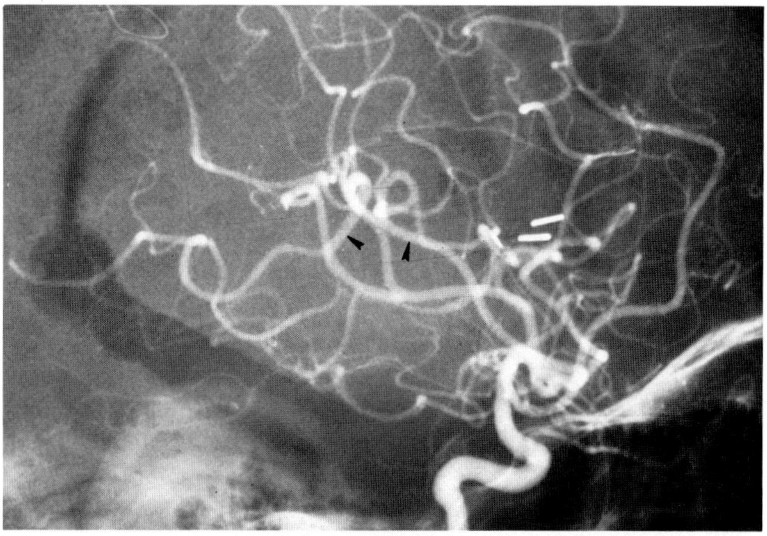

D

able benefit. It is at this stage that one encounters thin-walled vessels carrying arterialized blood in the white matter. If these vessels rupture, bleeding is troublesome and difficult to control. Hypotensive anesthesia and occlusion of the arterial feeders minimize these difficulties. If bleeding occurs during this time, "pack" the area with Gelfoam® (absorbable gelatin sponge, UpJohn) and cottonoids while turning attention to other aspects of the resection. Only when all the arterial feeders have been identified and divided may the last large draining vein be sacrificed.

When the malformation has been removed, the blood pressure is elevated above normal levels to test hemostasis and to identify residual malformation through the presence of arterialized veins. The precise control of hemostasis using the operation microscope has the disadvantage of permitting one to cut across a malformation and leave a portion behind. If arterialized veins are seen following a presumed total resection, it is indicative of residual malformation, which must be searched out and resected. This situation may exist in cases that are surgically treated shortly after an intracerebral hemorrhage in which the hemorrhage appears to split off portions of the malformation. In two of our surgical cases residual malformation was suspected by the presence of such veins at sur-

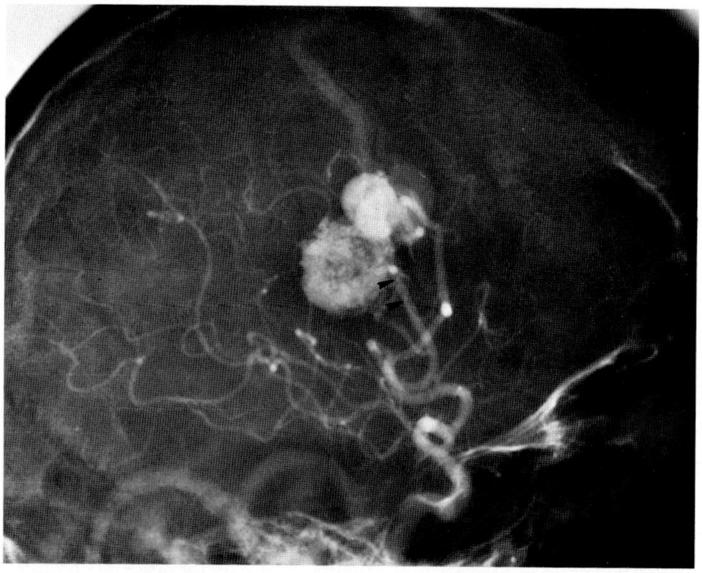

A

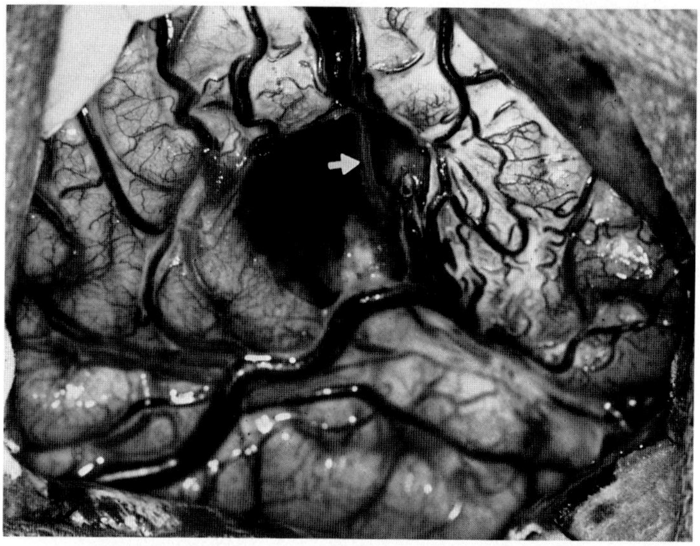

B

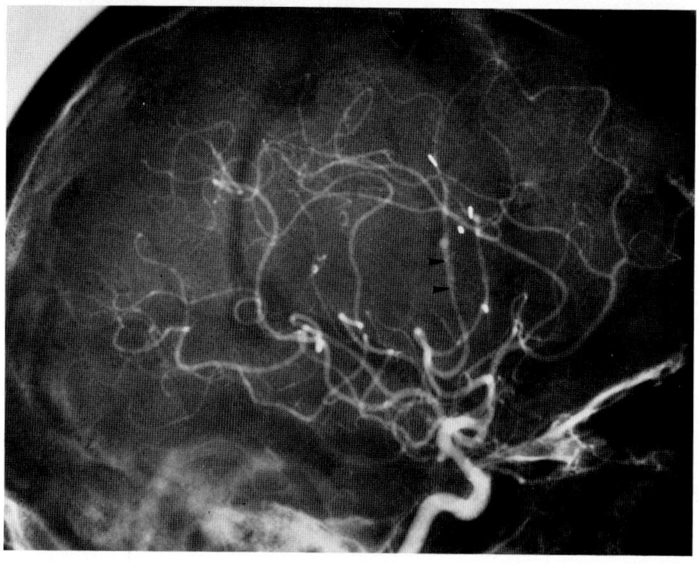

C

Fig. 2.16. **A.** Right carotid angiogram showing frontoparietal AVM. Important feeding artery (*arrows*) is intimate to AVM. Refer to Fig. 2.4 for operative appearance of this lesion. **B.** After resection of AVM. Note the important artery (*arrow*) preserved in the resection. **C.** Postoperative arteriogram showing preserved artery (*arrows*).

gery and confirmed by postoperative angiography. In both of these cases it was impossible to proceed further since one lesion was in the caudate nucleus and the other in the basal ganglia.

Arteriovenous malformations in certain locations require special techniques of exposure. In those lesions situated on the medial aspect of the temporal lobe adjacent to the incisura and quadrigeminal cistern (Fig. 2.13), the approach may be subtemporal, tracing the origin of the blood supply from the posterior cerebral and choroidal arteries. When a large portion lies paraventricular, the approach may be transcortical via the trigone or temporal horn. However, it is essential that the venous component not be disturbed until the arterial is under control. For malformations in the basal ganglia region it may be possible to separate them from the lenticulostriate arteries (Fig. 2.14). This determination may be made on the basis of the findings of a stereoscopic angiogram. The lesion is approached low by opening the Sylvian fissure, retracting the middle cerebral artery, and working under it. Midline lesions are approached parafalx with a craniotomy across the midline, the patient in a semisitting position. In all instances the principle of occluding arterial feeders at the margin of the AVM and dissecting close to the malformation must be followed.

In certain instances an important artery may run across the surface of an AVM, providing branches to the lesion. It is possible to detach and mobilize these arteries from the malformation. The malformation is then removed from under the involved artery leaving it to traverse the resultant cavity to supply normal brain (Figs. 2.15 and 2.16).

Following removal of the AVM we have been injecting the larger ones with methylmethacrylate for future corrosion of the soft tissue and three-dimensional anatomic study (Fig. 2.2).

In the postoperative period, depending on the location of the AVM, serious but usually temporary neurologic deficits may occur. These appear to be related to the dynamic shifts taking place in both the arterial and the venous circulations of the brain. Because of the occurrence of severe deficits, which invariably clear over a period of weeks, most of these problems apparently stem from venous stasis and thrombosis. Commensurate with this development we have noted slow resolution of vascular changes in comparing the pre- and postoperative angiograms on these patients. Residual vascular ectasia, stasis of contrast media, and retrograde thrombosis in some of the feeding arteries are common findings on angiograms done within a few weeks postoperatively.[39] It should be noted that all patients should have thorough postoperative angiography.

The results of a combined technique utilizing embolization as an adjuvant to surgery and resection of the lesions when feasible are recorded in Table 2.1.

Table 2.1. Cerebral AVM.

Operations (total)	No.	%
Total removals	170	—
Deaths	2	1.2
Morbidity		
Hemisensory/motor	8	4.7
Aphasia	2	1.2
Hemianopsia	15	8.8
Akinetic mute	1	0.6
Ataxia	1	0.6

References

1. Amacher AL, Allcock JM, Drake CG: Cerebral angiomas: the sequelae of surgical treatment. J Neurosurg 37:571–575, 1972
2. Boulos R, Kricheff I, Chase NE: Value of cerebral angiography in the embolization treatment of cerebral arteriovenous malformations. Radiology 97:65–70, 1970
3. Dandy WE: The Brain. Hoeber, Harper and Row, New York, 1969, pp 412–423
4. Dyck P: Spontaneous thrombosis of an arteriovenous malformation. Neurosurgery 1:287–290, 1977
5. Forster DMC, Steiner L, Hakanson S: Arteriovenous malformations of the brain. A long-term clinical study. J Neurosurg 37:562–570, 1972
6. French LA, Seljeskog EL: Arteriovenous malformations of the brain. In JR Youmans JR (ed): Neurological Surgery. WB Saunders, Philadelphia, 1973, p. 831
7. Garrido E, Stein BM: Removal of an arteriovenous malformation from the basal ganglion. J Neurol Neurosurg Psychiatry 41:992–995, 1978

8. Hamby WB: The pathology of supratentorial angiomas. N Neurosurgery 15:65–75, 1958
9. Heiss WD, Kvicala V, Prosenz P, Tschabitscher H: The importance of arterial shunting in areas of brain distant from an arteriovenous malformation. Neurology 20:376, 1970
10. Henderson WR, Gomez RDeRL: Natural history of cerebral angiomas. Br Med J 4:571–574, 1967
11. Höök O, Johanson C: Intracranial arteriovenous aneurysms: A follow up study with particular attention to their growth. Arch Neurol Psychiatry (Chicago) 80:39–54, 1958
12. Kaplan HA, Aronson SM, Browder EJ: Vascular malformations of the brain. An anatomical study. J Neurosurg 18:630–635, 1961
13. Kelly DL Jr, Alexander E Jr, Davis CH Jr, Maynard DC: Intracranial arteriovenous malformations: clinical review and evaluation of brain scans. J Neurosurg 31:422–428, 1969
14. Kerber C: Intracranial cyanoacrylate: A new catheter therapy for arteriovenous malformation. Invest Radiol 10:536–538, 1975
15. Kjellberg RN: Proton beam therapy of AVM. Presented at the Harvard Neurosurgery Postgraduate Course. November 13–17, 1978
16. Krayenbühl HA: Angiographic contribution to the problem of enlargement of cerebral arteriovenous malformations. Acta Neurochir (Wein) 36:215–242, 1977.
17. Künc Z: Surgery of arteriovenous malformations in the speech and motorsensory regions. J Neurosurg 40:293–303, 1974
18. Luessenhop AJ, Kachmann R, Shevlin W, Ferrero AA: Clinical evaluation of artificial embolization in the management of large cerebral arteriovenous malformations. J Neurosurg 23:400–417, 1965
19. Luessenhop AJ, Presper JH: Surgical embolization of cerebral arteriovenous malformations through internal carotid and vertebral arteries. J Neurosurg 42:443–451, 1975
20. MacKenzie I: The clinical presentation of the cerebral angioma: a review of 50 cases. Brain 76:184–214, 1953
21. McCormick WF: The pathology of vascular ("arteriovenous") malformations. J Neurosurg 24:807–816, 1966
22. McCormick WF, Nofzinger JD: "Cryptic" vascular malformations of the central nervous system. J Neurosurg 24:865–875, 1966
23. Morello G, Broghi GP: Cerebral angiomas. A report of 154 personal cases and a comparison between the results of surgical excision and conservative management. Acta Neurochir (Wein) 28:135–155, 1973
24. Newton TH, Troost BT: Arteriovenous malformation and fistula (Chapter 83). In Newton TH, Potts DG (eds) Vol 2, Book 4: Radiology of the Skull and Brain: Angiography. CV Mosby, St. Louis, 1974, pp 2490–2565
25. Norlén G: Arteriovenous aneurysms of the brain. Report of ten cases of total removal of the lesion. J Neurosurg 6:475–494, 1949
26. Olivecrona H, Ladenheim J: Congenital Arteriovenous Aneurysms of the Carotid and Vertebral Arterial Systems. Berlin, Springer Verlag, 1957, p 91
27. Olivecrona H, Riives J: Arteriovenous aneurysms of the brain: their diagnosis and treatment. Arch Neurol Psychiatry (Chicago) 59:567–602, 1948
28. Pascual Castroviejo I, Pascual Pascual JI, Blazquez MG, Lopez-Martin V: Spontaneous occlusion of an intracranial arteriovenous malformation. *Childs Brain* 3:169–179, 1977
29. Paterson JH, McKissock W: A clinical survey of intracranial angiomas with special reference to their mode of progression and surgical treatment: A report of 110 cases. Brain 79:233–266, 1956
30. Perret G, Nishioka H: Report on the cooperative study of intracranial aneurysms and subarachnoid hemorrhage. J Neurosurg 25:467–490, 1966
31. Pia HW, Gleave JRW, Grote E, Zierski J (eds): Cerebral Angiomas: Advances in Diagnosis and Therapy. Springer Verlag, New York, 1975
32. Pool JL: Treatment of arteriovenous malformations of the cerebral hemispheres. J Neurosurg 19:136–141, 1962
33. Pool JL, Potts DG: Aneurysms and Arteriovenous Anomalies of the Brain: Diagnosis and Treatment. Harper and Row, New York, 1965, p 463
34. Pool JL: Excision of cerebral arteriovenous malformations. J Neurosurg 29:312–321, 1968
35. Sano K: Intracranial arteriovenous malformation with special reference to its treatment. Neurol Med Chir 6:28–34, 1964
36. Sano K, Jimbo M, Saito I, Terao H, Hirakawa K: Artificial embolization with liquid plastic. Neurol Med Chir 8:198–201, 1966
37. Spetzler RF, Wilson CB: Enlargement of an arteriovenous malformation documented by angiography. J Neurosurg 43:767–769, 1975
38. Spetzler RF, Wilson CB, Weinstein P, Mehdorn M, Townsend J, Telles D: Normal perfusion pressure breakthrough theory. In Keever ED (ed) Vol 25: Clinical Neurosurgery. Williams & Wilkins, Baltimore, 1977, pp 651–672
39. Stein BM, Wolpert SM: Surgical and embolic treatment of cerebral arteriovenous malformations. Surg Neurol 7:359–369, 1977
40. Stein BM, Wolpert SM: Arteriovenous malfor-

mations of the brain I: Current concepts and treatment. Arch Neurol 37:1–5, 1980

41. Stein BM, Wolpert SM: Arteriovenous malformations of the brain II: Current concepts and treatment. Arch Neurol 37:69–75, 1980
42. Svien HJ, McRae JA: Arteriovenous anomalies of the brain. Fate of patients not having definitive surgery. J Neurosurg 23:23–28, 1965
43. Troupp H: Arteriovenous malformations of the brain: What are the indications for operation? In Morley TP (ed): Current Controversies in Neurosurgery, WB Saunders, Philadelphia, 1976, pp 210–216
44. Troupp H, Marttila I, Halonen V: Arteriovenous malformations of the brain: prognosis without operation. Acta Neurochir (Wein) 22:125–128, 1970
45. Waltimo O: The relationship of size, density and localization of intracranial arteriovenous malformations to the type of initial symptom. J Neurol Sci 19:13–19, 1973
46. Wendling LR, Moore JS, Kieffer SA, Goldberg HI, Latchaw RE: Intracerebral venous angioma. Radiology 119:141–147, 1976
47. Wilson CB, Hoi Sang U, Domingue, J: Microsurgical treatment of intracranial vascular malformations: J Neurosurg 51:446–454, October 1979
48. Wolpert SM, Stein BM: Catheter embolization of intracranial arteriovenous malformations as an aid to surgical excision. Neuroradiology 10:73–85, 1975
49. Wolpert SM, Stein BM: Factors governing the course of emboli in the therapeutic embolization of cerebral arteriovenous malformations. Radiology 131(1):125–131, 1979

3

Infratentorial Arteriovenous Malformations

Francis W. Gamache, Jr. and Russel Patterson, Jr.

Introduction

Vascular malformations anywhere in the cranial cavity threaten the patient and challenge the surgeon but none more so than those in the posterior fossa. Posterior fossa malformations are more likely to hemorrhage and generate neurologic deficits than their counterparts above the tentorium. Removing them is usually difficult and sometimes a feat. Fortunately, a better understanding of their pathologic anatomy plus better surgical techniques has improved the prospects of patients afflicted with them.

Pathology

Vascular malformations of the brain have been known for hundreds of years, and their classification has undergone continued modification. Virchow called those with no glia or nerve tissue between the cavernous spaces "cavernous angiomas," those with glia or nerve tissue between capillary structures "telangiectases," and those with glia or nerve tissue between arteries and veins "racemous angiomas."[94] Reflecting the uncertainty of their generation about the congenital or neoplastic origins of these lesions, Cushing and Bailey cataloged cavernous angiomas as tumors but telangiectases and racemous angiomas as malformations.[8] All thought of neoplasia was later discarded, and Bergstrand and co-workers in 1936 adopted and expanded Virchow's classification to include cavernous angiomas, telangiectasis, Sturge-Weber disease, arterial racemous angiomas, venous racemous angioma, and arteriovenous aneurysms.[5] Manuelidis in 1950 suggested the categories of telangiectases, cavernous hemangiomas, venous hemangiomas, and arteriovenous hemangiomas, and his schema saw modification at the hands of others.[44] The most widely used terminology today is that of McCormick, which divides them into telangiectasis (capillary angioma), varix, cavernous angioma (cavernoma), venous angioma, and arteriovenous malformation.[46,57,85] The important point is that arteriovenous malformations should not be lumped in one group but subdivided according to gross and microscopic findings because as will be shown, the prognosis varies between types.

The prototypical arteriovenous malformation of the cerebral or cerebellar hemispheres consists of dilated tortuous vascular channels that form a wedge-shaped mass, with the base of the wedge near the leptomeninges and the apex reaching the ventricle. Feeding arteries and draining veins are derived from both the superficial and choroidal circulations. The meninges are usually opacified and thickened, and calcification may be present. Microscopic examina-

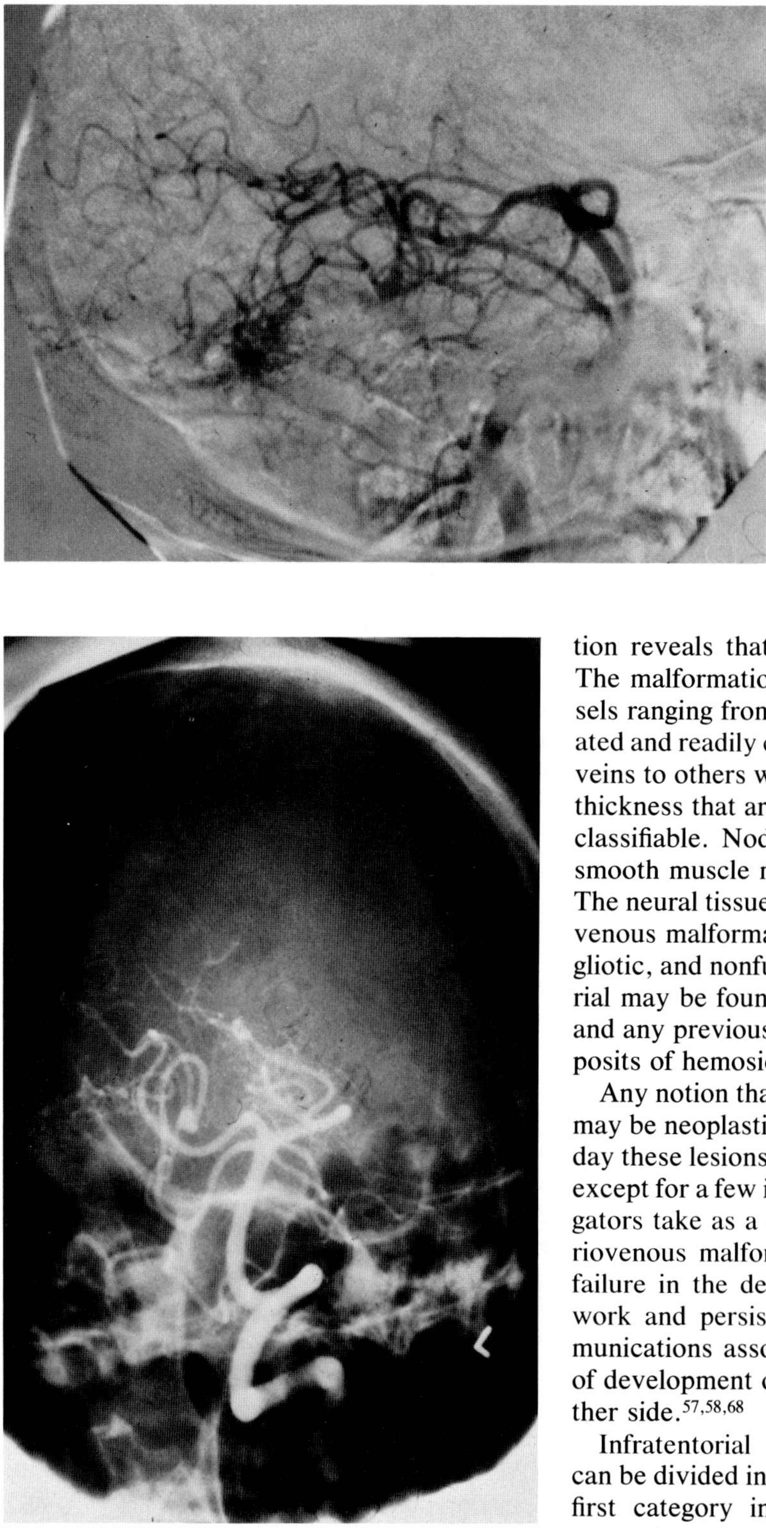

A

B

Fig. 3.1. **A.** Parenchymal arteriovenous malformations of the cerebellar hemisphere. **B.** Associated saccular aneurysm on one of the feeding arteries.

tion reveals that the lesion is quite complex. The malformation contains a spectrum of vessels ranging from some that are well differentiated and readily categorized as either arteries or veins to others with hyalinized walls of varying thickness that are poorly differentiated and not classifiable. Nodules of hyalinized intima and smooth muscle may project into their lumen.[46] The neural tissue within and around the arteriovenous malformation is generally degenerated, gliotic, and nonfunctioning. Amyloid-like material may be found at times in the vessel walls, and any previous hemorrhage will have left deposits of hemosiderin.[50,55,97]

Any notion that arteriovenous malformations may be neoplastic has long been discarded. Today these lesions are presumed to be congenital except for a few in the dura which some investigators take as a consequence of trauma. Arteriovenous malformations can be considered a failure in the development of a capillary network and persistent fetal arteriovenous communications associated with a variable degree of development of the arteries and veins on either side.[57,58,68]

Infratentorial arteriovenous malformations can be divided into one of three categories. The first category includes those that are *intraparanchymal* in the cerebellum, brainstem, or both (Fig. 3.1a,b). The second includes those that are *pial,* possibly with an intraparenchymal component, and the third are the *dural* arterio-

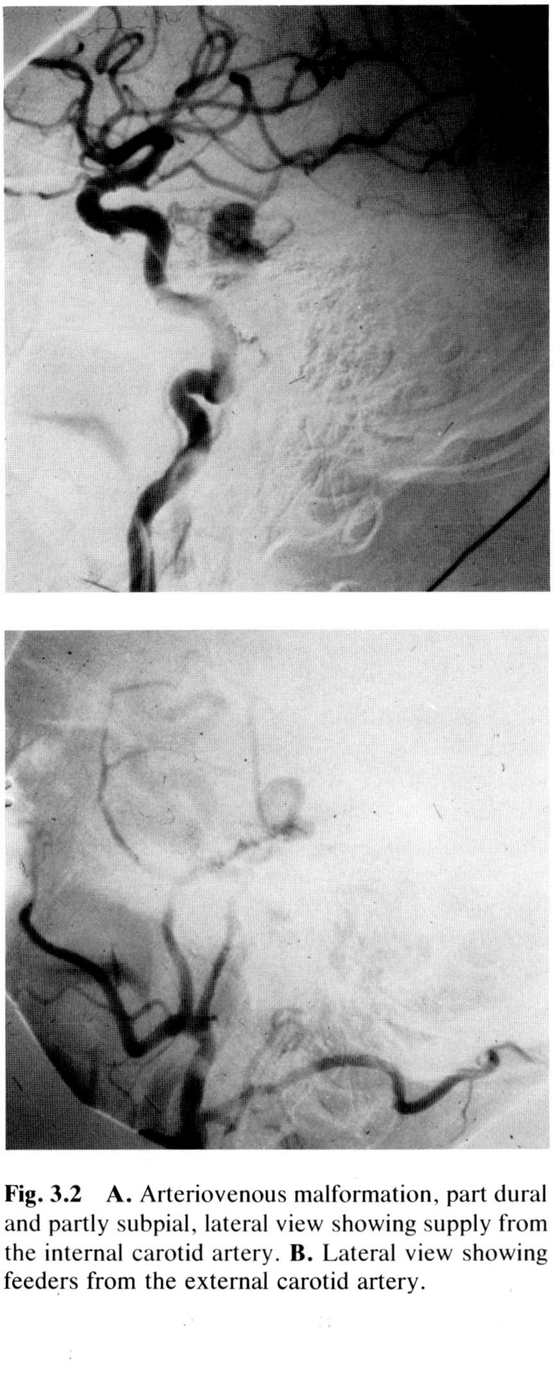

A

B

Fig. 3.2 **A.** Arteriovenous malformation, part dural and partly subpial, lateral view showing supply from the internal carotid artery. **B.** Lateral view showing feeders from the external carotid artery.

venous malformations (Fig. 3.2). This classification emphasizes that vascular anomalies in the posterior fossa can resemble the majority of supratentorial vascular anomalies and be primarily within the brain parenchyma or follow the pattern of many anomalies on the dorsal surface of the spinal cord and be primarily in the subarachnoid space.

Although infratentorial arteries may supply a vein of Galen malformation, the vein of Galen is anatomically a supratentorial structure and will not be considered in the following account.

Incidence

Infratentorial vascular malformations have generally been considered to be uncommon or even rare.* However, a review of infratentorial vascular anomalies by McCormick in 1968 led him to conclude this was not the case.[47] The first parenchymal malformation, in the pons, was reported by Virchow in 1851, and Sachs appears to have reported the first dural vascular anomaly in 1931, though Tonnis and Rottgen have been credited with an early description of a malformation involving the transverse sinus.[71,73,88,93] Perhaps as diagnostic radiologic methods have improved, especially with the introduction of computed tomography (CT), these anomalies are being recognized with greater frequency. Nevertheless, infratentorial malformations are less common than their supratentorial counterparts, except for the small, "cryptic" vascular malformations, which are distributed equally above and below the tentorium.[38,47,48,54,63,92] The participants in the cooperative study of subarachnoid hemorrhage found 7% of the 453 nondural vascular malformations occurred infratentorially.[63] Wappenschmidt and co-workers reported an incidence of 4.4% among 501 intracranial vascular malformations[95]. The incidence was 6.2% in the series of Krayenbuhl and Yasargil.[32] Laine in 1966 and Verbiest in 1968 reported an incidence of 20% though some dural malformations were included in Verbiest's review.[35,92] Matsumura in his review reported an incidence of 16.7%.[45] Houser et al found that 88% of vascular malformations were supratentorial, 10% infratentorial, and 2% straddled the tentorium.[27] In most series, lesions involving the brainstem have outnumbered those in the cerebellum, and in a few series the reverse has been the case.[38,45,47,63,66,69] The dura is the site of about 10% to 15% of intracranial malformations, and the majority of them occur near the transverse and sigmoid sinuses.[18,26,36,63,92] Occasionally, a

* References 1, 2, 4, 18, 20, 21, 57, 66, 69, 85, 92.

saccular aneurysm is associated with a vascular malformation.[1,6,47,59,63]

Malformations of the Cerebellum and Brainstem

Natural History

In a necropsy study of vascular malformations of the posterior fossa, McCormick and coworkers observed that the average age of patients with malformations above and below the tentorium were the same and that arteriovenous malformations predominated in the cerebellum whereas telangiectases predominated in the brainstem.[47] Telangiectases, of which 70% are found in the basis pontis, appear to be relatively innocuous, as a fatal hemorrhage had occurred in only one of their 38 cases. Hydrocephalus, either obstructive or communicating, was present in 6% of cases, less than the 15% which a survey of the surgical literature suggests.** Of the 51 malformations which had hemorrhaged in McCormick's study, 42 were arteriovenous malformations, demonstrating this type of anomaly is the one most likely to bleed.[48]

Supratentorial malformations can come to clinical attention by producing a variety of symptoms, but principally by causing convulsive seizures or by hemorrhaging. Convulsive seizures are not an expected symptom of infratentorial anomalies; they draw attention to themselves primarily through hemorrhage and, to a lesser extent, by inducing deficits in cranial nerve, cerebellar, and long tract function.[70] The report of the cooperative study showed that whereas only 68% of all malformations had bled by the time of entry into the study, 81% of infratentorial malformations had bled by that time.[63] The case fatality rate in the latter group for the initial bleed was 19%, and 6 of 13 patients managed conservatively died during the period of follow-up. Trumpy and Eldivik concluded that neither the location nor the size of the anomaly altered the risk of recurrent hemorrhage, which they estimated to result in a 10% mortality per decade for both supratentorial and infratentorial malformations combined.[90] Svien and McRae reported on 68 patients with predominantly supratentorial malformations who were not operated on and who were followed for an average of 10 to 14 years. In this group 16% died, 10% became invalids, and 22% developed a serious handicap.[80,81] Pool and Potts reviewed the course of 220 patients with mostly supratentorial malformations who were treated conservatively and estimated that 56% of them ultimately died or sustained an important neurologic deficit.[64,65] Although the data are scanty, the outlook for patients with vascular malformations of the cerebellum and brainstem may be more dismal than for those with malformations situated above the tentorium. Lusins and Sencer reported on nine patients who were untreated; during the period of follow-up, five of them died of rebleeding, one sustained a severe deficit, two a moderate deficit, and only one was functioning normally.[41]

** References 3, 7, 12, 16, 38, 41, 45, 64, 69, 72, 78, 91.

Clinical Syndromes

Approximately 60% of patients with posterior fossa vascular malformations have subarachnoid hemorrhage associated with multiple neurologic signs. Cerebellar signs include ataxia and dysesthesia. Brainstem signs such as hemiparesis, nystagmus, and even internuclear ophthalmoplegia have been reported. Cranial nerve signs are common, particularly extraocular palsies, deafness, and facial paralysis. Occasionally a medial longitudinal fasciculus syndrome develops.† If the patient displays only neurologic signs and gives no history of subarachnoid hemorrhage, which happens in 20% of cases, the clinical picture may be confused with other conditions such as multiple sclerosis.†† An occasional patient may present with trigeminal neuralgia, but vascular malformations are a rare cause of headache, except when they hemorrhage. Periodic headaches occur with approximately the same frequency in patients with vascular malformations as in the general population, which is 15%.[29,37,41,93]

Neurologic symptoms, in the absence of hemorrhage, are the consequence of the shunting of blood through the anomaly at the expense of the adjacent brain or perhaps an effect of compression of the brain by a progressively di-

† References 23, 29, 37, 38, 41, 75, 85, 92, 98.
†† References 23, 29, 37, 38, 41, 45, 63, 85, 92.

lating mass. The presence of a large malformation has widespread and important effects on cerebral blood flow and cerebral blood volume. For example, Tonnis and Lange-Cosack demonstrated that cerebral blood volume could decrease by 50% following extirpation of an arteriovenous malformation.[87] Heart failure as a consequence of the shunt occurs only in infants in whom the size of the shunt is large in proportion to cardiac output. However, in children, the removal of a large arteriovenous malformation may alter cardiovascular dynamics in such a way as to precipitate cardiac failure, as will be discussed later.[39,56,92]

About 20% of patients have subarachnoid hemorrhage without focal neurologic signs which suggest a posterior fossa locus.‡ Parenchymal anomalies may hemorrhage in the cerebellum, or less frequently, in the basis pontis. Possibly some of the examples of spontaneous cerebellar hemorrhage commonly associated with hypertension originate from cryptic anomalies that are below the resolution of the routine clinical tests.[48] Sometimes the hemorrhage will be in the subdural space, though this is distinctly uncommon.[92]

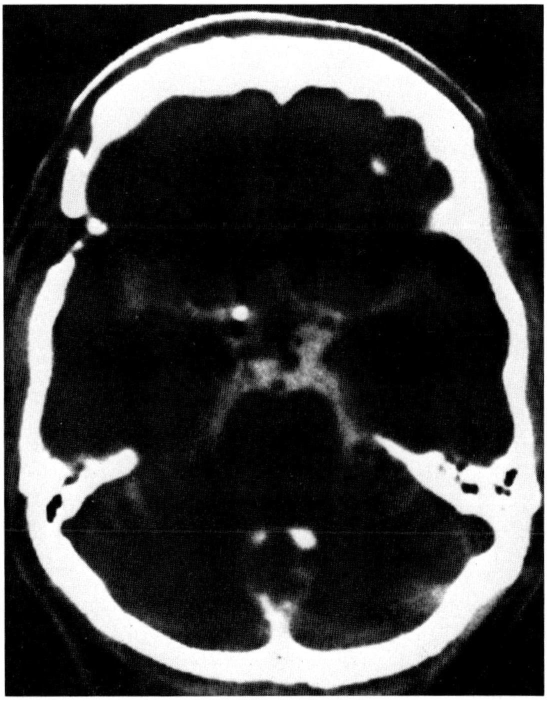

Fig. 3.3. CT scan after the subarachnoid injection of metrizamide demonstrates multiple filling defects due to a vascular malformation in the suprasellar cistern in part of the midbrain.

Diagnostic Tests

Plain skull films in as many as 60% of cases may show calcification within the anomaly, enlarged vascular foramina, or changes related to increased intracranial pressure such as erosion of the sella and thinning of the posterior clinoid processes or of the inner table of the skull.‡‡ None of these are pathognomonic of a vascular malformation.

CT studies may show areas of abnormal brain densities, usually increased, with poorly defined margins.[67,86] However, one-quarter to one-third of patients will have normal findings on the unenhanced scan. The sensitivity of the test is increased after contrast enhancement, but some vascular malformations will not be demonstrated, even with enhancement.[49,67] A CT scan is quite sensitive to fresh hemorrhage and is the best way of demonstrating that a parenchymal bleed has occurred. As in the case of ruptured saccular aneurysm, subarachnoid hemorrhage is proved by the presence of a xanthochromic supernatant after centrifuging the bloody spinal fluid obtained by lumbar puncture. Metrizamide CT scans may also be utilized to visualize the subarachnoid compartment of an arteriovenous malformation within the basal cisterns (Fig. 3.3)

Angiography with subtraction is the best tool for investigating vascular anomalies of the brain. Although small anomalies may be below the resolution of the technique, most anomalies of clinical significance will be demonstrated. Since the surgery of the malformation depends on a knowledge of its anatomy, the surgeon needs to see separate injection of all the major intracranial arteries and also of the external carotid artery[9,10,17,52,62] on the side of the lesion.[13] All the feeding vessels must be identified, if possible, and in 15% of patients the dural vessels will be found to contribute. Sometimes the effort to define the entire arterial and venous anatomy will fail despite films taken at a rate of 4 to 6 per second. A high rate of flow of blood, multiple feeders, a heavy stain in the anomaly

‡ References 16, 38, 41, 45, 69, 72, 78.

‡‡ References 2, 25, 38, 53, 56, 68, 69, 86, 92.

itself, and the shunting of blood from areas of lower flow all may make it impossible to obtain perfect films.[2,11,38,56,69,83,92] In children, the amount of contrast agent that can be safely injected may limit the study or require that the study be completed in stages.[39] Digital arteriography or NMR may provide additional helpful information about some of these (at times) difficult to define brainstem lesions.

Treatment

The effect that an arteriovenous malformation will have on a patient is unpredictable. As recounted earlier in this chapter, some patients tolerate them well for a lifetime, which is why neurosurgeons tend to be cautious about recommending excision if the lesion's size or location suggests that surgery carries substantial risk. Infratentorial vascular malformations differ from supratentorial vascular malformations in that they seem to have a significantly greater propensity for repeated hemorrhaging and inducing neurologic deficits. Because they carry a poor prognosis, we believe surgical excision should be attempted in most cases, with due consideration given for the condition of the patient, the location of the anomaly, and the experience of the surgeon. The following case is a striking example of the unpredictable outlook for patients with a posterior fossa arteriovenous malformation. An 85-year-old man sustained a subarachnoid hemorrhage associated with signs of malfunction of the left cerebellar hemisphere four years before. Angiogram at the time demonstrated an arteriovenous malformation in the left cerebellopontine angle (Fig. 3.4). He recovered well from the effects of the hemorrhage and remains well four years later.

A number of reports have suggested preoperative embolization of certain supratentorial vascular malformations may simplify a planned operation or sometimes even be curative. Reported experience to date is too scanty to define the role of embolization in the management of posterior fossa vascular malformations.[33,40,74] Fox and Al-Mefty reported the case of a 15-year-old boy with a large malformation near the midbrain that had caused hydrocephalus, quadriparesis, and oculomotor palsies. The lesion was almost entirely obliterated by embolization with 210 one-millimeter pellets. However, the patient died minutes later of an autopsy-confirmed midbrain hemorrhage, probably due to rupture of a residual portion of the arteriovenous malformation.[19]What role embolization will have in the management of these lesions is far from settled, but unless the malformation can be obliterated completely, which often is unlikely, the propensity for fatal hemorrhage may well be retained unless some other means is employed in conjunction to totally obliterate the AVM.

The location of the malformation determines the surgical approach. When a *suboccipital approach* is suitable, we prefer to position the patient prone and to fix the head in pins. This position allows the microscope to be vertical and gives the assistant easy access to the operating field. Others prefer the sitting position or the lateral decubitus position, both of which are quite acceptable. If the lesion is restricted to one cerebellar hemisphere or cerebellopontine angle, then we position the patient supine with the head turned so that the saggittal plane is horizontal. A unilateral opening that exposes the transverse sinus above and leaves the foramen magnum unopened is adequate for most lesions of the cerebellum. Rarely does the foramen magnum need opening or the lamina of C-1 have to be removed. Arteriovenous malformations in the midline of the cerebellum will require exposure of both cerebellar hemispheres and division of the occipital sinus.

A 60-year-old man sustained a severe headache and transient loss of consciousness. Examination revealed meningeal signs, ataxia of gait, and dysmetria of both upper limbs. Speech was slightly slurred. Angiography revealed an arteriovenous malformation in the right cerebellar hemisphere and what was taken as an aneurysm of the principal feeding artery (Figs. 3.5a,b). The anomaly was removed by a suboccipital approach, and the presumed aneurysm was found to be only a kink or loop in the artery. After a year he had some mild ataxia but was able to play golf and to work as a lawyer.

Hemorrhage from a telangiectasis in the pons is usually fatal, though if the hemorrhage is small, evacuation of the hematoma and biopsy of the malformation with recovery is possible.[78] We have had experience with four such cases, two of which were operated on to the patients' benefit. One case is cited here in detail.

Fig. 3.4. **A,B.** Lateral and AP angiogram of an 85 year old man who sustained an SAH at age 80 as his only symptom of a brainstem AVM.

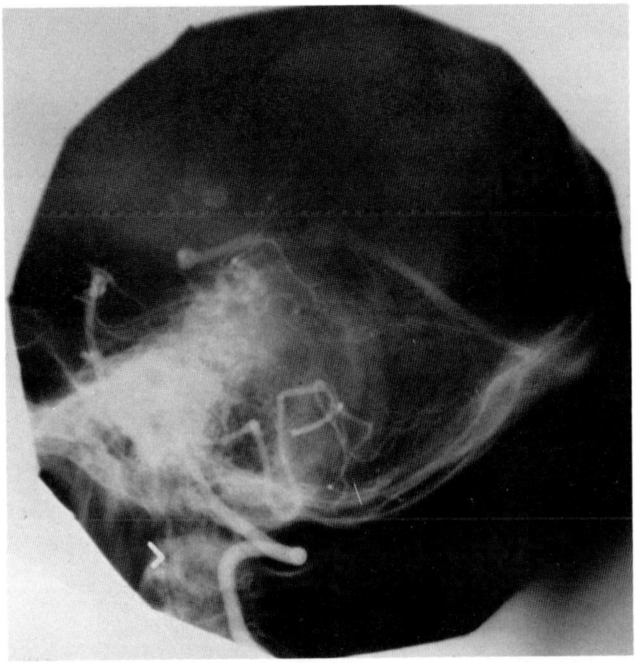

A

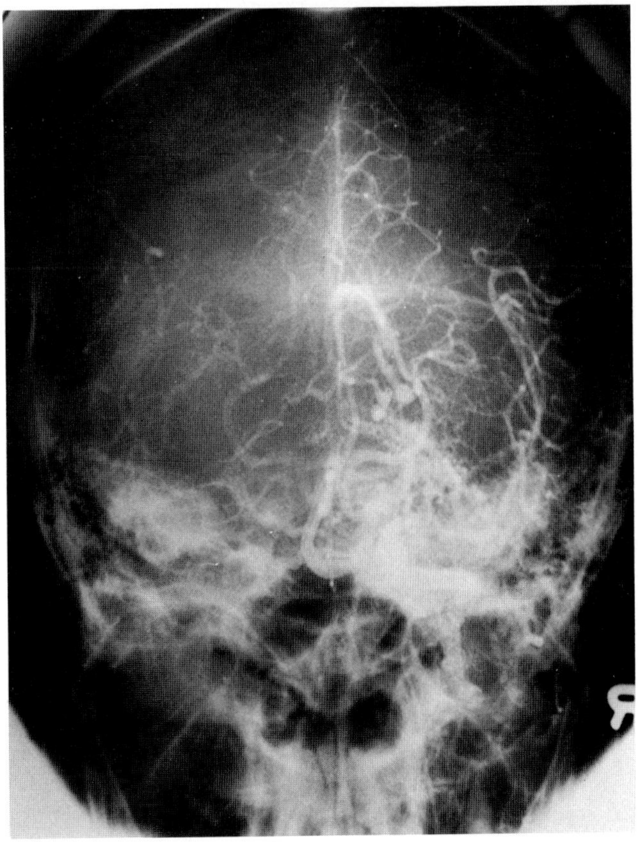

B

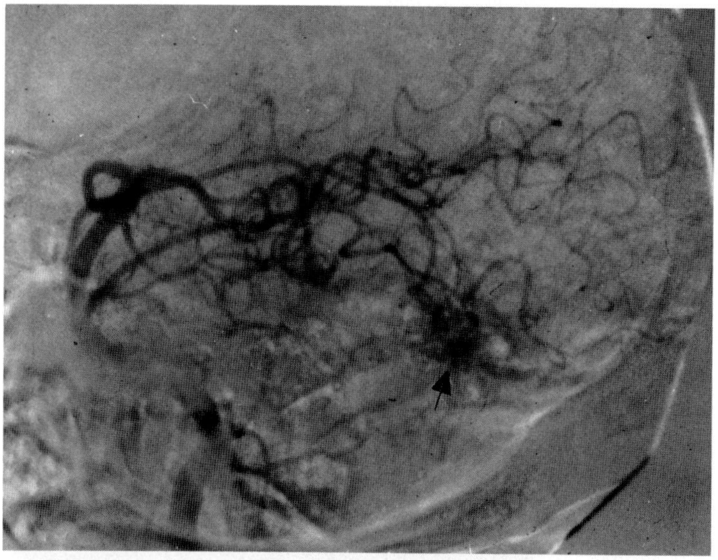

A

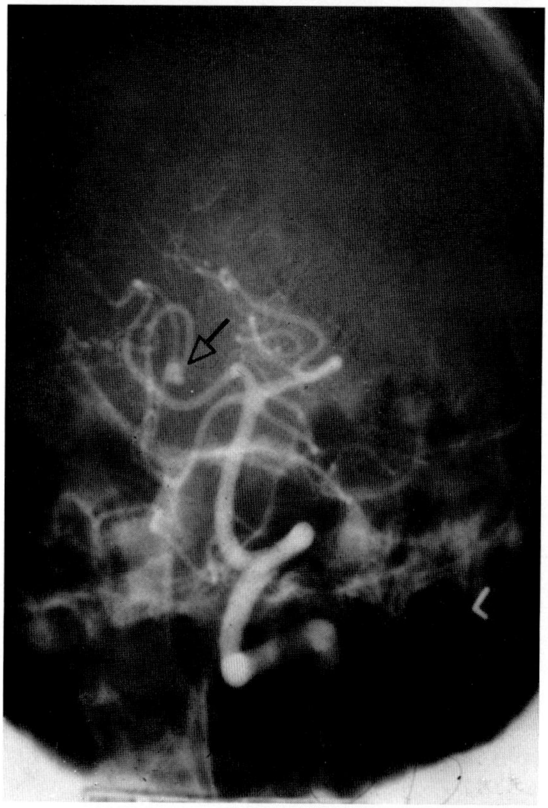

B

Fig. 3.5. A,B. AP and lateral angiogram of a 60 year old man with a cerebellar AVM that hemorrhaged and what was taken as a sacular aneurysm on a feeding artery. The aneurysm proved to be a loop in an ectatic artery.

A 24-year-old woman had two episodes of subarachnoid hemorrhage one year and again one month prior to surgery. She was left with a mild left hemiparesis, numbness of the right side of the face, and ataxia. A CT scan revealed a radiodense mass in the right side of the pons (Figs. 3.6a,b). At surgery the swollen pons was incised and a hematoma evacuated. Biopsies revealed gliosis with hemosiderin pigment. The neurologic signs cleared rapidly following surgery and were minimal after six months. Repeat CT scans one year later showed persistence of the radiodense lesion in the pons (Fig. 3.6c). Angiograms taken on two occasions were normal.

Anomalies on the *tentorial surface* of the cerebellum are difficult to manage by an approach which is exclusively suboccipital because the transverse sinus and upward slope of the tentorium obstructs the view. If the anomaly is not too large, exposure can be accomplished by a supratentorial craniotomy that exposes the superior sagittal and transverse sinuses (Fig. 3.7). The occipital lobe is elevated near the falx, preserving the lateral occipital vein. The tentorium then is opened by an L-shaped incision which parallels the straight sinus through the tentorial notch and then turns and parallels the transverse sinus. This gives good exposure of the superior surface of the hemisphere, and if all the veins between the cerebellum and the vein of Galen are divided, excellent exposure of the region of the quadrigeminal plate, pineal gland, and posterior choroidal arteries are obtained under the vein of Galen. In larger anomalies involving the superior surface of the cerebellum, we favor a *combined supratentorial and infratentorial craniotomy* extending from the midline laterally (Fig. 3.8). The transverse sinus

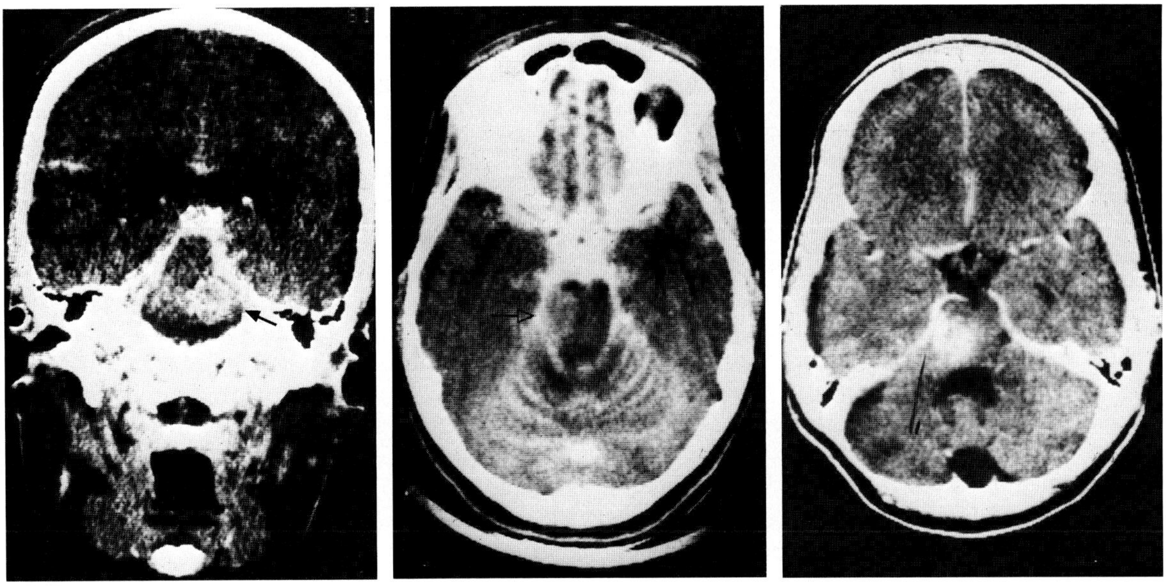

Fig. 3.6. A,B. Coronal and transaxial tomogram of a 24 year old woman with two episodes of brainstem hemorrhage from a telangectasis. **C.** 1 year following surgery.

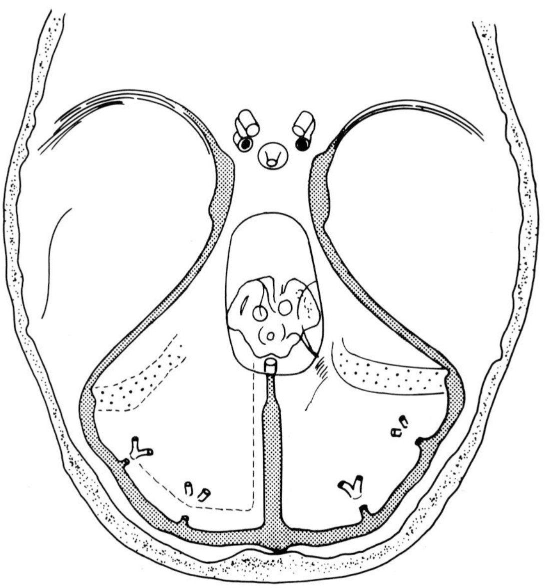

Fig. 3.7. Exposure of the superior surface of the cerebellum Occipital lobe is elevated and the tentorium divided along straight and transverse sinuses. Division of all veins connecting cerebellum to the Vein of Galen provides good exposure of the quadrigeminal plate, pineal gland, and posterior choroidal arteries.

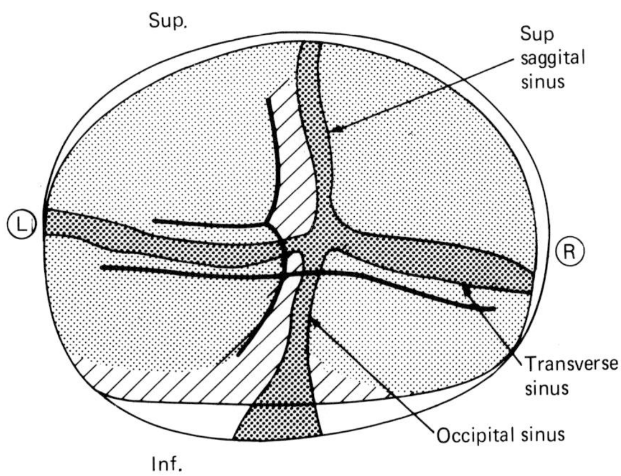

Fig. 3.8. Wide exposure of superior surface of cerebellum. Achieved by dividing one transverse and the occipital sinus, followed by division of the tentorium along the straight sinus. Division of cerebellar veins draining into the Vein of Galen also may be helpful. The tentorium and occipital lobe are retracted as a unit.

is divided just lateral to the torcular (Herophili) and the tentorium is opened through the tentorial notch. Angiograms taken prior to operation showing a patent contralateral transverse sinus are reassuring but the sinus should be clamped temporarily before being divided to ensure brain swelling does not occur. After division of the transverse sinus the tentorium and occipital lobe are elevated together. This preserves the draining veins from the cerebral hemisphere to the transverse sinus and thereby reduces the chances of dangerous postoperative cerebral edema or venous infarction.

Malformations of the brainstem involving the upper pons and midbrain are best exposed through a *subtemporal approach* with division of the tentorium through the tentorial notch, taking the usual precautions to save the trochlear nerve.

A 67-year-old woman sustained the sudden onset of nausea, vomiting, headache, and diplopia. Examination revealed disconjugate gaze with the right eye deviated inward and down. There was evidence of impairment in function of the right fifth, seventh, ninth, and twelfth cranial nerves, a right hemiparesis, and bilateral extensor plantar responses. Angiography revealed an arteriovenous malformation in the right side of the cerebellopontine angle (Figs. 3.9a,b). A right temporal craniotomy was performed, and the temporal lobe elevated. After division of the tentorium, the malformation was identified intimately involved with the trigeminal root and extending into the pons. The feeders which originated mostly from the superior cerebellar artery, were divided; then the veins, and finally the anomaly, could be entirely excised. The patient recovered well initially but developed a delayed venous infarct in the temporal lobe, producing a significant neurologic deficit. Some lesions were located on the anterior surface of the brainstem (Figs. 3.10, 3.11). These are best handled through an anterior temporal or pterional approach, which allows further access to the midline and to components on the opposite side of the stem (Fig. 3.12). If necessary the subtemporal approach can be combined with a lateral suboccipital craniotomy of the kind that is used for an acoustic tumor (Figs. 3.13a–c). The tentorial incision is carried parallel to the petrosal sinus through the transverse sinus, and the tentorium, including the posterior temporal lobe and the vein of Labbé, is retracted toward the vertex. An alternative is to burr away part of the mastoid bone and divide the petrosal sinus and sigmoid sinus. This allows elevation of the temporal lobe with preservation of the vein of Labbé in cases where the vein enters at the junction of the transverse and sigmoid sinuscs. In this circumstance, division of the transverse sinus laterally without jeopardizing the vein of Labbé can be difficult.

For the most part, brainstem malformations are in the subarachnoid or subpial space and are amenable to removal like their counterparts in the spinal cord. The feeding arteries, which can be multitudinous, are divided, and the anomaly is dissected off the brainstem in the subpial plane. In general the veins should be divided last, but if several draining veins can be identified, it may help to take one early and use the stump as a handle during the dissection.[16,60,61]

Infants with large anomalies provide a special problem. As Long and co-workers pointed out, their blood volume is expanded, and sudden obliteration of the shunt may increase peripheral resistance sufficiently to cause acute heart failure.[39] The monitoring of intra-arterial blood pressure, central venous pressure, or better, pulmonary wedge pressure provides helpful information about cardiac function and may signal that phlebotomy is necessary to protect the heart.

An occasional malformation will be of a size and location that surgical manipulations required to remove it may damage vital neural structures.[96] The damage results from efforts to control brisk hemorrhage with suction, bipolar coagulation, and pledgets of cotton. In this circumstance, profound hypothermia and circulatory arrest can provide a bloodless field in which vascular lesions can be removed atraumatically from the brainstem.[60] In the case of supratentorial lesions, the cannulations for the pump-oxygenator can be made through the femoral vessels without opening the chest. If a posterior fossa approach is necessary, it is more convenient to place the patient in a lateral position and expose the heart directly. The principal difficulty surgeons have with the technique is the persistent epidural bleeding after rewarming the patient and terminating cardiopulmonary bypass. This can be prevented by firmly tacking up the dura before going on bypass. If bleeding

Fig. 3.9. A,B. AVM in the subarachnoid space and pia mater of the brainstem at the tentorial notch.

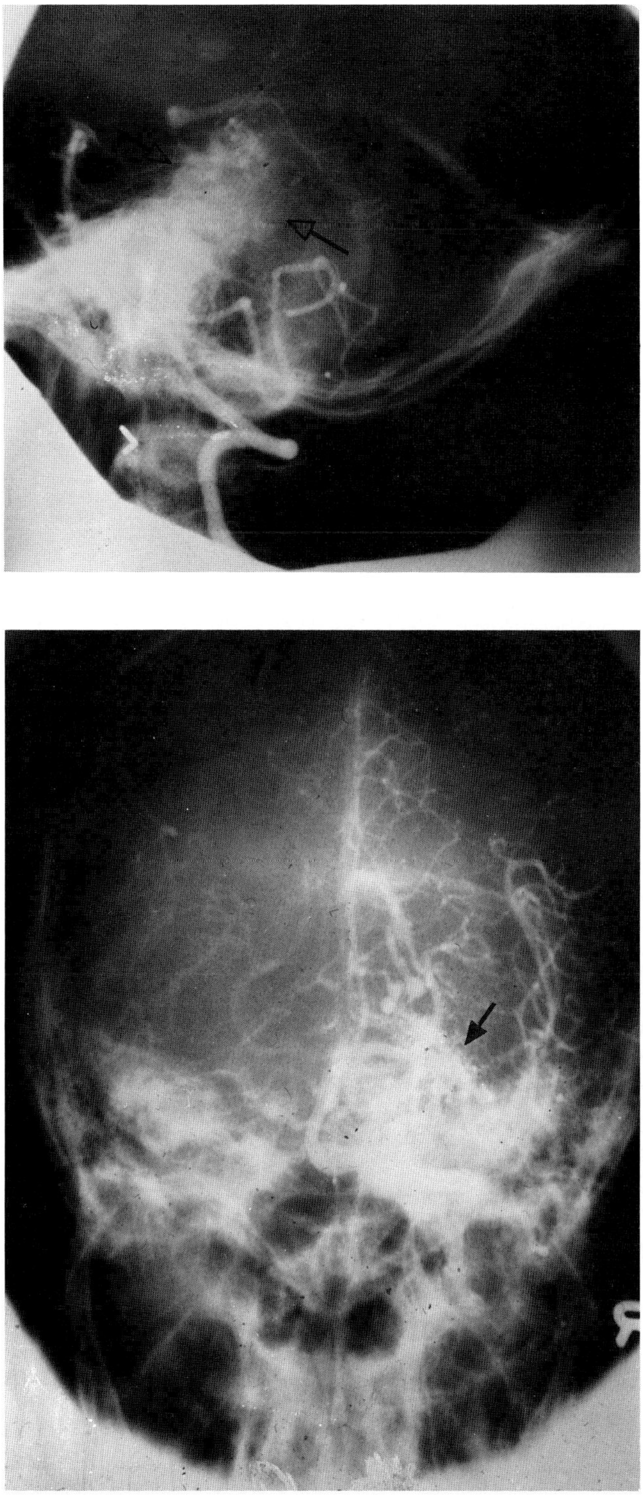

A

B

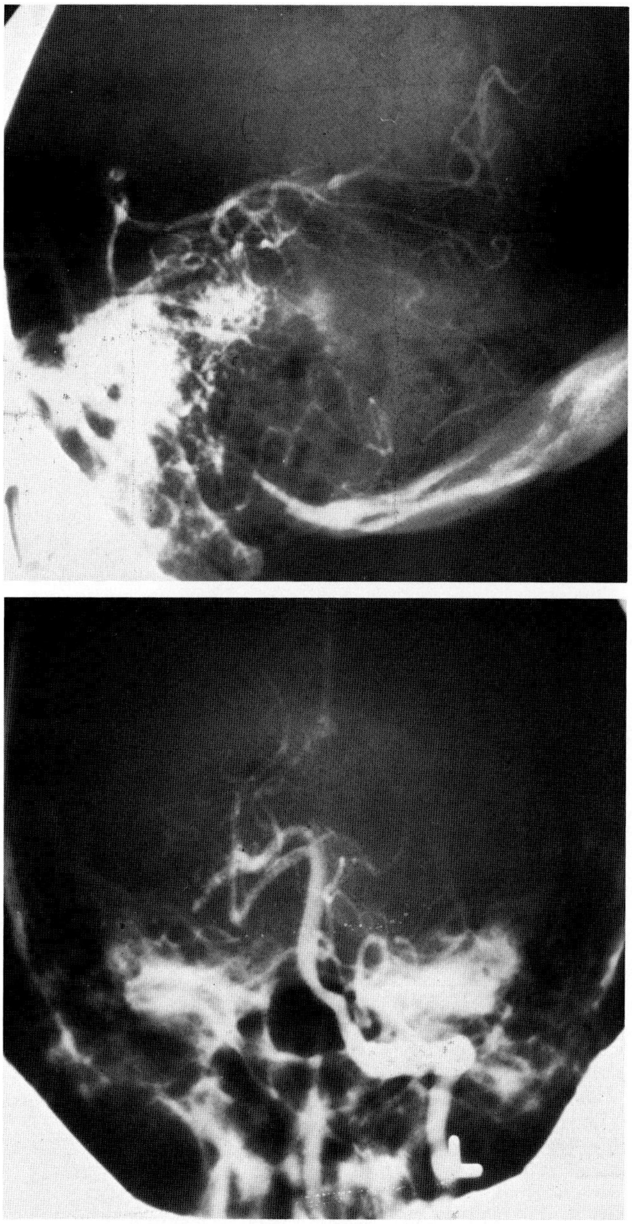

A

B

Fig. 3.10. **A.** Subpial arteriovenous malformation of the midbrain and pons, lateral view. **B.** Anterior posterior view.

still is troublesome at the end, the use of compounds such as ε-aminocaproic acid and factor IX concentrate are effective in restoring normal clotting, though, the latter carries the risk of inducing hepatitis. We find cooling takes 20 to 25 minutes and rewarming approximately 30 minutes. Thirty minutes of arrest time have proved safe, and reperfusion for a few minutes with cold blood will allow additional intervals of circulatory arrest.

While enthusiasm has been expressed regarding the use of lasers in excising AVMs, laser surgery of AVMs remains in experimental and developmental stages. The same may be said of radiation therapy of AVMs or the staged removal of AVMs.[30,76]

Dural Arteriovenous Malformations

The dura mater is a frequent component of an intracranial vascular malformation. Arteriovenous malformations of the brain itself receive a blood supply from the dura mater in about 15%

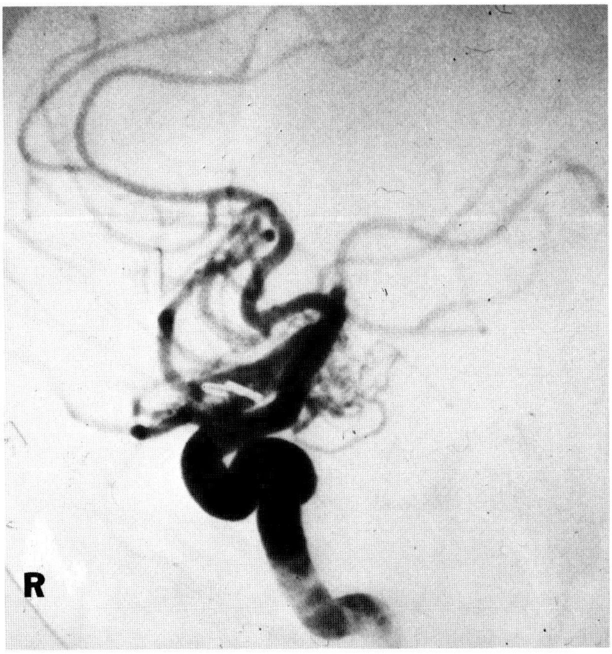

A

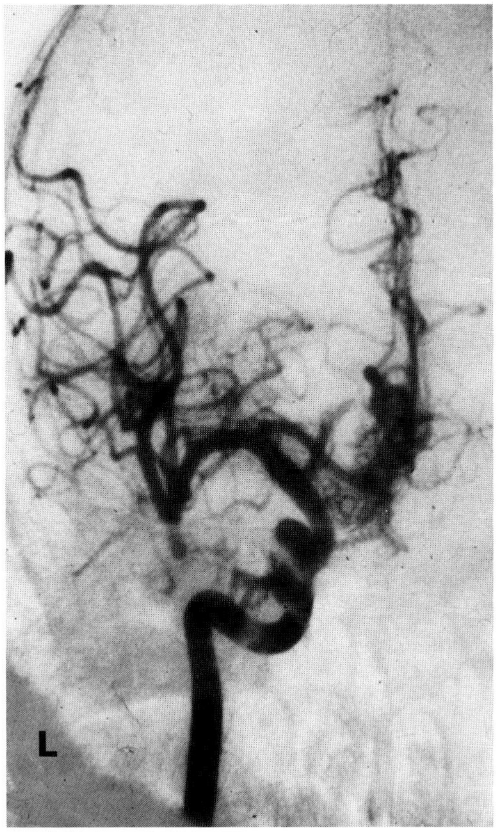

B

Fig. 3.11. **A.** Early arterial phase of an arteriovenous malformation in the suprachiasmatic and interpeduncular cisterns. **B.** Anteroposterior view. **C.** Late arterial venous phase lateral view. **D.** Late arterial venous phase anteroposterior view. (Fig. 3.11D see next page).

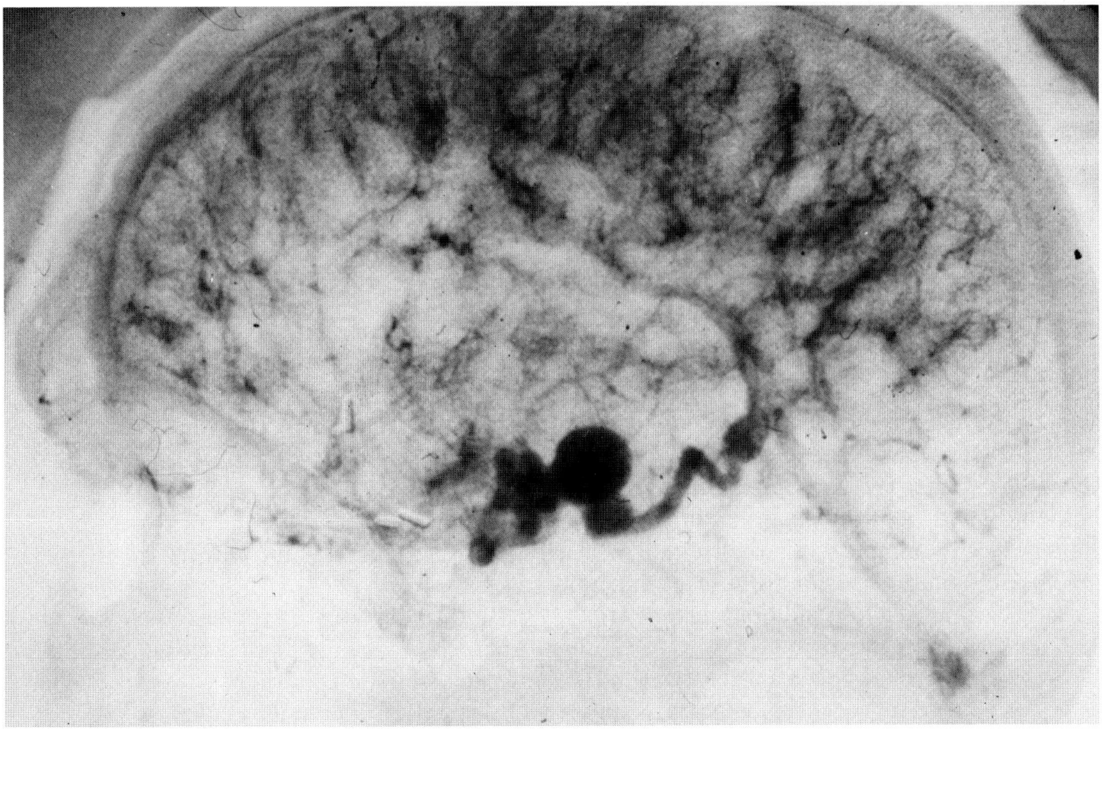

C

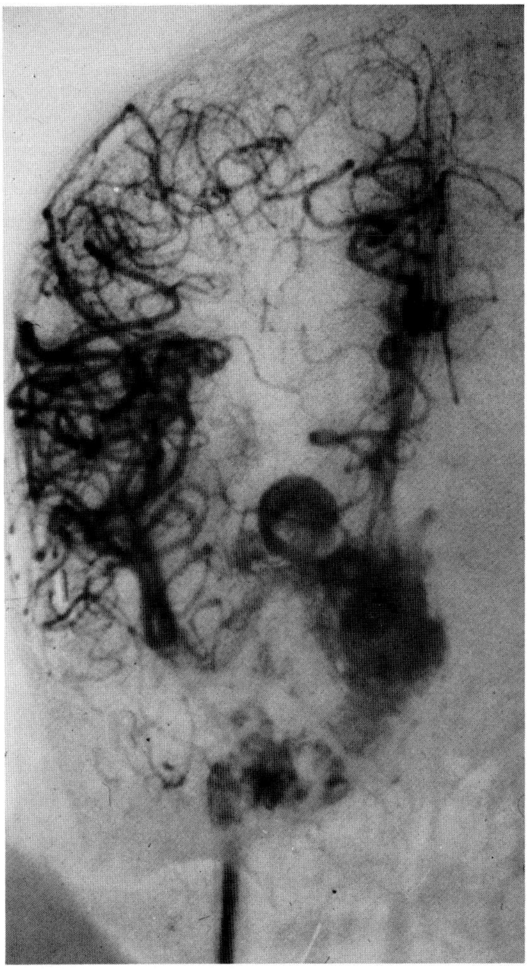

Fig. 3.11D

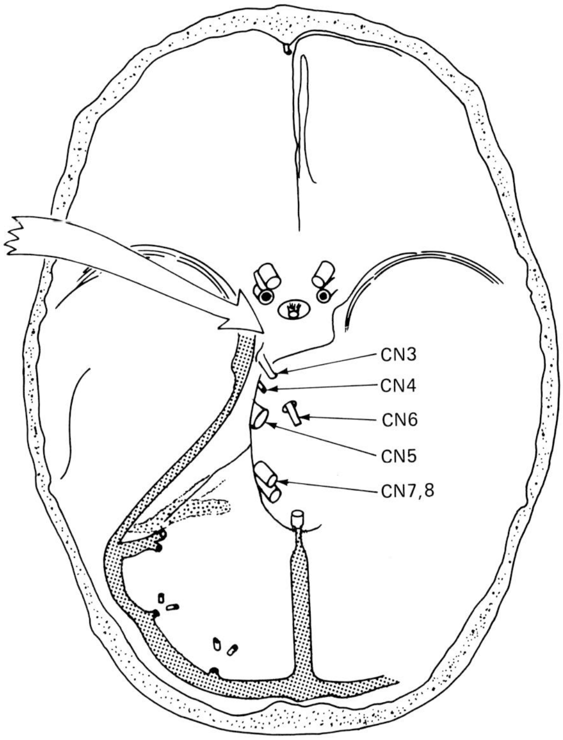

Fig. 3.12. Anterior brainstem anomilies are best exposed by the pterional approach splitting the Sylvian fissure widely and freeing temporal lobe from the third nerve. The medical anterior temporal lobe may have to be resected or improved exposure. The tentorium can be divided sparing the trachlear nerve. The advantage of this approach is that the cranial nerves are lateral and out of the field. Exposure of cerebello pontine angle is limited.

of cases, and the dura alone is the seat of a vascular malformation in another 10%.[51] Perhaps one-third to one-half of this latter group are located around the sella turcica, middle fossa, and cerebral convexity. However, the preponderance are in proximity to the transverse and sigmoid sinuses, into which they drain (Fig. 3.2).

Anatomical Considerations

The dura in the region of the transverse and sigmoid sinuses receives an arterial blood supply from the internal carotid, external carotid, and vertebral arteries. The meningohypophyseal trunk and the lateral and marginal tentorial arteries of Bernasconi and Cassinari originate from the internal carotid artery. The external carotid artery provides the posterior branch of the middle meningeal artery; the ascending pharyngeal artery, which supplies the dura near the foramen magnum; and the meningeal branches of the occipital artery, which penetrate the occipital bone and supply the dura of the posterior fossa. The vertebral artery provides the posterior meningeal artery, which anastomoses with branches of the middle meningeal artery. Occasionally, cervical branches of the subclavian artery also supply the dura near the foramen magnum and feed these anomalies.[9,10,17,52,62,84]

Houser and others reported that the arterial supply in 15 patients with occipitomastoid anomalies was predominately from multiple regional dural arteries but that in some cases a

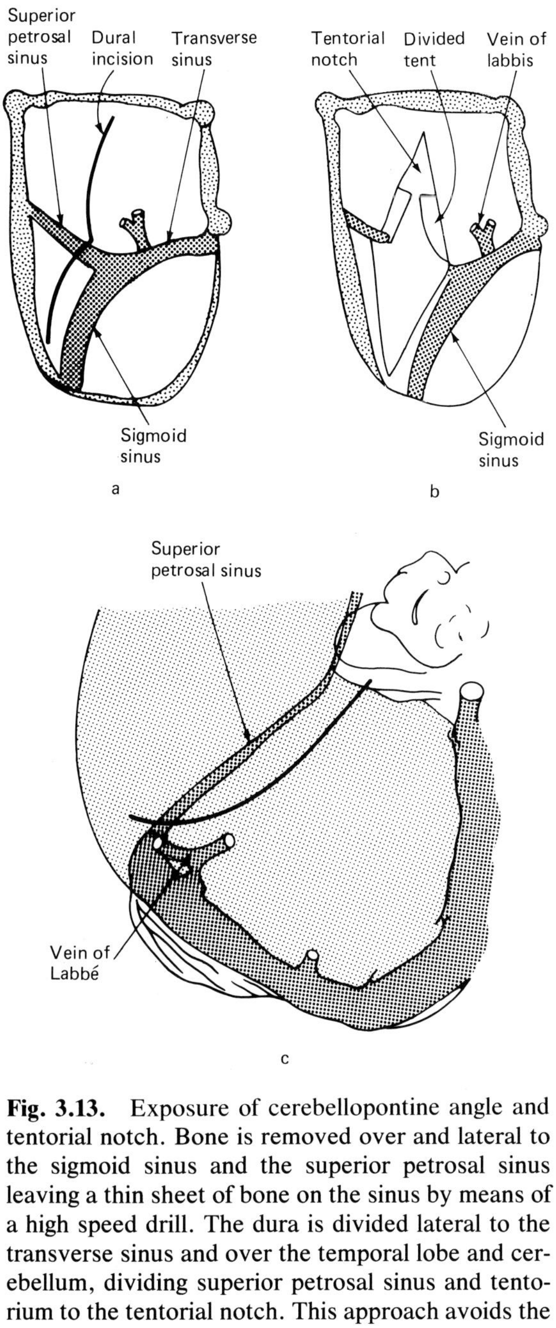

Fig. 3.13. Exposure of cerebellopontine angle and tentorial notch. Bone is removed over and lateral to the sigmoid sinus and the superior petrosal sinus leaving a thin sheet of bone on the sinus by means of a high speed drill. The dura is divided lateral to the transverse sinus and over the temporal lobe and cerebellum, dividing superior petrosal sinus and tentorium to the tentorial notch. This approach avoids the Vein of labbe, which enters the transverse sinus near the junction with the petrosal sinus.

single artery was involved.[26] In the series of 31 cases reviewed by Debrun et al, some were reported to be supplied exclusively by the occipital branch of the external carotid artery, but careful angiography is likely to prove such cases to be exceptional.[11] Dural vascular malformations may have a pial component or even extend through the cranium to the scalp. Venous drainage can be through either dural or pial channels, with about two-thirds draining exclusively into dural sinuses.[26] A shunt of large volume may reverse the flow of blood from the transverse sinus into the superficial cerebral veins, such as the vein of Labbé and the lateral occipital vein.

Thrombosis of the transverse or sigmoid sinus has been reported in many cases of vascular anomaly of the dura. The fact that the sigmoid sinus is so often blocked suggested to Sundt an inflammatory process which obstructs the sinus. An inflammatory hypervascularity then develops into an arteriovenous fistula.[79] Older speculations centered on an embryologic cause, possibly a delay in the embryologic development of the external carotid artery and the coexistence of a large number of emissary veins at the skull base.[26,82] Others see the close anatomic relationship between dural arteries and veins as a cradle for the easy development of dural vascular malformations.[2]

Pathophysiology

Parenchymal vascular malformations become symptomatic because the malformation diverts blood from the brain with consequent brain ischemia, or the dilating mass may compress the brain, or the fragile vessels may rupture and cause hemorrhage.[11,18,22,56] On the other hand, dural vascular malformations, commonly located at the skull base, distress the patient by being a source of thrills or bruits. Sinus thrombosis may overload venous reserve and cause intracranial hypertension manifest by headaches and papilledema.[18,22,31,56] Papilledema may be present without an elevated spinal fluid pressure. Nicola and Nizzoli observed patients with dural vascular malformations of the posterior fossa with venous congestion and hypertension at the level of the torcular but with normal pressure on lumbar puncture.[54] Rarely, a dural AVM may even spontaneously close and thrombus.[42]

In those patients who manifest subarachnoid hemorrhage, probably a pial component is present, and it is this part of the anomaly that is responsible for the bleed.

Symptoms

The first symptom of a dural vascular malformation is bruit in about two-thirds of cases. Headache is present in 40%, and one-third have papilledema or, less commonly, exopthalmus. As many as 20% may have subarachnoid hemorrhage. Occasionally they are asymptomatic in life and found incidentally at necropsy.* Seizures are rare, but may occur owing to reversed flow in the cerebral veins, resulting in passive congestion of the brain.

Obrador and co-workers[56] reviewed 115 cases and found that symptoms fell into one of six patterns. The patients in the first group, which contained 35% of cases, complained only of bruit. A second group of 17% of cases had headache, papilledema, and visual failure due to increased venous pressure. The third group of 17% of patients was composed of those who experienced subarachnoid hemorrhage. A fourth group, 10%, had neurologic signs attributed to ischemia, and a fifth group was composed of infants with hydrocephalus and bruit and accounted for 4%. The last group of 15% of patients combined the symptoms of two of the groups above, which were commonly the second and fourth.[56]

Treatment

Early efforts to treat these lesions consisted of ligation of the external carotid or occipital artery. In some cases long-term improvement was observed, but more often the bruit either persisted or disappeared only transiently.[31,56]

A number of authors have reported success with embolization of dural vascular malformations using silicone pellets, Gelfoam, and silastic glue.[14,24,43,77] We have had experience with embolization using fragments of plastic sponge in three cases involving the transverse and sigmoid sinus. In each case the malformation was cured, as judged by postoperative angiograms, and the patients tolerated the procedure well. Experience is still too limited to say what percentage of patients can be treated this way, and the number may be limited, as the arterial feeders in many cases are multiple, small, and may originate from the internal carotid artery.

* References 2, 18, 22, 31, 34, 36, 37, 56, 92.

Another therapeutic option is to excise the entire anomaly, although this may be risky in some cases. If the transverse sinus is primarily involved, excision is possible without much difficulty. The upper part of the sigmoid sinus can be removed, particularly if the overlying mastoid bone is taken away first. A number of arterial feeders from the external carotid artery usually are found penetrating the mastoid and draining into the first part of the sigmoid sinus. One might not expect excision of a transverse sinus involved with a dural vascular malformation to interfere with the venous drainage of the cerebral hemisphere, as pressure in the sinus is elevated, and reverse flow is often present from the sinus into the cerebral veins. However, we observed one patient who tolerated division of the draining veins and excision of the sinus well for three days and then developed a venous infarct in the parietal lobe. Probably the flow was fast in the veins when the anomaly was present and became stagnant after the anomaly was removed, leading to thrombosis.[31] Consequently, we have reservations about the wisdom of removing the transverse sinus in these cases.

Hugosson and Bergstrom proposed a method of treatment which preserves cerebral venous drainage and yet obliterates the fistula.[28,34] The principle is to isolate the transverse and sigmoid sinus from all blood vessels except the draining veins. Sufficient bone is removed to expose the dura over the occipital lobe and cerebellum. Lumbar drainage of cerebrospinal fluid may be necessary to reduce the intracranial pressure prior to opening the dura, as the brain is often swollen. An incision is made in the dura above the parallel to the transverse sinus from the midline to the superior petrosal sinus laterally. A second incision is made in the tentorium from the torcula to the superior petrosal sinus, and this sinus is ligated, divided, and the dura coagulated. If the draining cerebral veins make this difficult, the tentorium can be divided from below. A third incision in the dura is made below the transverse sinus and follows the transverse and sigmoid sinuses down to the region of the jugular foramen. The dura is divided on either side of the sigmoid sinus. Part of the mastoid bone is then removed to divide penetrating feeders from the posterior auricular and occipital arteries. The authors point out that feeders may remain in the dura that is not divided

A 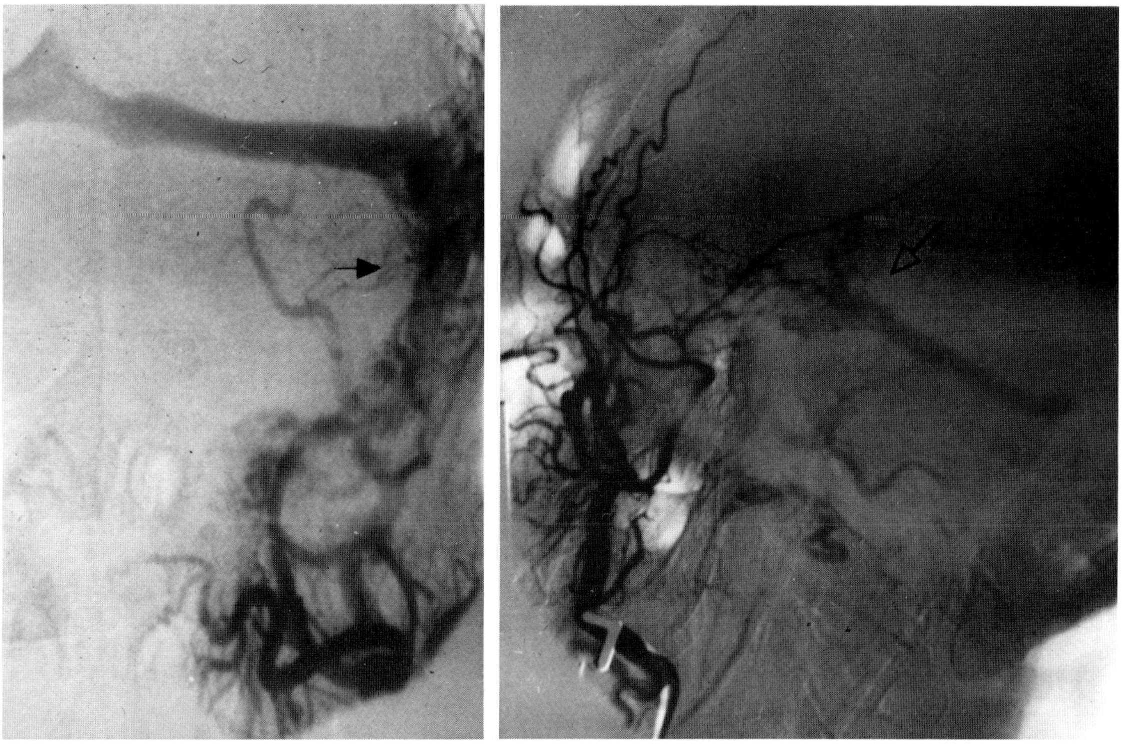 B

Fig. 3.14. A. AP and **B** oblique view of a dural AVM near the mastoid process associated with thrombosis of the sigmoid sinus.

around the jugular foramen. If a bruit still persists, then the ascending pharyngeal artery should be divided in the neck.

A 55-year-old woman developed intermittent left suboccipital headache eight months prior to surgery. Six weeks prior to surgery a pulsing sound appeared in both ears, more in the left side. Pressing around the left mastoid process obliterated the noise. In addition, she noted numbness of the right limbs, and examination revealed a mild right hemiparesis and incoordination of the left upper and lower limbs. Angiography revealed a dural arteriovenous malformation around the transverse and sigmoid sinus with thrombosis of the sigmoid sinus near its origin. The main feeding artery appeared to be the greater auricular artery (Figs. 3.14a,b). At surgery the transverse and sigmoid sinuses were excised, and the mastoid process partially removed to obliterate the feeding artery. On the third postoperative day she developed right homonymous hemianopsia and receptive aphasia associated with seizure activity on the EEG. The Symptoms may have been due to venous compromise of the tempero-occipital region of the brain, but they subsided entirely, and she remains well.

Results—Infratentorial Arterial Malformations

In the past six years we have seen 22 patients with vascular abnormalities in the posterior fossa. Fifteen of them were operated on, with satisfactory results in twelve of them, but death followed surgery in two cases, and a severe hemiplegia developed in a third case (Table 3.1). Three of the patients with dural arteriovenous malformations involving the transverse sinus have been embolized with satisfactory results.

We believe many posterior fossa vascular anomalies pose no particular problem at surgery. Those involving the cerebellum are quite comparable to their supratentorial counterparts. The dural anomalies appear to be treatable by embolization for the most part. Surgery

Table 3.1. Vascular malformations of the posterior fossa (the New York Hospital).

Location	No.	Operations	Embolization	Results
Brainstem telangectasia	4	2	—	Good
Cavernous angioma, CBll	1	1	—	Good
AVM, CBll	4	3	—	Good
Venous angioma CBll	2	1	—	Good
AVM, angle	5	3	—	1 Death 1 Hemiparesis
Dura	6	2	3	1 Death

AVM, arteriovenous malformation; CBll, cerebellum.

for malformations within the brainstem itself seems to be limited to the evacuation of hematomas, which also is quite straightforward though this may be the place for treatment of small AVM's.

The difficulties lie mostly with malformations in the subarachnoid space and pia mater. These lesions can be difficult to manage because they may be difficult to expose, or be partly buried in the brainstem, or have an unfortunate relationship to the cranial nerves, or be rather extensive. Like malformations of the spinal cord, the actual shunt may be quite small and may even be located in the dura mater. In this case, dilated, red draining veins can be mistaken as part of the anomaly. However, only the arterial component should be removed, and the draining veins should be left in place in so far as possible. Extensive removal of draining veins can lead to venous infarction of the brainstem.

References

1. Ameli NO: Brain angiomata and intracerebral hematoma. Prog Brain Res 30:427–431, 1968
2. Aminoff MJ: Vascular anomalies in the intracranial dura mater. Brain 96:601–612, 1973
3. Askenasy H, Herzberger EE, Wijsenbeek HS: Hydrocephalus with vascular malformations of the brain. Neurology 3:213–220, 1953
4. Bergman PS: Hemangioma of the pons. Case report and review of the literature. J Mt Sinai Hosp 17:119–131, 1950
5. Bergstrand H, Olivecrona H, Tonnis W: Gefässmissbildungen and Gefässgeschwülste des Gehirns. Georg Thieme, Leipzig, 1936
6. Boyd-Wilson JS: The association of cerebral angiomas with intracranial aneurysms. J Neurol Neurosurg Psychiatry 22:218–223, 1959
7. Chou SN, Erickson DL, Ortez-Suarez HJ: Surgical treatment of vascular lesions in the brain stem. J Neurosurg 42:23–31, 1975
8. Cushing H, Bailey P: Tumors arising from blood vessels of the brain, angiomatous malformation and hemangioblastoma. Thomas, Springfield, Ill, 1928
9. Dahl RE, Kline DG: Intraparenchymal arteriovenous malformations with predominant external carotid artery contribution. J Nuerosurg 41:681–686, 1974
10. Danzinger J, Bloch S: The value of the external carotid circulation in the assessment of intracranial disease. Clin Radiol 26:261–266, 1975
11. Debrun G, Chartres A: Ingra and supratentorial arteriovenous malformation. A general review. Neuroradiology 3:184–192, 1972
12. DeFeo DR, Kusske JA, Rush JL, et al: Aqueductal occlusion by midline arteriovenous malformation. Surg Neurol 5:59–62, 1976
13. DiChiro G: Relative value of air studies, angiography, and radioisotope scanning in the diagnosis of glial intracranial tumors. In Krayenbühl H, Maspes PE, Sweet WH (eds.): Progress in Neurological Surgery, Vol 2, S Karger, Basel/New York, 1968, pp 312–315
14. Djindjian R, Cophignon J, Rey A, et al: Superselective arteriographic embolization by the femoral route in neuroradiology. Study of 50 cases. III. Embolization in craniocerebral pathology, p 143 Neuroradiology 6(1):143–163, 1973
15. Djindjian R, Cophignon J, Theron J, et al: Embolization by superselective arteriography from the femoral route. Review of 60 cases. 1. Technique, indications, complications. Neuroradiology 6:20–26, 1973

16. Drake CG: Surgical removal of arteriovenous malformations from the brain stem and cerebellopontine angle. J Neurosurg 43:661–670, 1975
17. Fadhli HA: Congenital arteriovenous fistula involving the occipital artery and lateral venous sinus. J Neurosurg 30:299–300, 1969
18. Fernandez-Urdanibia J, Silvela J, Soto M: Occipital dural arteriovenous malformations. Neuroradiology 7:57–64, 1974
19. Fox JL, Al-Mefty O: Embolization of an arteriovenous malformation of the brain stem. Surg Neurol 8:7–9, 1977
20. Green JR, Vaughn RF: Blood vessel tumors and hematomas of the posterior fossa in adolescence. Angiology 23:474–487, 1972
21. Grotts BF: Spontaneous hemorrhage from a hemangioma of the pons. J Pediatr 37:98–101, 1950
22. Handa J, Yoneda S, Handa H: Venous sinus occlusion with a dural arteriovenous malformation of the posterior fossa. Surg Neurol 4:433–437, 1975
23. Henderson WR, Gomez R: Natural history of cerebral angiomas. Br Med J 4:571–574, 1967
24. Hilal SK, Michelsen JW: Therapeutic percutaneous embolization for extra-axial vascular lesions of the head, neck, and spine. J Neurosurg 43:275–287, 1975
25. Hoare RD: Arteriovenous aneurysm of the posterior fossa. Acta Radiol 40:96–102, 1953
26. Houser OW, Baker HL, Rhoton AL, et al: Intracranial dural arteriovenous malformations. Radiology 105:55–64, 1972
27. Houser OW, Cambell JK, Campbell RJ, Sundt TM Jr: Arteriovenous malformation affecting the transverse dural venous sinus—an acquired lesion. Mayo Clin Proc 54:651–661, 1979
28. Hugosson R, Bergstrom K: Surgical treatment of dural arteriovenous malformations in the region of the sigmoid sinus. J Neurol Neurosurg Psychiatry 37:97–101, 1974
29. Johnson MC, Salmon JH: Arteriovenous malformation presenting as trigeminal neuralgia. J Neurosurg 29:287, 1968
30. Kjellberg RN, Hanamura T, Davis KR, Lyons SL, Adams RD: Bragg-Peak proton beam therapy for arteriovenous malformations of the brain. N Engl J Med 309:269–274, 1983.
31. Kosnik EJ, Hunt WF, Miller CA: Dural arteriovenous malformations. J Neurosurg 40:322–329, 1974
32. Krayenbühl H, Yasargil MG: Das Hirnaneurysma. Series Chirurg Geigy, Basel, 1958
33. Kricheff II, Madayag M, Braunstein P: Transfemoral catheter embolization of cerebral and posterior fossa arteriovenous malformations. Radiology 103:107–111, 1972
34. Kuhner A, Krastel A, Stoll W: Arteriovenous malformations of the transverse drual sinus. J Neurosurg 45:12–19, 1976
35. Laine E, Galibert P: Aneurysmes arterioveineux et cirsoides de la fosse posterieure. Rev Neurol 115:276–288, 1966.
36. Lamas E, Lobato RD, Esparza J, et al: Dural posterior fossa AVM producing raised saggital sinus pressure. J Neurosurg 46:804–809, 1977
37. Lessell S, Ferris EJ, Feldman RG, Hoyt WF: Brainstem arteriovenous malformations. Arch Opthalmol 86:255–259, 1971
38. Logue V, Monckton G: Posterior fossa angiomas. Brain 77:252–273, 1954
39. Long DM, Seljeskog EL, Chou SN, et al: Giant arteriovenous malformations of infancy and childhood. J Neurosurg 40:304–312, 1974
40. Luessenhop AJ: Artificial embolization for cerebral arteriovenous malformation. Prog Neurol Surg 3:320–362, 1969
41. Lusins J, Sencer W: Posterior fossa vascular malformations. NY State J Med 76:416–420, 1976
42. Magidson MA, Weinberg PE: Spontaneous closure of a dural AVM. Surg Neurol 6:107–110, 1976
43. Manaka S, Izawa M, Nawata H: Dural arteriovenous malformation treated by artificial embolization with liquid silicone. Surg Neurol 7:63–65, 1977
44. Manuelidis EE: Uber Hamangiome des Gehirns. Arch Psychol 184:601, 1950
45. Matsumura H, Makita Y, Someda K, et al: Arteriovenous malformations in the posterior fossa. J Neurosurg 47:50–56, 1977
46. McCormick WF: The pathology of vascular ("arteriovenous") malformations. J Neurosurg 24:807–816, 1966
47. McCormick WF, Hardman JM, Boulter TR: Vascular malformations ("angiomas") of the brain, with special reference to those occurring in the posterior fossa. J Neurosurg 28:241–251, 1968
48. McCormick WF, Nofzinger JD: "Cryptic" vascular malformations of the central nervous system. J Neurosurg 24:865–875, 1966
49. Naidich TP, Leeds NE, Kricheff II, et al: The tentorium in axial section. Normal CT appearance and non-neoplastic pathology. Radiology 123:631–8, 1977
50. Neumann MA: Combined amyloid vascular changes and argyrophilic plaques in the central nervous system. J Neuropathol Exp Neurol 19:370–382, 1960
51. Newton TH, Cronquist S: Involvement of dural arteries in intracranial arteriovenous malformations. Radiol 90:27–35, 1968

52. Newton TH, Greitz T: Arteriovenous communication between the occipital artery and transverse sinus. Radiology 87:824–828, 1966
53. Newton TH, Weidner W, Greitz T: Dural arteriovenous malformations in the posterior fossa. Radiology 90:27–35, 1968
54. Nicola GC, Nizzoli V: Dural arteriovenous malformations of the posterior fossa. J Neurol Neurosurg Psychiatry 31:514–518, 1968
55. Nystrom SHM: Cytological Aspects of the Pathogenesis of Intracranial Aneurysms in Intracranial Aneurysms and Subarachnoid Hemorrhage. Fields WS, Sahs AL (eds.). CC Thomas, Springfield, Ill, 1965, pp 40–69
56. Obrador S, Soto M, Silvela J: Clinical syndromes of arteriovenous malformations of the transverse-sigmoid sinus. J Neurol Neurosurg Psychiatry 38:436–451, 1975
57. Olivecrona H, Ladenhoim J: Congenital arteriovenous aneurysms of the carotid and vertebral arterial systems. Springer Verlag, Berlin, 1957, IV, 91 pp
58. Olivecrona H, Riives J: AV aneurysms of the brain. Arch Neurol Psychiatry 59:567–602, 1948
59. Paterson JH, McKissock W: A clinical survey of intracranial angiomas with speical reference to their mode of progression and surgical treatment. A report of 110 cases. Brain 79:233–266, 1956
60. Patterson RH Jr, Fraser RAR: Vascular neoplasms of the brainstem: A place for profound hypothermia and criculatory arrest. Advances in Neurosurgery 3:425–428, 1975
61. Patterson RH Jr, Voorhies RM: Surgical approachs to intracranial and intraspinal arteriovenous malformation. Clin Neurosurg 25:412–424, 1978
62. Pecker J, Bonnal J, Javalet A: Deux nonveaux cas d'anevrismes arterioveineaux intra-duraux de la fossa posterieure par la carotide externe. Neurochirurgie 4:327–332, 1965
63. Perret G, Nishioka H: Report on the cooperative study of intracranial aneurysms and subarachnoid hemorrhage. VI arteriovenous malformations. J Neurosurg 25:467–490, 1966
64. Pool JL: Treatment of arteriovenous malformations of the cerebral hemispheres. J Neurosurg 19:136–141, 1962
65. Pool JL, Potts DG: Aneurysms and arteriovenous anomalies of the brain. Harper and Row, New York, 1965
66. Poppen JL: Vascular surgery of the posterior fossa. Clin Neurosurg 6:198–210, 1958
67. Pressman BD, Kirkwood JR, Davis DO: Computerized transverse tomography of vascular lesions of the brain. Part I. Am J Roentgenol 124: 208–214, 1975
68. Ray BS: Cerebral AV aneurysm. Surg Gynecol Obstet 73: 615–648, 1941
69. Reuter SR, Newton TH, Greitzt: Arteriovenous malformations of the posterior foss. Radiology 87:1080–1088, 1966
70. Richardson J, Bagnall AW: Recurrent subarachnoid hemorrhage due to an arterial angioma of the cerebellum and brainstem. Can Med Assoc J 43:111–115, 1940
71. Rottgen P: Weitere Erfahrungen an Kongenitaten Arterio-Venosen Aneurysmen des Schadelinnern. Zbl Neurochir 2:18–33, 1937
72. Russo RH, Dicks RE: Arteriovenous malformation of the brain stem in childhood. Surg Neurol 8:167–171, 1977
73. Sachs F: The Diagnosis and Treatment of Brain Tumors. Kimpton, London, 1931
74. Sano K: Intracranial arteriovenous malformation with special reference to its treatment. Neurol Med Chir 6:28–34, 1964
75. Sharpe JA, Rosenberg MA, Hoyt WF, et al: Paralytic pontine exotrupia. A sign of acute unilateral pontine gaze palsy and internuclear opthalmoplegia. Neurology 24:1076–1081, 1974
76. Steiner L, Leksell L, Greitz T, Furster DM, Backlund EO: Stereotactic radiosurgery in intracranial arteriovenous malformations. Acta Neurochir [Suppl] 21:195–209, 1974
77. Storrs DG, King RB: Management of extracranial congenital arteriovenous malformations of the head and neck. J Neurosurg 38:584–590, 1973
78. Sundaresan N, Galicich JH: Successful surgical treatment of pontine vascular malformation in a 3 year old. Case report. Child's Brain 5:131–136, 1979
79. Sundt TH Jr, Piepgras DG: The surgical approach to arteriovenous malformations of the lateral and sigmoid dural sinuses. J Neurosurg 59:32–39, 1983
80. Svien HJ, McRae JA: Arteriovenous anomalies of the brain. J Neurosurg 23:23–28, 1956
81. Svien HJ, Olive I, Angulo-Rivero P: The fate of patients who have cerebral arteriovenous anomalies without definitive surgical treatments. J Neurosurg 13:293–299, 1956
82. Svien AJ, Peserico L: Regression in size of arteriovenous anomaly. J Neurosurg 17:493–496, 1960
83. Takekawa SD, Holman CB: Roentgenologic diagnosis of anomalous communications between the external carotid artery and intracranial veins. Am J Roentgen 95:822–825, 1965
84. Tamaki N, Fujita K, Yamashita H: Multiple arteriovenous malformations involving the scalp, dura, retina, cerebrum and posterior fossa. J Neurosurg 34:95–98, 1971

85. Teilmann K: Hemangiomas of the pons. Arch Neurol Psychol 69:208–223, 1953
86. Terbrugge K, Scotti G, Ethier R, et al: Computed tomography in intracranial arteriovenous malformations. Radiology 122:703–705, 1977
87. Tonnis W: Aneurysma arteriovenoosum. In Bergstrand H, Olivecrona H, Tonnis W (eds.): Gefässmissbildungen und Gefässgeschwülste des Gehirns. Georg Thieme, Leipzig, 1936, pp 88–134
88. Tonnis W, Lange-Cosack H: Klinik, Operative Behandlung und Prognose der arteriovenousen Angiome des Gehirns und seiner Häute. Dtsch Z Nervenheilk 170:460–485, 1953
89. Troupp H, Marttila I, Halonen V: Arteriovenous malformations of the brain. Prognosis without operation. Acta Neurochir 22:125–128, 1970
90. Trumpy JA, Eldevik P: Intracranial arteriovenous malformations: Conservative or surgical treatment? Surg Neurol 8:171–175, 1977
91. Verbiest H: Arteriovenous aneurysms of the posterior fossa. Analysis of 6 cases. Acta Neurochir 9:171–195, 1961
92. Verbiest H: Arteriovenous aneurysms of the posterior fossa. Prog Br Res 30:383–396, 1968
93. Virchow R: Über die Erweiterung kleiner Gefässe. Arch Pathol Anat 3:427, 1851
94. Virchow R: Die krankhaften Geschwülste. Vol 3. A Hirschwald, Berlin, 1863, p 306
95. Wappenschmidt J, Grote W, Holbach KH: Diagnosis and therapy of arteriovenous malformations shown by vertebral angiography. Adv Neurosurgery 7:52–57, 1979
96. Warren JE, Tsueda K, Young B: Respiratory pattern changes during repair of posterior fossa arteriovenous malformation. Anesthesiology 45:690–693, 1976
97. White R, Wood N, Kernohan JW: A Study of 50 intracranial vascular tumors found incidentally at necropsy. J Neuropathol Exp Neurol 17:392–398, 1958
98. Zeller RS, Chutorian AM: Vascular malformations of the pons in children, Neurology 25:776–780, 1975

4

Venous Angiomas of the Brain

Hajime Handa and Kouzo Moritake

Introduction

Vascular malformations are often classified into four groups: telangiectasis, cavernous angioma, arteriovenous malformation, and venous angioma.[19,20,33] Although venous angiomas of the brain are not uncommon incidental lesions at autopsy,[20,25] clinically they have been considered rare vascular malformations.[4,11] Until the introduction of computed tomography (CT), a few angiographically demonstrated cases had been reported.[5,7,13,31,35,37,42,43] Most of the clinically diagnosed cases were discovered on CT examinations.*

The term venous angioma refers to a vascular malformation consisting only of a venous component histologically and no arterial component either histologically or angiographically. Recent neuroradiologic progress, however, has shown that the profile of the disease is complicated. Angiographic findings in reported cases are varied, and the hemodynamics of the lesion have not been investigated thoroughly. Disagreement continues concerning the angiographic criteria for diagnosing this type of vascular malformation, and in some cases there is confusion with other vascular malformations.[2,8,14,17,32] Based on a review of the literature, the definition of venous angioma of the brain is discussed in relation to other forms of vascular malformations.

* References 1, 3, 9, 10, 12, 15, 16, 18, 21, 22, 24, 26–30, 36, 38, 39, 40, 41.

Clinical Characteristics

The patients reported in the literature ranged in age from 8 to 76 years (average, 35.3 years) (Table 4.1). A slight male predominance can be noted. Clinically, venous angioma is considered usually asymptomatic, only rarely causing seizures, symptoms, signs of subarachnoid hemorrhage, or intracerebral hematoma. Of 75 patients, 21 had only epileptic seizures, 18 had headache or miscellaneous symptoms or signs that did not seem to be directly related to their venous angiomas (Table 4.2). In four other patients the clinical diagnosis was postconcussion syndrome. In 8 patients clinical manifestations were caused by concomitant cerebral disorders, namely, ruptured cerebral aneurysm, arteriovenous malformation, and pituitary adenoma in two patients each and hepatic coma and amyotrophic lateral sclerosis in one each. In these cases venous angioma was discovered incidentally during examination for the other lesions. Hemorrhage from venous angiomas occurred in 13 patients.

Venous angioma can occur anywhere in the venous system. The angiomas reported in the

Table 4.1. Sex and age distribution of patients with venous angiomas of the brain.[a]

	Age (yr)							
	0–9	10–19	20–29	30–39	40–49	50–59	60–	Total
Male	1	3	10	10	9	9	1	43
Female	1	2	10	7	8	3	1	32
Total	2	5	20	17	17	12	2	75

[a] Range, 8 to 76 years; average, 35.3 years.

brain, however, were located most commonly in the frontal lobe (28 cases) or the parietal lobe (5 cases), where the medullary veins are more numerous (Table 4.3).[3] Twenty-one of the lesions were in the deep cerebrum and another 21 in the cerebellum. The incidence of hemorrhage of the lesions occurring in the deep cerebrum or in the cerebellum was higher than that in the cerebral hemisphere.

Venous angiomas were arbitrarily divided into three groups—small, medium, and large—defined, respectively, by diameters of less than 2 cm, 2 to 4 cm, and more than 4 cm (Table 4.4). The incidence of hemorrhage was highest in medium-sized angiomas.

Table 4.2. Clinical manifestations in 75 cases.

Manifestation	No. of patients
Hemorrhagic attack caused by venous angioma	13
Epilepsy	21
Cerebellar ataxia	7
Headache and/or miscellaneous	18
Exophthalmos	1
Cerebral ischemic attack	3
Posttraumatic syndrome	4
Cerebral aneurysm (ruptured)	2
Arteriovenous malformation	2
Pituitary adenoma	2
Hepatic coma	1
Amyotrophic lateral sclerosis	1

Table 4.3. Location of venous angiomas.

Site of lesion	No. of angiomas	Hemorrhage +	Hemorrhage −	Not mentioned
Frontal lobe	28	2	25	1
Parietal lobe	5	1	4	0
Deep cerebrum	21	6	15	0
Cerebellum	21	5	16	0
Temporal lobe	1	0	1	0
Occipital lobe	1	1	0	0

Table 4.4. Size of lesions.

Size of lesion	No. of angiomas	Hemorrhage +	Hemorrhage −	Not mentioned
Large	23	2	21	0
Medium	36	9	26	1
Small	11	2	9	0
Not mentioned	7	0	7	0

Radiologic Studies

CT Findings

CT studies were performed in 55 patients, 52 without and 55 with contrast material (Table 4.5). In plain CT scans, positive findings were obtained in 25 of 52 angiomas: high density in

Table 4.5. Findings on CT studies of venous angiomas.

	No. of lesions studied	Positive	Negative
Plain	52	25[a]	27
Contrast enhancement	55	44	11

[a] High density, 12; low density, 8; mixed, 2; calcification, 3.

12, low density in 8, mixed in 2, and calcified mass in 3. With contrast material, enhancement of the angioma was seen in 44 of 55 lesions.

Figure 4.1 shows CT scans in a 39-year-old man with venous angioma of the right frontal lobe. CT scan without contrast material revealed a diffuse low-density area in the right frontal lobe (Fig. 4.1 left). A small lucent focus was also found in the left basal ganglia. With contrast, cord-like enhancement, probably consisting of dilated deep cerebral veins, was found deep in the right frontal lobe. No evidence of local edema or mass effect was discovered (Fig. 4.1 right).

Figure 4.2 shows CT scans in a 50-year-old man with venous angioma of the left cerebellar hemisphere. CT scan without contrast enhancement revealed no abnormality (Fig. 4.2 left). With contrast infusion, however, a small, well-demarcated, high-density area was visualized in the left cerebellar hemisphere accompanied by a perifocal low-density area on the lower section (Fig. 4.2 right).

Fierstien et al[9] compared the information obtained by CT scans and cerebral angiography. Six of eight angiographically diagnosed cerebral venous angiomas were visualized in CT scans, and four of them were seen only on scans with contrast; in none was there sufficient information to make a specific diagnosis. No mass effect, local edema, or hydrocephalus was identified on the scans. These authors stressed that small angiomas tend to be overlooked by CT study with or without contrast, and a definite diagnosis cannot be made by CT. They concluded that CT adds no information to that obtained by angiography. However, our overall survey indicates that although CT findings are nonspecific, they are very useful for detecting a venous angioma when it is small and does not accompany another major cerebral lesion and for demonstrating associated changes, namely hematoma and edema. The recent increase in reported cases of cerebral venous angioma is undoubtedly due to the introduction of CT scanning, through which the lesion is often found incidentally.

Angiographic Findings

Technical improvement in angiography is of most importance in the identification of venous angioma. The angiographic appearance of venous angioma is reported to be characteristic. It usually consists of numerous radiating transcerebral or transcerebellar medullary veins (Figs. 4.3c, 4.4). These veins converge into a relatively large and centrally located vein that then pursues a transcerebral or transcerebellar course to reach a superficial cerebral or cerebellar vein and hence to dural sinuses or, at times, deep cerebral or cerebellar veins. Venous angiomas could represent dilatations of normal veins of the white matter. The result of analysis of draining veins in venous angiomas is shown in Table 4.6. Of 75 venous angiomas, 47 drained only into dural sinuses, mostly the superior sagittal sinus. Another 13 drained exclusively into the deep venous system and seven into both the dural sinuses and deep cerebral veins. And another two drained into the large aberrant vein.

Table 4.6. Draining veins of venous angiomas.

Vein	No. of angiomas
Dural sinuses:	47
Superior sagittal	22
Sigmoid	3
Transverse	6
Straight	9
Superior petrosal	7
Deep cerebral	13
Combined	7
Superficial cortical	5
Aberrant	2
Unknown	1

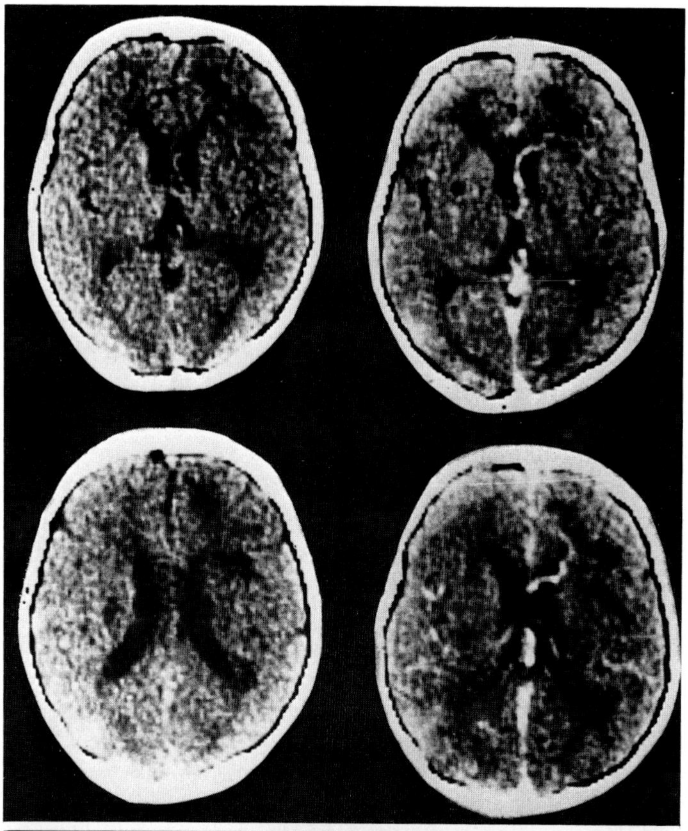

Fig. 4.1. A 39-year-old man with venous angioma of the right frontal lobe (case 1). CT scans without contrast material (*left*) reveal a diffuse low-density area in right frontal lobe and small lucent foci in left basal ganglion, lying medially with respect to the putamen and in the left corona radiata. With contrast (*right*), cord-like enhancement in right frontal lobe is revealed. From Moritake K, et al: Venous angiomas of the brain. Surg Neurol 14:95–105, 1980.

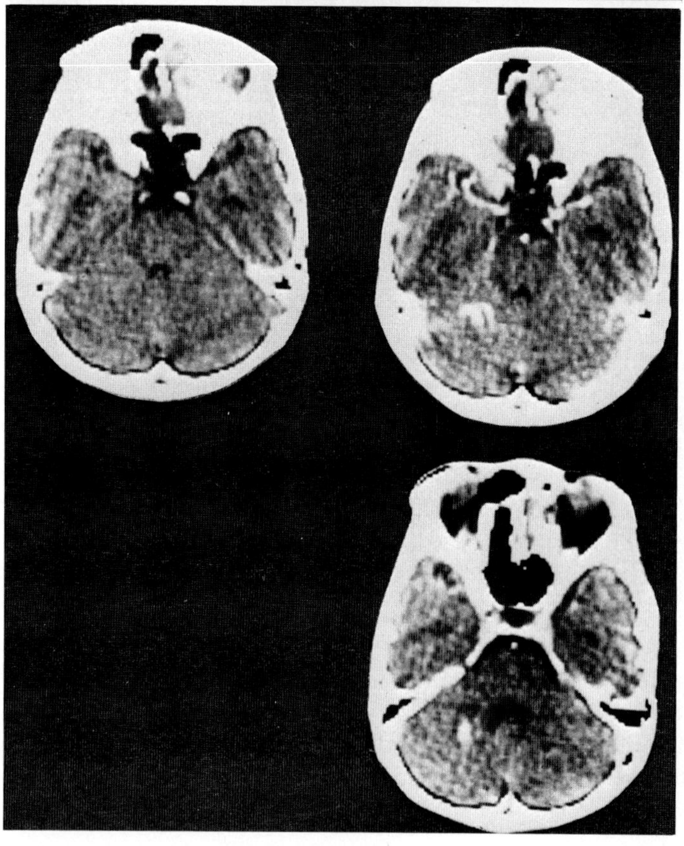

Fig. 4.2. A 50-year-old man with venous angioma of the left cerebellar hemisphere (case 2). Plain CT scan (*left*) is normal. After contrast infusion (*right*) a small, well-demarcated high-density area is visualized in left cerebellar hemisphere (*upper right*), accompanied by a perifocal low-density area on the lower section (*lower right*), which was not seen on the plain scan. From Moritake K, et al: Venous angiomas of the brain. Surg Neurol 14:95–105, 1980.

Venous angioma is considered to have a normal circulation time and normal arterial phase angiographically. Some authors[9,18] stress this criterion, namely, lack of gross abnormality in the arterial phase, in the differential diagnosis of venous angiomas. By use of rapid serial angiography in combination with magnification angiography, it should be possible to examine in greater detail the arterial and capillary phases as well as the venous phases to detect the subtle angiographic changes related to venous angiomas. Wolf et al[43] reported a patient with a hypertrophic parietal branch of the middle cerebral artery traced to the malformation. Wendling et al[42] also indicated slightly enlarged perforating arteries and a homogeneous blush on magnification subtraction arteriography in two cases. Although similar findings have not always been made in other reported cases of venous angioma, their two cases may support the hypothesis that this lesion represents an arteriovenous shunt and thus can be considered a form of arteriovenous malformation with venous prominence. Fierstien et al,[9] however, suggested that without a head of pressure high enough to be seen angiographically in the form

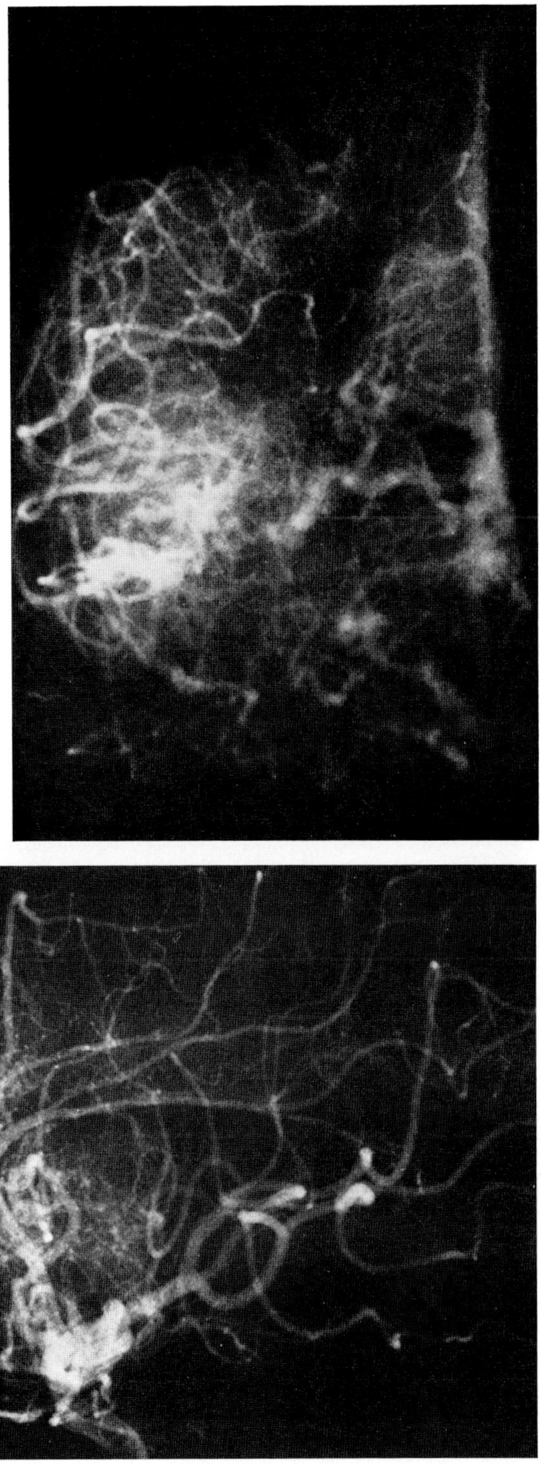

A

B

Fig. 4.3. Case 1: Late arterial phase, right carotid angiogram. **A.** Anteroposterior and **B**, lateral views. Early-filling veins radiate transcortically. Diffuse capillary blush is evident. No remarkable arterial dilatation or mass effect can be seen. **C.** Capillary phase. Several noticeably enlarged transcortical veins, fed by numerous medullary veins, drain into the anterior part of the superior sagittal sinus, internal cerebral vein, and basal vein of Rosenthal. From Moritake K, et al: Venous angiomas of the brain. Surg Neurol 14:95–105, 1980.

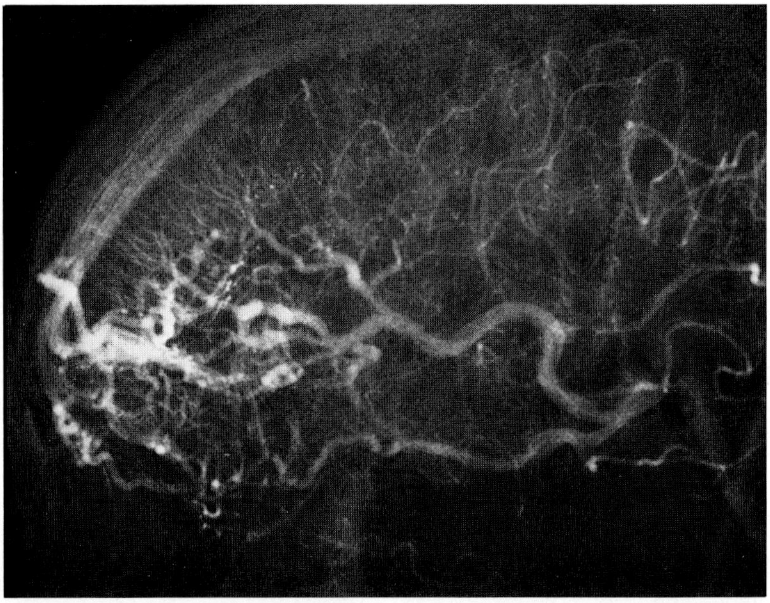

Fig. 4.3C

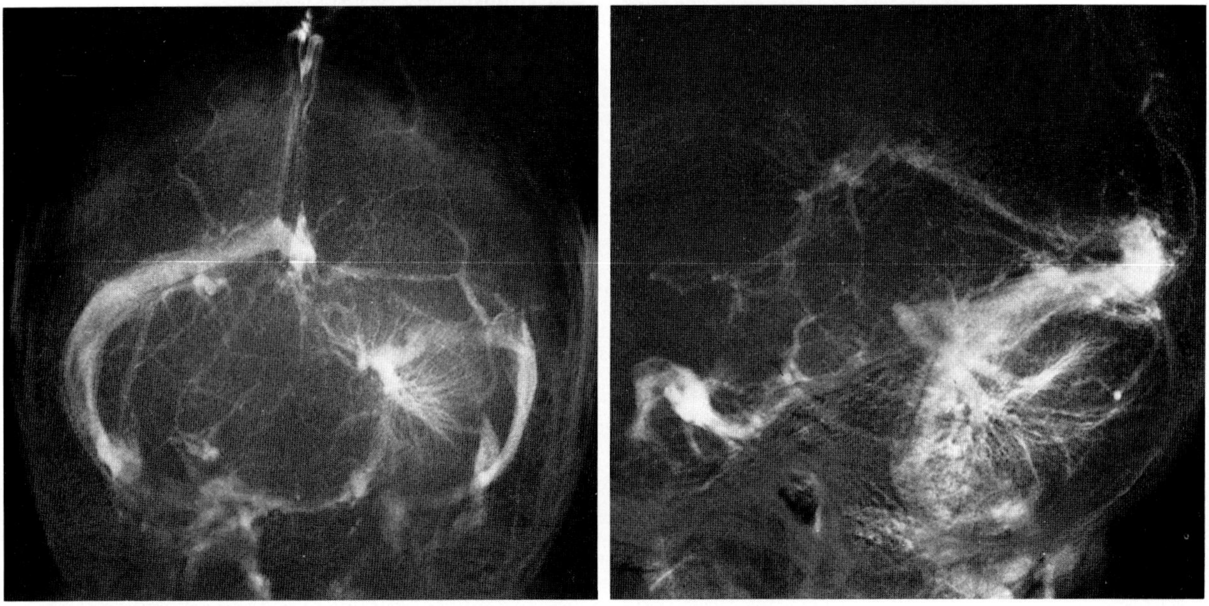

A

Fig. 4.4. Case 2: Venous phase, left vertebral angiogram. **A.** Anteroposterior and **B,** lateral views. Medium-sized venous angioma located deep in left cerebellar hemisphere is seen draining into left sigmoid sinus. From Moritake K, et al: Venous angiomas of the brain. Surg Neurol 14:95–105, 1980.

of increased arterial size, as in arteriovenous shunting, the venous size of an arteriovenous malformation would not stay enlarged. Therefore, they believed that these malformations were separate entities. Sarwar and McCormick[36] commented that in previously reported patients in whom the malformation satisfied the criteria of venous angioma histologically, demonstration of an arterial contribution on angiography did not seem acceptable as a bona fide finding. They described a case with no arterial contribution but early venous filling and capillary blush in the arterial phase.

In at least 21 of the 77 reported venous angiomas, early-filling vessels were seen in the late arterial to capillary phases, sometimes accompanied by a poorly marginated homogeneous capillary blush (Table 4.7). All except three venous angiomas with early-filling vessels were located in the frontal lobe. Strictly speaking, it is inappropriate to classify those with early-filling vessels as venous angiomas. From angiographic and histologic appearance, Cabanes et al[3] described venous angiomas as capillary venous malformations. Lesions very similar to the venous angiomas presented in Figs. 4.3 and 4.4 have been diagnosed by some authors as other types of vascular malformations that are thought to have a higher tendency to bleed than venous angiomas. For example, case 4 of Bogren et al,[2] a case from Jonutis et al,[14] and four cases of Liliequist,[17] were presented as cavernous angiomas, whereas a case of Roberson et al[32] and two cases of Diamond et al[8] were reported as telangiectases accompanied by cavernous angiomas. These cases could be accepted as cerebral venous angioma, however, they are not included in the clinical analysis in this article. Miyahara et al[23] reported a pathologically proved case of cerebral venous angioma which showed no angiographic abnormality, except for arterial displacement by calcified mass. We did not include this case in the present survey either, because the calcified nature of the specimen made it difficult to rule out other vascular malformations.

From the analysis of reported cases, bleeding tendency is higher in venous angiomas without early-appearing vessels than those with early-appearing vessels (Table 4.7). From the results of regional cerebral blood flow studies, radionuclide angiography, and Doppler flow studies, it is apparent that the hemodynamic differences exist between venous angiomas with and without early-filling vessels. For the purpose of clarifying the various angiographic features of venous angiomas and avoiding confusion in the differential diagnosis of vascular malformations, we propose classifying venous angiomas angiographically into two subgroups, namely, venous angiomas with early-filling vessels and those without them.

Table 4.7. Incidence of hemorrhage with venous angiomas with and without early-appearing vessels in angiographic study.

Type of malformation		Hemorrhage +	Hemorrhage −	Not mentioned
With early-appearing vessels	21	1	20	0
Without early-appearing vessels	44	10	33	1
Not mentioned	12	3	9	0
Total	77	14	62	1

Radionuclide Scintigraphy

Cabanes et al[3] emphasized the value of angioscintigraphic analysis with regard to the modifications that these angiomas cause in cerebral circulation. In quantitative angioscintigraphic analysis, they found increased activity in the region of the angioma in their case 1 but could not confirm any blood steal by the angiomatous lesion.

Of 77 lesions, radionuclide angiography was performed on 15 and was positive for 11 (Table 4.8). Two of the remaining 4 lesions were located in the posterior fossa. Although radioisotope studies are usually less demonstrative of lesions in the posterior fossa, a venous angioma was depicted by radionuclide angiography in our patient (Fig. 4.5) with a lesion in that region. The angioma appears as a focus of increased activity in the late arterial and venous phases. There was no definite correlation between findings from radionuclide studies and angiography.

In contrast to radionuclide angiography, static radionuclide brain scan in venous angioma is generally negative, probably because the blood-brain barrier is not disturbed. Static ra-

Table 4.8. Findings of radionuclide scintigraphy studies.

	No. of lesions studied	Positive	Negative
Radionuclide angiography	15	11	4
Static radionuclide brain scan	25	7	18

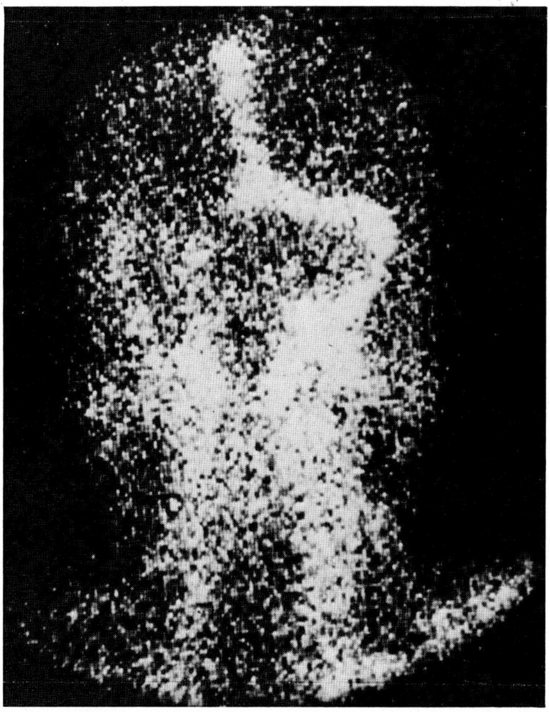
A

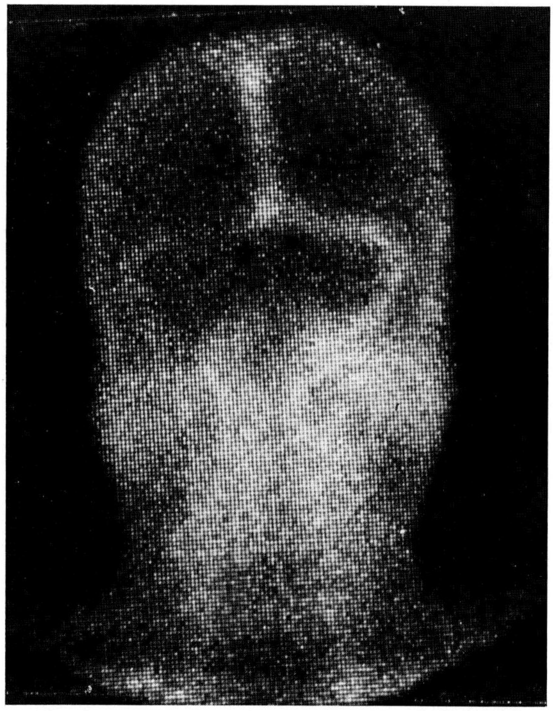
B

Fig. 4.5. **A.** Case 2: Angioscintigram 18 to 22 seconds after iv injection of a bolus of diethylenetriamine pentaacetic acid (DTPA) technetium 99m, showing a focus of increased activity in left cerebellar hemisphere. Transverse sinus is hypoplastic on the left, the side of the lesion. From Moritake K, et al: Venous angiomas of the brain. Surg Neurol 14:95–105, 1980. **B.** Case 2: Technetium 99m pertechnetate brain scan shows nonvisualization of left transverse sinus. Otherwise no apparent abnormalities are found. From Moritake K, et al: Venous angiomas of the brain. Surg Neurol 14:95–105, 1980.

dionuclide brain scan was performed for 25 of the 77 reported lesions, only seven of which showed positive uptake (Table 4.8).

Other Hemodynamic Assessments

Regional cerebral blood flow studies by xenon 133 carotid injection and transcutaneous Doppler flow measurements are sometimes useful in assessing the hemodynamics of this lesion. In cases in which angiography demonstrated early-filling vessels (Fig. 4.3), these studies revealed a significant increase in blood flow on the side of the lesion (Fig. 4.6). Stealing from other parts of the brain was suspected.

Preissig et al[31] observed a "red vein" during operation, such as is commonly observed in arteriovenous malformations. On the other hand, in a case of Scotti et al,[37] vascular structures were entirely venous, and enlarged feeding arteries or capillaries were not found. No evi-

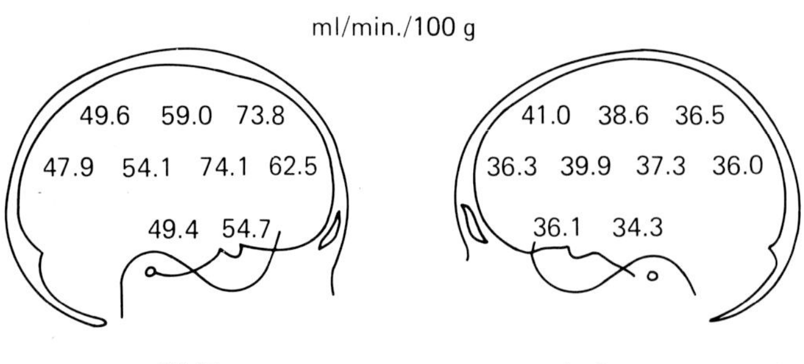

Fig. 4.6. Case 1: Regional cerebral blood flow ($rCBF_{10}$), calculated using height-over-area method by Xenon 133 intracarotid injection. Normal $rCBF_{10}$ is about 40 ml/min/100 g of tissue. Cerebral blood flow is increased in the right hemisphere, especially in the frontal region. Steal of blood flow from left to right hemispheres is suspected. From Moritake K, et al: Venous angiomas of the brain. Surg Neurol 14:95–105, 1980.

dence was discovered of increased pressure or flow within the malformation. On angiography a case of Preissig et al[31] was found to have a capillary blush whereas that of Scotti et al[37] did not.

The results of these hemodynamic studies and of the radionuclide dynamic studies by Cabanes et al,[3] together with the intraoperative findings of some authors just described, suggest that more blood is fed to venous angiomas with early-filling vessels than those without. However, the increase in blood supply is not large enough to cause angiographically detectable dilatation of feeding vessels.

To elucidate the hemodynamics of venous angiomas in relation to other types of cerebral vascular malformation, further investigations, including Doppler flow studies, regional cerebral blood flow studies, and dynamic radionuclide studies, should be conducted not only before and after operation, but also intraoperatively.

Histology

Some authors stress the importance of pathologic findings in the diagnosis of venous angiomas.[25] The vessels comprising venous angiomas are devoid of large quantities of smooth muscle and elastic tissue. Hyalinization and thickening of the walls are common.[43] As with arteriovenous malformations and telangiectases, but not with cavernous angiomas, neural parenchyma is found between the vascular elements in this malformation. The findings, however, have not been consistent. Cabanes et al[3] noted that proliferation of capillary-like structures may be seen in venous angiomas, and they stressed the need for careful study of size and arrangement of the vessels in the entire specimen to differentiate venous angiomas from telangiectases and cavernous angiomas.

Fierstien et al[9] noted that lack of arteries on histologic examination may be related to the location of the feeding arteries on the periphery of the malformation—outside the area of the pathologists' interest. We consider that histologic findings are not necessarily definitive in the diagnosis of vascular malformations, as such a complete histologic study as mentioned here is very difficult.

Of 77 lesions, only 12 were proved pathologically. In most clinical cases vascular malformations must be diagnosed without histologic evidence. Therefore, it is necessary and pragmatically useful to define the criteria for diagnosis of venous angioma from angiographic findings.

Therapy and Clinical Outcome

Impressions of the clinical significance of venous angiomas have been controversial. Most venous angiomas are thought to be clinically silent.[6] Cerebral venous angiomas are usually disclosed incidentally during the investigation of other lesions or in clinical manifestations unrelated to the venous angiomas. Based on the results of observation of six cases of their own and of studies of 26 previously reported cases, Saito et al[34] concluded that venous angioma has little clinical significance and that the small, dilated veins that develop secondarily are due to an abnormality in venous development during embryogenesis. However, the results of the other studies, including our own, indicate that this is not always true and emphasize the clinical importance of these lesions. Because the incidence of bleeding from these angiomas is not as low as was once thought, surgical removal seems advisable, as with arteriovenous malformations, if the lesion is accessible, despite angiographic findings.

Of the 77 reported venous angiomas, 14 were treated surgically. Ten of them were extirpated, and hematomas were removed in the remaining four. Of the 14 patients treated surgically, five were operated on for hemorrhage from the venous angioma, six for epilepsy, one for cerebellar ataxia, and four for headache and miscellaneous symptoms and signs that seemed not to be directly related to the venous angioma.

Of the 75 patients, follow-up studies were undertaken on 56, 10 of whom had been operated on (Table 4.9). Of the patients not operated on, three died, one from hepatic coma, one from massive bleeding from the angioma, one from bleeding in pituitary adenoma, and two deteriorated. Of 10 patients who had been operated on, eight improved after surgical removal of the angioma but the remaining two with angioma in the cerebellum died. These results suggest that the indication of surgical treatment should be

Table 4.9. Clinical outcome in 56 cases.

	Operated group	Nonoperated group
Asymptomatic or improved	8	28
Unchanged	0	13
Deteriorated	0	2
Died	2	3

determined more cautiously in patients with lesions in the cerebellum. Senegor et al[38] reported a patient with a venous angioma of the cerebellum and fourth ventricle who died after clipping of the major tributaries of the lesion. They concluded that surgical intervention can be disastrous in the treatment of those lesions occurring in the posterior fossa because venous angiomas in this region are developmental anatomic anomalies with enlargement of certain venous structures as a result of inadequate alternative venous drainage.

References

1. Ahnen A, Koivisto E, Kuikka J, Laitinen J, Tolonen U: Radionuclide diagnosis of venous angioma. Eur J Nucl Med 3:67–68, 1978
2. Bogren C, Svalander C, Wickbom I: Angiography in intracranial cavernous angioma. Acta Radiol 10:81–89, 1970
3. Cabanes J, Blasco R, Garcia M, Tamarit L: Cerebral venous angiomas. Surg Neurol 11:385–389, 1979
4. Campbell H, Ballance CA: A case of venous angioma of the cerebral cortex. Lancet 202:10–11, 1922
5. Constans JP, Dilenge D, Védrenne C: Angiomes veineux cérébraux. Neurochirurgie 14:641–650, 1968
6. Courville CB: Morphology of small vascular malformations of the brain, with particular reference to the mechanism of their drainage. J Neuropathol Exp Neurol 22:274–284, 1963
7. Crevits L, De Reuck J, van de Velde E, vander Eecken H: Venous malformation drained by the precentral cerebellar vein. An angiographic and post-mortem study. Clin Neurol Neurosurg 80:149–155, 1978
8. Diamond C, Torvik A, Amundsen P: Angiographic diagnosis of teleangiectases with cavernous angioma of the posterior fossa. Report of two cases. Acta Radiol [Diagn] 17:281–288, 1976
9. Fierstien SB, Pribram HW, Hieshima G: Angiography and computed tomography in the evaluation of cerebral venous malformations. Neuroradiology 17:137–148, 1979
10. Hacker DA, Latchaw RE, Chou SN, Gold LHA: Bilateral cerebellar venous angioma. J Comput Assist Tomogr 5:424–426, 1981
11. Hamby WB: The pathology of supratentorial angiomas. J Neurosurg 15:65–75, 1958
12. Hammer B, Pohlhammer H: Das venose Angiom des Gehirns. Diagnostik im Computer-Tomogramm und in der Angiographie. Radiologe 20:113–117, 1980
13. Iraci G, Galligioni F, Gerosa M, et al: Intracerebral venous angiomas as a cause of exophthalmos. Ann Ophthalmol 11:603–612, 1979
14. Jonutis AJ, Sondheimer FK, Klein HZ, Wise BL: Intracerebral cavernous hemangioma with angiographically demonstrated pathological vasculature. Neuroradiology 3:57–63, 1971
15. Kasamo S, Kobayashi E, Awa H, et al: A case of cerebral venous angioma as an epileptogenic lesion detected by CT scan and surgically treated. Neurol Med Chir (Tokyo) 20:865–873, 1980
16. Kobayashi K, Nakamura T, Aki T, Iwata T, Toya S, Shiga I: Two cases of cerebral venous angioma—with special reference to the neuroradiological diagnosis. Neurol Surg (Tokyo) 9:424–431, 1981
17. Liliequist B: Angiography in intracerebral cavernous hemangioma. Neuroradiology 9:69–72, 1975
18. Maehara T, Tasaka A: Cerebral venous angioma: Computerized tomography and angiographic diagnosis. Neuroradiology 16:296–298, 1978
19. McCormick WF: The pathology of vascular ("arteriovenous") malformations. J Neurosurg 24:807–816, 1966
20. McCormick WF, Hardman JM, Boulter TR: Vascular malformations ("angioma") of the brain, with special reference to those occurring in the posterior fossa. J Neurosurg 28:241–251, 1968
21. Meyer JD, Baghai P, Latchaw RE: Cerebral varix and probable venous angioma. An unusual isolated anomaly. AJNR 4:85–87, 1983.
22. Michels LG, Benson JR, Winter J: Computed tomography of venous angiomas. J Comput Assist Tomogr 1:149–154, 1977
23. Miyahara S, Kuromatsu C, Kim PY: Calcified cerebral venous angioma with negative by serial angiography—A case report. Neurol Med Chir (Tokyo) 19:523–527, 1979

24. Moritake K, Handa H, Mori K, Ishikawa M, Morimoto M, Takebe Y: Venous angiomas of the brain. Surg Neurol 14:95–105, 1980
25. Noran HH: Intracranial vascular tumors and malformations. Arch Pathol 39:393–416, 1945
26. Numaguchi Y, Kitamura K, Fukui M, Ikeda J, Hasuo K, Kishikawa T, Okudera T, Uemura K, Matsuura K: Intracranial venous angiomas. Surg Neurol 18:193–202, 1982
27. Pak H, Patel SC, Malik GM, Ausman JI: Successful evacuation of a pontine hematoma secondary to rupture of a venous angioma. Surg Neurol 15:164–167, 1980
28. Pardatsher K, Fiore DL, Galligioni F, Iraci G: Diagnosis of cerebral venous angioma by rapidly enhanced CT scan. Surg Neurol 14:111–113, 1980
29. Partain CL, Guinto FC, Scatliff JH, Limbacher J, Janicki P, Heindel CC: Cerebral venous angioma: Correlation of radionuclide brain scan, transmission computed tomography and angiography. J Nucl Med 20:1166–1169, 1979
30. Pelz DM, Vinuela F, Fox AJ: Unusual radiologic and clinical presentation of posterior fossa venous angiomas. AJNR 4:81–84, 1983
31. Preissig RS, Preissig SH, Goree JA: Angiographic demonstration of a cerebral venous angioma. J Neurosurg 44:628–631, 1976
32. Roberson GH, Kase CS, Wolpow ER: Telangiectases and cavernous angiomas of the brain stem: "Cryptic" vascular malformations. Neuroradiology 8:83–89, 1974
33. Russel DS, Rubinstein LJ: Pathology of Tumors of the Nervous System. ed 2. Edward Arnold, London, 1971, pp 99
34. Saito Y, Kobayashi N: Cerebral venous angioma: clinical evaluation and possible etiology. Radiology 139:87–94, 1981
35. Sartor VK, Fliedner E, Weber K: Venöse Angiome des Gehirns. ROFO 128:171–176, 1978
36. Sarwar M, McCormick WF: Intracerebral venous angioma. Arch Neurol 35:323–325, 1978
37. Scotti LN, Goldman RL, Rao GR, Heinz ER: Cavernous venous angioma. Neuroradiology 9:125–128, 1975
38. Senegor M, Dohrmann GJ, Wollmann RL: Venous angiomas of the posterior fossa should be considered as anomalous venous drainage. Surg Neurol 19:26–32, 1983
39. Solomon EH, Bonstelle CT, Modic MT, Kaufman B: Angiographic and computed tomographic correlation in cerebral venous angiomas. CT 4:217–221, 1980
40. Suganuma Y, Oie K, Tanigawa K, Matsushima Y, Inaba Y: A case of cerebral venous angioma. Neurol Surg (Tokyo) 1:77–83, 1978
41. Tomaccini D, Venturi C, Scarfo GB: Cerebral venous angioma, cutaneous angioma, facial asymmetry and recurrent stroke. Eur Neurol 20:29–32, 1981
42. Wendling LR, Moore JS, Kieffer SA, Goldberg HI, Latchaw RE: Intracerebral venous angioma. Radiology 119:141–147, 1976
43. Wolf PA, Rosman NP, New PFJ: Multiple small cryptic venous angioma of the brain mimicking cerebral metastases. Neurology 17:491–501, 1967

5

Embolization of Cerebral Arteriovenous Malformations

W. Jost Michelsen and Sadek K. Hilal

Introduction

A revolution of some proportion has occurred during the past two decades in the therapeutic approach to a patient harboring an intracranial arteriovenous malformation (AVM). It has become clear during this time that the natural history of this disorder is considerably worse than previously thought.[16] Coincident with this knowledge, a new field in medicine, interventional radiology, has come out of infancy and into early maturity. Stimulated by the pioneering and continuing efforts of Luessenhop,[15] vascular radiologists have developed techniques for studying and actually passing catheters into very small blood vessels.[1,4,8–10] Multiple materials have been released into the vascular tree from these catheters as emboli for treatment.[9] Thus, the ability of the neurosurgeon to deal with difficult vascular problems has been greatly enhanced. This is particularly true of cerebral AVMs. This chapter reflects our experience with somewhat more than 450 patients with intracranial AVMs. Of these patients, 22 had vein of Galen lesions.

History

Brooks, a surgeon in Tennessee,[3] first used muscle in embolizing a carotid-cavernous fistula. However, real credit must be given to Luessenhop, who in 1960 and thereafter[13–15] reported his experience in surgical embolization of large AVMs. His conclusions, which are still valid today, noted that embolization of large malformations reduced the frequency of seizures, often made an operative approach easier, and probably had no effect in terms of preventing future hemorrhage. His approach required an operative exposure of the carotid artery and general anesthesia. With the development of catheter techniques, radiologists in the late 1960s were able to place large catheters into the carotid and vertebral arteries, allowing embolization to be performed in the x-ray suite, using sedation and local anesthesia.[10] This technique allowed multiple embolization procedures.

More recently, further developments have allowed the use of small balloon catheters either for temporary obstruction of normal vessels or for controlled release of rapidly solidifying plastics.[1,7,19] These tiny balloon catheters are able to travel to distant portions of the intracranial vascular tree *with great safety*.[1,8–10,20]

Coincident with rapidly evolving catheter technology is the continuing hunt for a perfect embolic material. Silastic spheres probably remain the safest material to use intracranially, but recent reports suggest that bucrylate may well be the material of the future.[1,10,18]

At this time, all of the rapidly solidifying plastics must still be considered experimental.[5,18] The use of Gelfoam or muscle is not indicated except as a temporizing measure, as they are both rapidly resorbed. Thus, silastic spheres remain the mainstay in our institution for embolizing intracranial malformations.

Technical Considerations

Embolization is virtually always performed percutaneously and through a catheter placed in the femoral artery. This is done in the x-ray department. All patients are premedicated 24 hours prior to the procedure with dexamethasone. In the x-ray department, droperidol and fentanyl in appropriate doses are used for sedation. Catheters, measuring 9 through 12 French are used and inserted through a Mylar sheath. Small balloon catheters may be inserted through the large catheters as necessary. Because large catheters are used, and the flush solution is heparinized, great care must be taken in compressing the arterial puncture site after the procedure.

Patients are discharged 48 hours after the procedure. It is important not to perform the initial arteriogram on the same day as the embolization, as it is too time-consuming. It is equally important to perform postembolization angiograms three to six months after embolization, as progressive thrombosis of the malformation may occur.

Embolization of Intracranial Arteriovenous Malformations

Embolization is exceedingly useful in the treatment of intracranial AVMs.[14] Fundamentally, the goal of treatment in every case is total obliteration of the malformation. Embolization will rarely produce this goal, but it is helpful. Embolization is useful in the following five categories of lesions:

1. Large malformations with high-flow characteristics that are being considered for surgical excision. In this situation embolization will slowly reduce the flow through the lesion, allowing the normal brain circulation to accommodate, thus reducing the risk of "normal perfusion pressure breakthrough."[17] It will also simplify the operative procedure, as a considerably smaller lesion will be present.
2. Large malformations in the motor area where the primary manifestations are repeated and uncontrolled seizures.
3. Malformations when the primary manifestation is a relentlessly progressive neurologic deficit.
4. Large malformations when headache is the primary symptom.
5. Vein of Galen malformations, particularly in patients with heart failure.

Embolization is not a consideration when a malformation has a single feeding vessel unless the malformation is deep within the brain and total obliteration becomes a possibility.

A new group of patients have become candidates for embolization as a result of new techniques using balloon catheters. These are the basal ganglia lesions, heretofore untreatable by virtually any technique, and lesions involving the distal anterior cerebral artery.[1,13]

The remainder of this chapter will be devoted to examples of cases where embolization is helpful and of those where it is of little use. It is well to put the entire situation into perspective. Fewer than 25% (47) of the AVMs operated on by the author during the past decade (total 201) have undergone embolization preoperatively (see Table 5.1). Conversely, 150 patients have undergone embolization *alone* as a primary treatment of their malformation.

Lesions of the Anterior Cerebral Artery

When the only feeding vessels to an AVM are from the anterior cerebral artery, embolization is unnecessary and is potentially harmful. These lesions usually lie anterior to the coronal suture (Fig. 5.1), are fed by branches of the

Table 5.1. Distribution of lesions with pre-operative embolization.

Anterior cerebral artery	1
Middle cerebral artery	21
Middle cerebral-posterior cerebral	14
Posterior cerebral	11

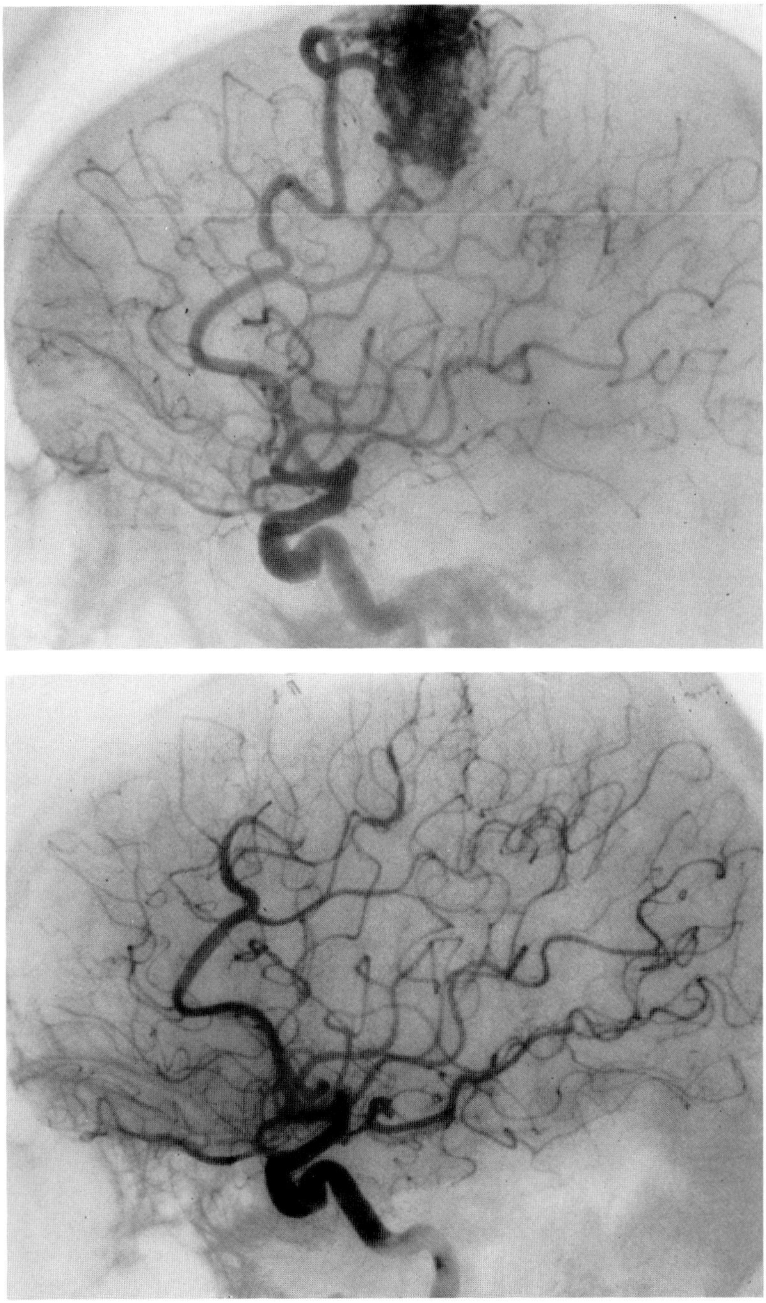

A

B

Fig. 5.1. AVM supplied only by the anterior cerebral artery; **A,** preoperative, **B,** postoperative. Note preservation of normal branches of the parent artery.

pericallosal or callosomarginal artery, both of which then supply normal brain tissue. The malformation is easily excised with no compromise of the parent artery.

Malformation Involving the Anterior and Middle Cerebral Artery

These malformations are among the most commonly encountered by the clinician. They may be anywhere on the convexity, from the coronal area to the lambdoid. As the malformation is placed more posteriorly, the middle cerebral artery becomes more prominent in the vascular pattern. The more anterior the malformation, the less the need to embolize the lesion, as the middle cerebral flow is slow and less important. As the lesions approach the parietal area, (Fig. 5.2), larger middle cerebral feeders are the rule, and the lesions are of the high-flow variety.[16] In

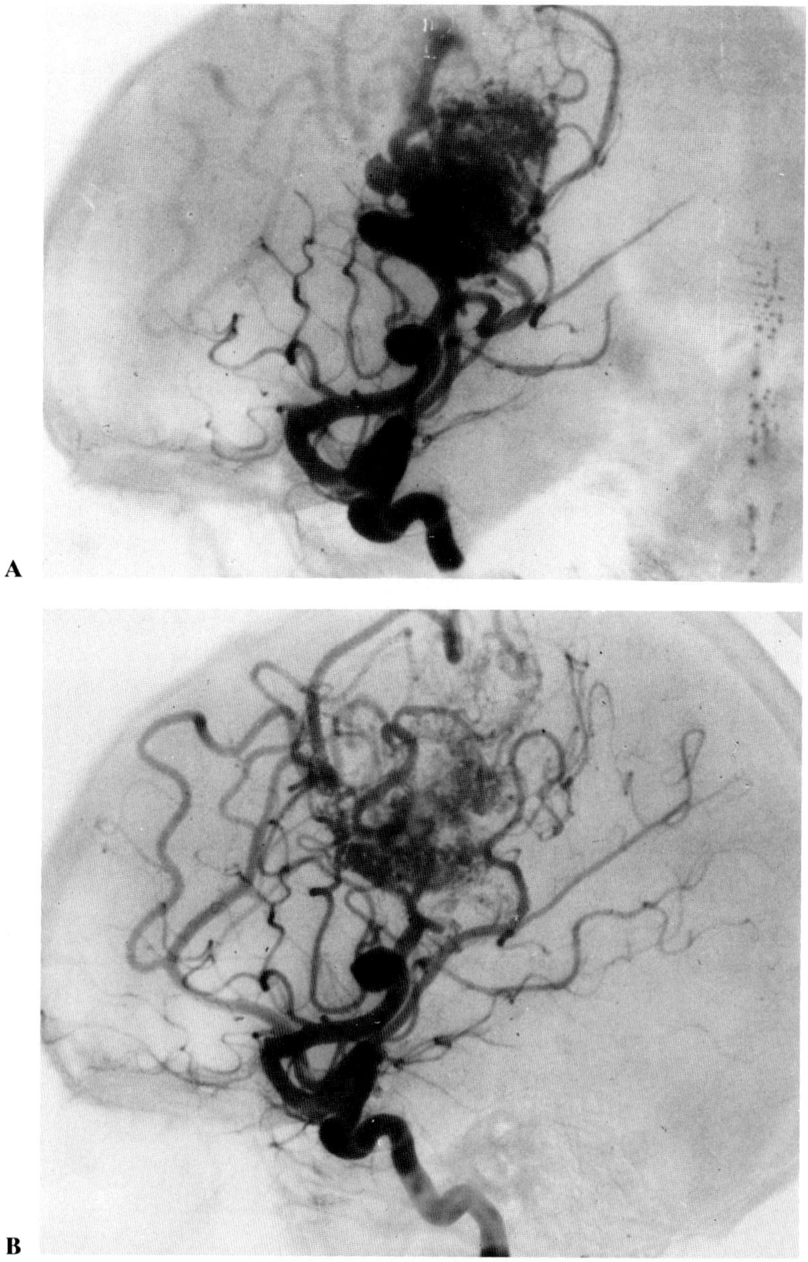

Fig. 5.2. Large AVM involving anterior and middle cerebral artery, before **(A)** and after **(B)** embolization. Note appearance of the anterior cerebral artery after embolization.

this case embolization is very important and helpful. Flow is markedly reduced, the lesion is rendered "softer," and excision is safer. Embolization may be repeated safely.

Middle Cerebral Artery Only

If an AVM involves only small branches of the middle cerebral artery, excision is probably the best technique. However, if it is a high-flow lesion involving several large branches, embolization (Fig. 5.3) will greatly reduce its size. It is well to keep in mind, however, that in large lesions there is always a deep feeder or feeders that cannot be adequately treated with embolization.

Middle Cerebral and Posterior Cerebral Artery

These malformations are most often on the lateral surface of the temporal lobe or occipital

Fig. 5.3. High-flow lesion in middle cerebral artery distribution, before **(A)** and after **(B)** embolization. Note virtual disappearance of the lesion and normalization of circulation.

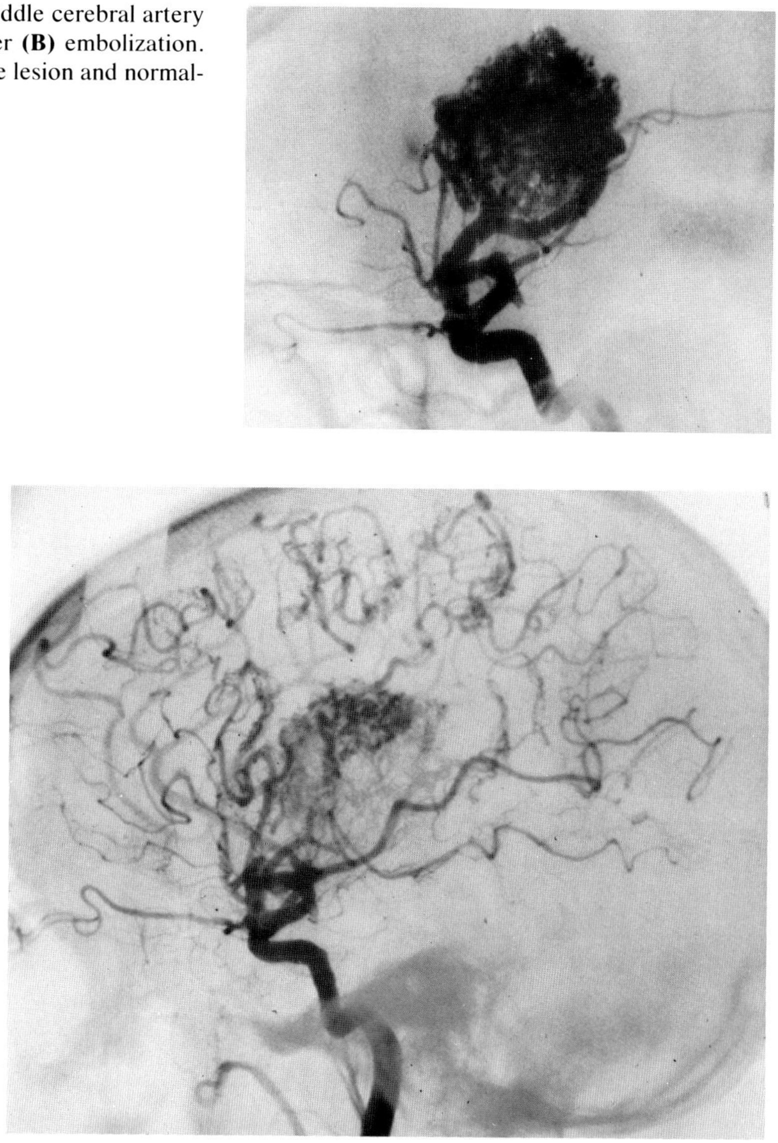

A

B

lobe. The lesions of the temporal lobe are fed by the posterior temporal branch of the posterior cerebral artery and the middle cerebral group. Direct operation is preferable. If the lesion is on the lateral surface of the occipital lobe (Fig. 5.4), embolization of the posterior cerebral artery prior to operation makes surgery considerably easier. Total obliteration of the posterior cerebral artery supplying an AVM produces visual field defects in less than 15% of cases.

If a lesion of the temporal lobe has deeper feeders, e.g., a large anterior choroidal vessel, embolization is possible. This is accomplished by placing a balloon catheter at the bifurcation of the intracranial carotid artery, expanding the balloon, and then embolizing proximal to the catheter (Fig. 5.5). This results in obliteration of the deep feeders.

Lesions of the Posterior Cerebral Artery

When the malformation is fed by the distal branches of an enlarged posterior cerebral artery, embolization may reduce flow and ease operation. If, however, the choroidal vessels are the primary feeding vessels, a direct opera-

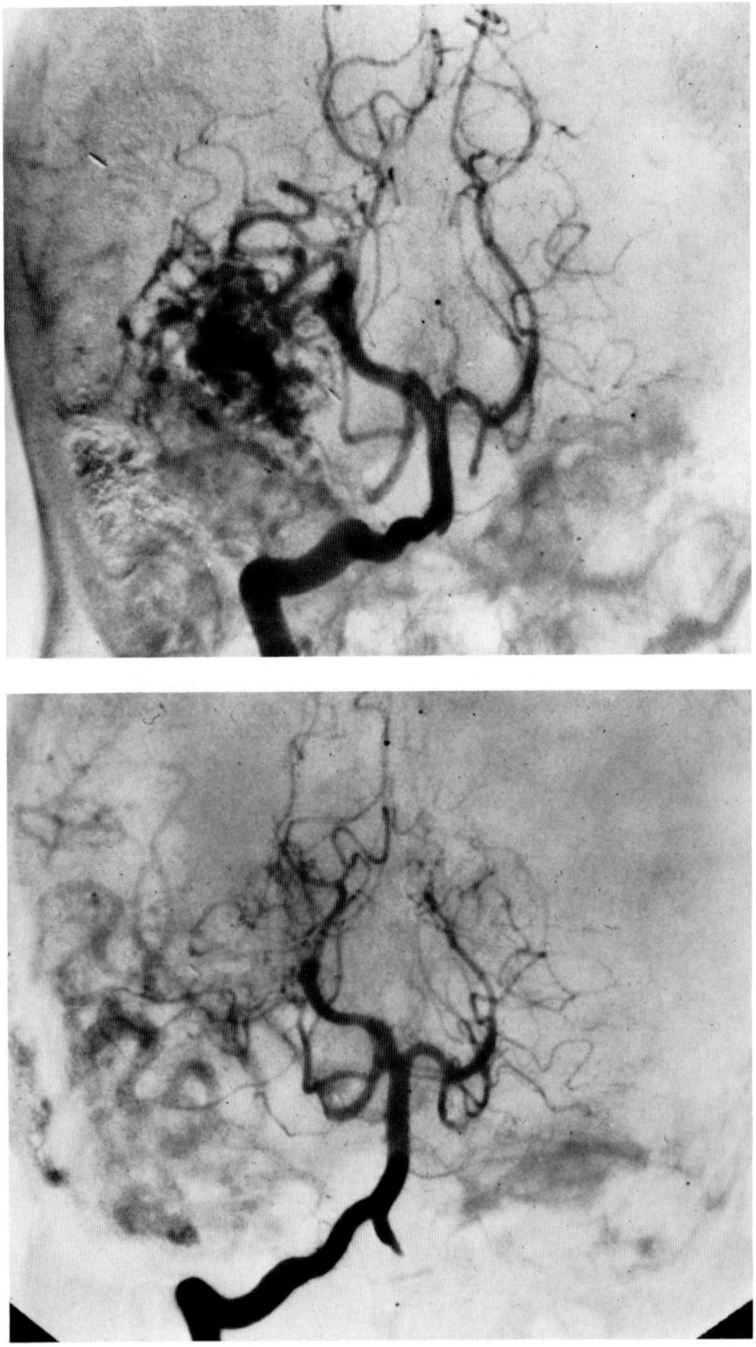

A

B

Fig. 5.4. Branches of posterior cerebral artery going to lateral occipital lobe lesion, before **(A)** and after **(B)** embolization.

tive approach is usually best. Here the primary consideration is preservation of the parent vessel.

Midline Lesions: Corpus Callosum and Vein of Galen

Corpus callosum malformations are best dealt with by direct operation. On occasion, preoperative embolization of the posterior feeding vessels may be useful.

Vein of Galen AVMs

AVMs of the brain situated deeply and in the midline have a common venous drainage into the great vein of Galen, hence the name vein of Galen malformations. The arterial supply is var-

Fig. 5.5. Large perforating vessels of the carotid artery eliminated with embolization using balloon catheter to obstruct the distal flow **(A,B)**.

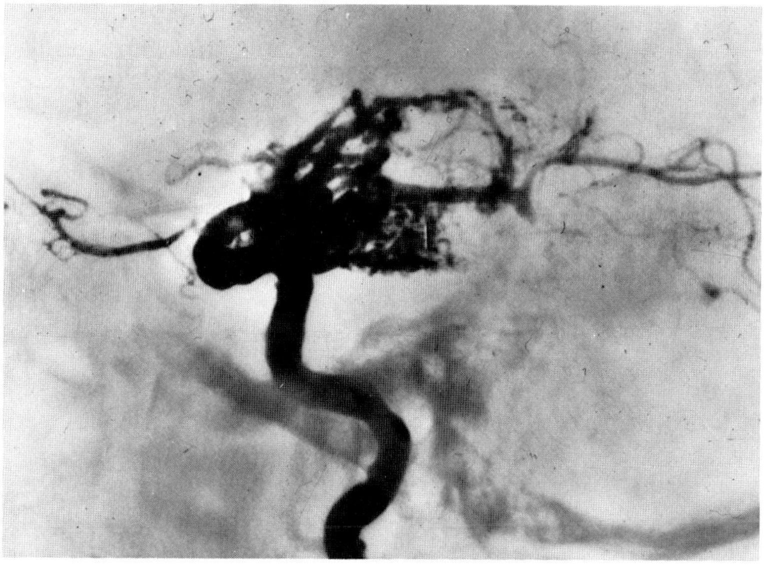

A

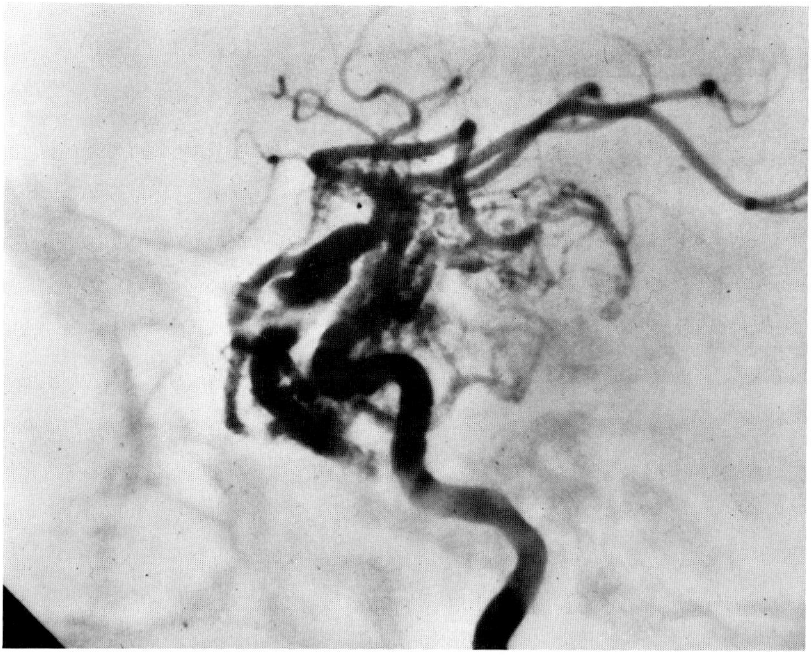

B

iable and may include all the major intracranial arteries, both deep and hemispheric. More commonly, the posterior cerebral arteries and the deep perforating vessels supply the malformation. More than 60% of patients with this malformation also have a major anomaly of the cerebral venous sinuses, most frequently the lateral sinus but also the superior saggital sinus and others in combination. This fact is responsible for some of the symptoms.

Clinical manifestations of this lesion depend on the age of the patient, the size of the shunt, and the adequacy of venous drainage. A newborn infant with a large arteriovenous shunt may be sending more than 60% of his cardiac output intracranially, resulting in intractable heart failure. A smaller lesion at birth may cause only cardiomegaly. Hydrocephalus is due to aqueductal compression from the enlarged vein of Galen. Megancephaly is also common in these patients.

The type of malformation most suitable for embolization (Fig. 5.6) is the racemase variety, where many small, deep perforating vessels are

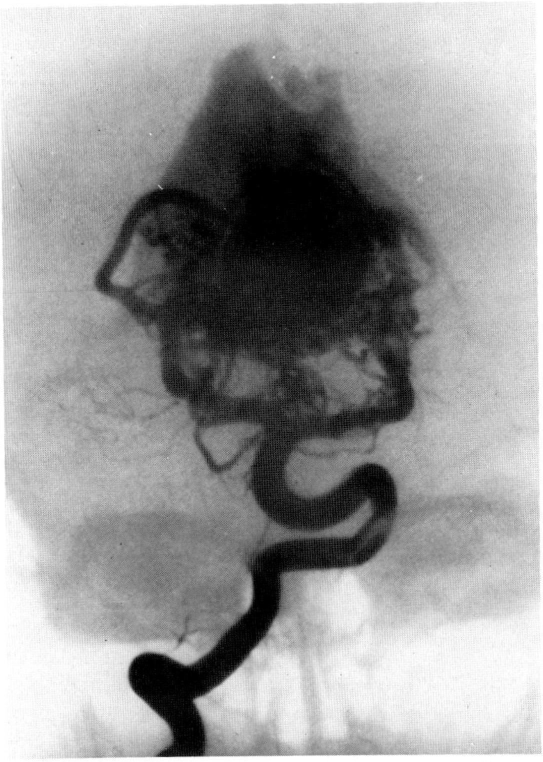

A

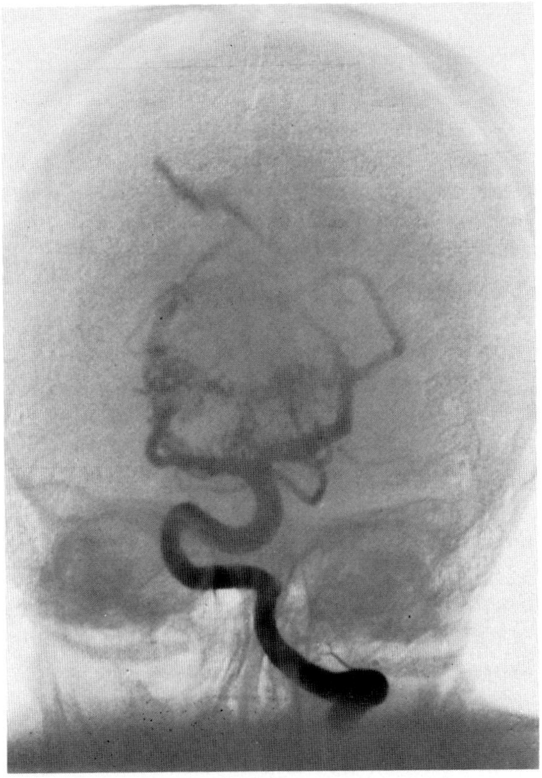

B

Fig. 5.6. Large vein of Galen malformation, before **(A)** and after **(B)** embolization. Patient awakened from coma after embolization.

present rather than the direct large posterior cerebral feeders.

Embolization has been an exceedingly useful procedure in the management of this rare malformation. We have embolized 20 pateints with this malformation during the past 12 years (in one patient reversing heart failure in the neonatal age group. The results of embolization are difficult to quantitate except symptomatically. Headaches have been relieved, heart failure reversed, and blood flow to normal brain improved.[16]

A problem of major proportions occurs when embolizing these malformations in small children (neonates). Open exposure of the carotid artery and vertebral artery may be necessary so that a catheter of sufficient size for embolization may be introduced.

Seizure Control

Long-term follow-up of patients whose primary manifestation of their AVM has been seizures is not yet available. In our group of paitents there has been a definite reduction in seizure tendency. A group of patients were studied before and after embolization using xenon 133 blood flow techniques. One of these patients had up to 20 seizures a day. After the malformation was embolized, the seizures stopped rather abruptly. The cerebral blood flow studies revealed a marked increase in cerebral blood flow to the brain surrounding the malformation, lending credence to the theory that a "steal of blood" from the normal brain is responsible for the seizures.[6] Feindel has found similar results in an operated patient. Embolization would therefore seem ideal for this problem.

Progressive Neurologic Deficit

This is a rare manifestation of convexity AVMs, but a common problem with basal ganglia lesions. Reversal or stabilization of neurologic deficit occurs with embolization of convexity lesions. These are usually very large lesions and not suitable for operative resection.

Basal ganglia lesions may now be treated with embolization using silastic spheres. The technique involves obstruction of the distal middle cerebral artery using a balloon and proximal embolization with small 1- to 1.5-mm spheres. Although we have only used this technique for one year, the results are exceedingly promising. Similar results are possible using bucrylate, but with a somewhat greater risk.[1]

Headache

The most frequent type of headache we have encountered that can unequivocally be ascribed to an AVM is the migraine type of headache seen with large occipital AVMs. These headaches differ from typical migraine in that the visual symptoms are elementary visual sensations rather than jagged lines. These patients do not have increased intracranial pressure. Embolization will virtually eliminate these headaches. Resection will also do this.

Intracranial embolization at the time of craniotomy with bucrylate is undergoing evaluation.[18] Excellent results have been reported with total obliteration of the malformation in some cases. The ultimate role of this technique is not clear.

New Techniques

The advent of small balloon catheters, 1 mm in diameter, has allowed a new dimension in embolization.[10] These catheters have been used in two distinctly separate fashions. In one application a double-lumen catheter is used with a calibrated leak balloon. A rapidly polymerizing plastic such as isobutyl-2-cyanoacrylate is injected and arteries are blocked. Often, a large part of a malformation can be obliterated using this technique. A small portion most often remains, and surgical excision is required. A major objection to this technique is that arterial obstruction takes place often at a distance from the lesion. A second problem is that polymerization timing must be precise and the balloon catheter rapidly removed from the area.

We have preferred a different approach. We use the balloon catheter to obstruct the normal arteries so that silastic spheres can pass only into the abnormal circulation. This has allowed safe embolization of the anterior choroidal and lenticulostriate vessels, something never before possible, without blocking major vessels.[13] Similarly, one posterior cerebral artery can be blocked and the other embolized.

Therefore, embolization with silastic spheres has very little dependence on geometry or vessel size. The balloon may be inflated or deflated at will, allowing normal circulation for most of the procedure.

It is clear from the foregoing that further advances are "on the drawing board" as miniaturization occurs.

Contraindications

Most of the contraindications have been mentioned previously. One situation that is not infrequent involves large malformations of the middle cerebral artery. A stenosis of the proximal middle cerebral artery may be present. This is well seen only if special views are taken of the artery at its bifurcation. This anatomic fact absolutely contraindicates embolization. Its etiology is obscure. Other contraindications include lack of size differential between feeding and nonfeeding arteries, poor vascular geometry, and generalized cerebrovascular disease.[19]

Complications

Complications of embolization using silastic spheres are few. Minor neurologic deficits may appear after the procedure but are rarely permanent. Two patients have suffered an intracerebral hemorrhage in our series with one death.[11]

Coincidental aneurysms may rupture as a result of embolization. Complications due to arteriography itself must be considered. Large-diameter catheters in the femoral artery have not, to date, caused a problem.

Conclusions

Embolization of cerebral AVMs is a very useful adjunct in their treatment. Although rarely a cure in itself, the treatment may render surgery easier and therefore safer, may reduce seizure frequency, reverse or stabilize progressive neurologic deficit, and eliminate headache. In infants, heart failure may be reversed.

Complications of the procedure are rare when performed by experienced personnel, but may be disastrous. Future developments involve the search for better materials and their safe delivery.

References

1. Berenstein A: Techniques of catheterization and embolization of the lenticulostriate arteries. J Neurosurg 54:783–789, 1981
2. Boulos R, Kricheff II, Chase NE: Value of cerebral angiography in the embolization treatment of cerebral arteriovenous malformations. Radiology 97:65, 1970
3. Brooks B: Discussions of paper by L. Noland and A. S. Taylor. Trans South Surg Assoc 43:171, 1931
4. Cares HI, Hale JR, Montgomery DB: Laboratory experience with a magnetically guided intravascular catheter system.
5. Cromwell L, Harris AB: Treatment of cerebral arteriovenous malformations; a combined neurosurgical and neuroradiological approach. J Neurosurg 52:705–708, 1980
6. Hilal SK, Johnson PM, Cannon P, Michelsen WJ, Brust J: Changes in the cerebral perfusion before and after percutaneous embolization of arteriovenous malformations. Invest Radiol 8:268, 1973
7. Hilal SK, Michelsen WJ: Therapeutic percutaneous embolization for extra axial vascular lesions of the head, neck and spine. J Neurosurgery 43:275–287, 1975
8. Hilal SK, Michelsen WJ, Driller J: POD catheter; a means for small vessel exploration, J Appl Physics 40:1046, 1969
9. Hilal SK, Michelsen WJ, Driller J, Leonard E: Magnetically Guided devices for vascular exploration and treatment. Radiology 113:529–540, 1974
10. Kerber C: Use of Balloon catheters in the treatment of Cranial arterial abnormalities, Stroke 11:210–216, 1980
11. Kricheff I, Madayag M, Braenstein O: Transfemoral catheter embolization of cerebral and posterior fossa arteriovenous malformations; Radiology 103:107–118, 1972
12. Kvam D, Michelsen WJ, Quest DO: Intracerebral hemorrhage as a complication of artificial embolization of arteriovenous malformations, Neurosurgery 7:491–493,
13. Luessenhop AJ, Majica PH: Embolization of segments of the circle of Willis and adjacent branches for management of certain inoperable cerebral arteriovenous malformations. J Neurosurg 54:573–583, 1981
14. Luessenhop AJ, Presper JJ: Surgical embolization of cerebral arteriovenous malformations through internal carotid and vertebral arteries, Long term results. J Neurosurgery 42:443–451, 1975
15. Luessenhop AJ, Spence WT: Artificial embolization of cerebral arteries; report of use in a case of arteriovenous malformation. JAMA 172:1153, 1960
16. Michelsen WJ: The pathophysiology of arteriovenous malformations. Clin Neurosurg 25:307–313, 1979
17. Nornes H, Grip A: Hemodynamic aspects of cerebral arteriovenous malformations. J Neurosurg 53:456–464, 1980
18. Samson D, Ditmore M, Beyes CW: Intravascular use of isobutyl 2-cyanoacrylate part I. Neurosurgery 8:43–51, 1981
19. Stein BM, Wolpert SM: Arteriovenous malformations of the brain; Current concepts and treatment. Arch Neurol 37:1–5, 69–75, 1980
20. Vinters HV, Delrun G, Kaufman JCE, Drake CG: Pathology of arteriovenous malformations embolized with isobutyl-2-cyanocrylate. J Neurosurg 55:819–825, 1981

6

Radiosurgery in Cerebral Arteriovenous Malformations

Ladislau Steiner

. . . and there is nothing new under the sun. Is there anything of which one can say, "look, this is new"? No, it has already existed, long ago before our time.
Ecclesiastes 1, 10.

Introduction

In 1951 Leksell coined the provocative concept of "radiosurgery," a technique of stereotactically focusing narrow beams of ionizing radiation to a target within the brain. Initially he used relatively low-energy x-rays but subsequently a cobalt 60 (Co 60) gamma unit was specially designed to be included in Leksell's stereotactic system.[57] The technique was primarily developed for functional neurosurgery, i.e., capsulotomy or thalamotomy.

In 1970 I used for the first time the narrow beams from the ^{60}Co gamma unit at the Karolinska Hospital to irradiate cerebral arteriovenous malformations (AVM). In the first two cases treated, the AVM no longer filled on the subsequent angiograms.[103,104] Follow-up of the patients since treated has been carefully planned and carried out strictly, and the results are given in this chapter.

With good selected cases a permanent cure of AVM with stereotactic gamma irradiation is currently possible. Though there are still unsolved problems and failures, radiosurgery seems to have already acquired an established place in the treatment of AVM. Therefore, the presentation in this book of the closed treatment method of AVM will be of benefit to the group of patients judged to be unsuitable for conventional surgery. The selection of patients for radiosurgery should be in the hands of a neurosurgeon experienced in the treatment of cerebrovascular lesions. His decision will be determined by a balanced evaluation of the case from the position of a specialist equally familiarized with both conventional surgery and radiosurgery. Stereotactic procedures, notwithstanding the physical agent used (heat, chemicals, or beams), are an integral part of the neurosurgic technique and have to be performed by the neurosurgeon. The fact remains, however, that for an overwhelming number of neurosurgeons, radiosurgery is still a fairly exotic topic. Therefore, although it is beyond the aim of this chapter to give a detailed presentation of the fundamentals of radiophysics and vascular radiobiology, the following are included:

1. Some elementary facts of radiologic physics to provide a better understanding of the tools and the procedures described here
2. A crude summary of the state of play as far as radiobiology of the vessels is concerned
3. A historical sketch on irradiation therapy for AVM.

Radiologic Physics

In presenting these few fundamentals of radiologic physics, the works of 34 and 118 have been used for references.

The Atom

The basic unit of matter is the atom, built up of a positively charged nucleus and a number of negatively charged electrons orbiting around the nucleus. Because of their diffuse nature and despite their reduced mass as compared with the nucleus, the electrons determine the size of the atom. Nuclei are made up of protons and neutrons. Protons carry a positive charge, neutrons have no charge, and both have nearly the same mass. Since there is one proton in the nucleus for every electron outside the nucleus, the atom as a whole is electrically neutral. The atomic number Z is the number of protons in the nucleus as well as the number of electrons outside the nucleus and defines the element to which the atom belongs, i.e., hydrogen with the atomic number 1 has one proton, helium with the atomic number 2 has two protons. Neutrons do not influence the atomic number although they determine the mass number (A) of the atom, which is the total number of protons and neutrons in the nucleus.

Work with high-energy machines have revealed further particles like, e.g., the positron; the neutrino; mu, pi, and K mesons; and the antiproton. The photon, which was originally considered to be a similar particle, is actually a bundle of energy. Nevertheless, in many interactions it acts as a particle. Photons are usually referred to as quanta or gamma rays.

The pattern in the arrangement of the electrons in the atom depends on the value of Z. Thus, in hydrogen a single electron moves in an orbit about the nucleus. In the atom of helium two electrons revolve in opposite direction in the same orbit. As one proceeds to higher values of Z, the increasing number of electrons must be added to new orbits as required by quantum mechanical reasoning. The next orbits, referred to as L, M, and N orbits or shells, gradually fill up in the given order.

The stability of an atom depends on the number of electrons in its outermost shell. If the outer shell is not completely filled or has an excess of electrons, the atom will have a propensity to react with any element that can give or take electrons.

Electromagnetic radiation is a form of energy that is propagated by wave motion. The wavelength determines the properties of the radiation, and the electromagnetic spectrum includes radiations from the long radiowaves to the short, penetrating gamma rays.

According to Planck's concept of the quantal properties of radiation, high-energy x and gamma rays are small bundles of a given amount of energy moving with a specific velocity and are called quanta or photons. Moreover, Bohr stated that electrons only emit radiation when shifting between two shells. These two concepts are indispensable for the understanding of x and gamma radiations.

If a high-speed electron collides with an atom of another element, it may remove a K, M, L, or N electron and for that an energy equal to the binding energy of the dislodged electron will be required. After a short time, an electron from one of the outer shells will fill the empty space and when this occurs, radiation will be emitted in the form of a quantum of energy. The energy of the emitted quantum in electron volts is the difference between the two binding energies.

An electron is the amount of energy released when an electron volt falls through a potential difference of 1 volt.

$$1 \text{ MeV} = 1{,}000 \text{ kev} = 10^6 \text{ ev} = 160 \times 10^{-13} \text{ joules.}$$

Einstein coined the concept of interchangeability of mass and energy and stated that mass is only another form of energy. Furthermore, according to his theory of relativity, an increase in velocity to or near that of light appears as an increase in mass rather than as an increase in velocity. Actually, experiments with high-speed nuclear particles show that the mass of a particle increases with velocity. Electromagnetic radiation can also be converted into "mass," provided the "photon" has sufficient energy. A photon of energy greater than 1 meV can produce an electron-positron pair.

Roentgen or X-rays

Whenever high-speed electrons impinge on various substances, especially heavy metals, x-rays (first observed by Roentgen in an evacuated discharge tube) are produced, and their nature is determined by the speed of the electrons. X-rays have a marked penetrating power, they induce fluorescence, affect photographic plates, and ionize tissues through which they pass.

Naturally Occurring Radioactive Substances

Henri Becquerel 1896 discovered that uranium compounds emitted penetrating rays. Schmidt and Madame Curie subsequently showed that thorium, polonium, and radium compounds produced the same effect and were described as being radioactive. All elements with an atomic number greater than 82 (lead) are radioactive.

Elements composed of nuclei with the same number of protons but unequal number of neutrons are called isotopes, assuming they have the same atomic number but a different atomic mass. Because of an unbalanced number of protons and neutrons, the isotope may be unstable, and this leads to "disintegration," until a more stable form evolves. All isotopes of cobalt are unstable until they evolve into $^{59}_{27}Co$.

Artificial Radioactivity

New unstable isotopes can be obtained either in an accelerator by bombarding stable nuclei with neutrons, high-energy protons, deuterons, alpha particles and gamma rays, or by splitting heavy nuclei. This last process is known as nuclear fission.

Disintegration

In a stable nucleus, despite a continual motion and collision of nuclear particles with a resulting transfer of energy, no particle ever acquires enough energy to escape by overcoming the strong forces of attraction between the nuclear particles. Such an escape, however, may occur in a radioactive nucleus. In the disintegration process, energy in the form of alpha, beta, and gamma rays is emitted. The alpha rays—doubly charged helium atoms—are deflected in electric and magnetic fields as if they were positively charged. Beta rays consist of high-energy electrons and behave as if negatively charged. They are more penetrating than alpha rays. Both gamma rays and x-rays are an electromagnetic radiation. Their only difference is the source. X-rays are generated by x-ray machines, whereas gamma rays are emitted from radioactive nuclei. Both gamma and x-rays remain undeflected by electric or magnetic fields and are very much more penetrating than the alpha and beta rays.

Exponential Decay

The time required for one-half the original amount of atoms in a radioactive element to disintegrate is called the half-life. The number of atoms decreases geometrically after every half-life (i.e., three half-lives leave an eighth of the original number of atoms). This rate of disintegration can be illustrated by an exponential decay curve.

Disintegration, i.e., the activity of a radioactive element, may be measured in any number of units. However, a special unit, the curie, has been defined as follows:

1 curie (Ci) = 3.7000 $\times$ 10^{10} disintegration/second
1 millicurie (mCi) = 3.7000 $\times$ 10^{7} disintegration/second
1 microcurie (μCi) = 3.7000 $\times$ 10^{4} disintegration second
1 curie (Ci) = 37 G becquerel (GB_2)

High-Energy and Teletherapy Machines

Roentgen obtained his x-rays in 1895 using an evacuated discharge tube. In a modern x-ray tube, the source of electrons is the cathode made of a spiral of tungsten wire and heated by a small electrical current. The anod is a copper rod, including a tungsten disk, which is the target for the high-speed electrons. The electrons are accelerated under the action of the electric field induced between the cathode and the anod. In high-energy machines or particle accelerators, the particles are given repeated increments of energy instead of direct acceleration by high-voltage source. The accelerators may be divided into two groups according to whether the particles travel in a straight line or in a circular or spiral orbit during acceleration.

Linear Accelerators

Electrons are accelerated in a straight line by a moving high-frequency radiowave.

Cyclotron and Synchrocyclotron

Protons and deuterons, respectively, are maintained in a circular orbit by a magnetic field and given energy by repeatedly being accelerated by an electric field at the right instant.

Deuteron and alpha particle radiation has been used by Tobias et al.; proton beams have been used by Lawrence et al.,[54] by Kjellberg and Kliman[37] for pituitary tumors, by Minakova[74] for pituitary destruction in cases of cancer.

The proton beam of the 185 meV synchrocyclotron in Uppsala was used for stereotaxic radiosurgery in animal studies and in single cases of parkinsonism.[1,49,50,56,60,70,92]

Betatron

Electrons are accelerated and held in a circular orbit by an alternating magnetic field. In the teleisotope machine, the source of radiation is an isotope, usually ^{60}Co, which emits penetrating gamma rays.

Many different types of ^{60}Co units have been designed. The ^{60}Co gamma units, used at the Karolinska Institute in Stockholm, were designed by Leksell. The technical details have been published,[16,52,61,95] and the clinical use of these machines has been described.[6,7,8,24,57,59,79,90,99,100,101,102,103,104]

The Interaction of X and Y Radiation With Matter

When a beam of x or gamma radiation passes through matter, some of the radiation is scattered and some is absorbed. In the process of absorption, emission of long wavelength x-rays may occur; this is termed secondary radiation. Thus, the total radiation intensity at any point along the track of the beam is determined by both primary as well as secondary radiation.

The characteristics of the absorption and scattering processes that finally may reduce the intensity of the beam depend on the quantitative relation between the energy of the incident photon on one hand and the binding energies of the electrons in the absorbing medium on the other hand.

When the photon energy is less than the binding energy of the electrons in the atom, only *classical scattering* occurs. The incident photon changes direction without losing energy. Photoelectric absorption occurs when the energy of the photon exceeds the binding energy of an inner shell electron. This electron is knocked out of its shell and an outer electron fills the vacancy, and secondary rays characteristic of the absorber are produced. The ejected electron is a photoelectron.

Compton scattering occurs when a quantum with great energy collides with an electron "that is free or unbound," as its binding energy is much less than that of the incident photon. Part of the energy of the photon is given up to the electron, causing it to recoil while part is scattered in the form of lower energy.

When the energy of the incident photon exceeds 1.02 meV, the energy of the photon may be converted into an electron and a positron as a result of the interaction between the photon and the nucleus. This is called *pair production.* The positron combines with a free electron and produces two photons of radiation.

The *linear attenuation coefficient* is equal to the fraction of energy removed from the beam per centimeter of absorber.

The *half value layer (HVL)* of a beam is the thickness of an absorber required to attenuate half the intensity of the incident radiation. HLV is usually in millimeters of aluminium for x-rays generated below about 120 kilovolt (peak) in millimeters of copper for 120 to 140 kV(p) and in millimeters of lead for higher voltages.

The *electronic attenuation coefficient* is the fractional reduction in x-ray intensity produced by a layer of thickness 1 electron/cm^2.

The *energy transfer coefficient* is the fraction of photon energy that is converted in kinetic energy (KE) of charged particles per centimeter of absorber.

The *energy absorption coefficient* is the fraction of photon energy that is completely absorbed from the motion of charged particles per centimeter of absorber.

Measurement of Radiation: The Roentgen and the Rad

The roentgen is an international unit used to measure the output of an x-ray source or the emission from a radioactive material. It is the quantity of x or gamma radiation such that the associated corpuscular emission per 0.001293 g of air produces in air ions carrying 1 electrostatic unit of electrical charge of either sign. (0.001293 g) is the mass of 1 mL of dry air at 0° C and 760 mm pressure. The number of roentgens of radiation delivered per unit time to a given region is proportional to the rate at which energy would be absorbed by air in that region and is called the dose rate in air or the dose rate in the region.

The definition of the roentgen makes it impossible to measure radiation if the beam of radiation has an energy of more than about 3 meV. Furthermore, roentgen is only defined for electromagnetic radiation and may not be used for particles such as electrons, protons, and neutrons.

The fact that in biology one is interested also in the amount of energy that is absorbed by the biologic material and not only in that which passes through it, makes it practical to speak of exposure and dose or absorbed dose. Exposure describes a property of the beam—its ability to ionize (air). Absorption depends on exposure as well as specific type of biologic material at the given point (soft tissue, bone, brain). Exposure in roentgens is related to the flow of energy through unit area taken at right angles to the beam. The "absorbed dose" is defined as the energy delivered to matter by ionizing particles per unit mass of irradiated material at the selected site. This is measured in *rads*. One rad denotes an energy absorption of 100 ergs/g.

In Gray's comparison, the relation between exposure in roentgens and dose in rads is the same as between a lecturer's "flux of words," which pass through the listener from ear to ear, and the small portion of acquired knowledge retained in his brain.

The total energy absorbed by the patient during a treatment is called the *integral dose*. The integral dose to a mass of tissue is the product of the mass of tissue and the dose that it receives. The unit of integral dose is the gram rad.

$$1 \text{ g rad} = 100 \text{ ergs}$$
$$1 \text{ rad} = 0.01 \text{ gray (Gy)}$$
$$1 \text{ Gy} = 100 \text{ rad}$$

Depth dose is the intensity of radiation received by tissues below the skin expressed in percentage of that received at a reference point such as body surface. When points having the same depth dose are jointed together, an *isodose curve* is obtained. The distribution of dose rate can be determined experimentally and isodose charts showing the distribution in one or more planes through the central axis can be prepared as required.

As demonstrated by Wilson,[116] the initial velocity and energy of the high-energy particles decrease gradually along their track through the absorbant medium, and the irradiation is influenced by pair production and Compton scattering. Near the end of the range, when the particle has little energy and is traveling slowly, the rate of energy loss suddenly increases. The intense ionization at the end or range of the beam is called the *Bragg peak,* and it is assumed that it occurs as a result of photoelectric absorption processes. Kjellberg et al utilized the Bragg peak of a proton beam from the 160 meV Harvard cyclotron to concentrate radiation to intracranial targets.

The reader is referred to the works of Johns and Cunningham[34] and Young[118] for further discussion of the fundamentals of radiologic physics.

Radiobiology of the Vessels

Charged particles passing through any material induce ionization and a state of molecular excitation. Because of the secondary electron absorption, one quantum of x or gamma rays yields many ionizations. The amount of energy in a given distance along the beam track varies with the different types of ionizing radiation and the so-called linear energy transfer (LET) is measured in kiloelectron volt per μ of track. Highly penetrating beams, such as gamma rays, have a relatively low LET, the energy being released over a long distance and causing a low ion yield. The greater the charge and the lower the velocity of the particle, the greater is its LET.

When ionizing radiation penetrates the cell, it triggers a variety of physical and chemical events. Most of the energy is absorbed by the intracellular water. The water molecule may be ionized and the process will yield (1) a solvated or aqueous electron e − aq; (2) an uncharged hydroxyl radical, −OH; (3) a hydrogen radical −H. The initial chemical effects induce subsequent chemical or biochemical reactions. Breakdown products may recombine as reactive radicals with oxidative or reduction reactions. These reactive radicals may interact with the intracellular structures and functions. Double-strand breaks, single-strand breaks, and base damage occur at the molecular levels, one of the most sensitive targets being the genetic material, DNA.

Since the organelles of cells have a rather well-defined organization and localization, the relative biologic effectiveness (RBE) depends on the LET of the radiation. The effects of radiation on cells are primarily destructive. However, there is sometimes an increased activity of the cell secondary to a preceding injury. The manifestations of radiation damage at cell level are nonspecific. Moreover, they differ only quantitatively but not qualitatively when produced by differing ionizing radiations. Differences in the degree of responsiveness of biologic cells to ionizing radiation led to the concepts of radiation sensitivity and radiation resistance.

Radiation Pathology of Vessels

It is now generally agreed that vessels are moderately sensitive to radiation. Small–vessel damage by radiation has long been recognized in the skin[117,119] and later in other organs as well as in larger pulmonary vessels and in the aorta of man.[109]

Electron radiation in the dog[62,63] and x-radiation in the dog produced lesions similar to those seen in arteriosclerosis. Smith[97] observed a slight constriction of the arterial wall and an immediate reduction in blood flow in the vasavasorum within the first minute when isolated carotid arteries in swine and dog were exposed to ^{60}Co gamma rays. These are only a few examples of the large body of evidence indicating that vessels, generally speaking, are sensitive to ionizing radiation.

Endothelial tissue of small blood vessels appears to be more responsive to radiation than that of vessels of a larger caliber. Whether this fact suggests a difference in conditional sensitivity or in some indirect mechanisms remains to be determined. The fact that greater degrees of endothelial change are seen in the small vessels of irradiated organs containing radio-sensitive parenchymal cells as compared with the small vessels found in organs with radio-resistant parenchymal cells may indicate a dependence of the radiation-induced endothelial changes upon the degree of vascular inflammatory response to the radiation damage in the parenchymal cells. The reason for the difference between the radiation effect on both the large and the small vessels is that the lumen of small vessels tolerates only rather small endothelial changes before being occluded, whereas the patency of the large vessels with a wide lumen has a greater margin. Alterations in vessel walls occur in early as well as in late postirradiation phases.

Pathology of the Early Period

Early radiation-induced changes in small vessels involve variable degrees of swelling, degeneration, and necrosis of endothelial cells with subsequent hyperemia, blood congestion, thrombi, fissuring of the walls, and consequent development of punctate hemorrhages. These changes were found also in animal experiments after radiation of the brain by electron beams,[4] narrow beams of high-energy protons,[60] narrow ^{60}Co gamma rays,[77] and in the spinal cord by using high-energy protons.[48] Wennerstrand and Ungerstedt[115] found similar histologic changes in patients treated for pain with the gamma unit. Rubin and Casarett[94] pointed out that following the perivascular or subendothelial edema induced by radiation, there may be increased interstitial colloid. In such regions, the fibroblastic activity increases with subsequent fibrosis.

Early changes after irradiation may be subtle and scattered. With progressive vascular damage, increasing areas of the small vessel bed undergo degenerative and fibrotic change. Medium-sized muscular arteries also show degenerative intimal, medial, and adventitial changes in the early periods after irradiation, although these and the large arteries are not as severely damaged as are arterioles and capillaries.

Marcial-Royas and Castro[71] described microscopic changes in aorta and carotid arteries in patients who died following rupture of these large elastic arteries during or within five weeks after radiation therapy for neoplastic disease. Associated infection and the presence of tumor infiltration of the vessels in these cases made a pathologic interpretation of the lesion difficult. The microscopic study revealed an intima covered by fibrin and subendothelial and subintimal edema, vacuolization and necrosis with infiltration by polimorphonuclear leucocytes and fat-laden macrophages. Edema, some inflammatory cells, separation, and fragmentation of elastic fibers were observed in the media. The adventitia was fibrotic and thickened and contained large "radiation fibroblasts." Finally, fibrin thrombi were seen in the lumen. Organized fibrosis occurred in the vasa vasorum.

Pathology of the Late Periods

An excessive proliferation of the endothelial cells and the subendothelial connective tissue following irradiation with narrowing or total occlusion of small-vessel lumens may occur. In the large vessels proliferation of medial elements, in addition to proliferation of endothelial lining, may be observed. These changes are usually progressive.

Andersson et al[1] described the late histopathologic effects in the goat brain after cross-fire irradiation with high-energy proton beams. Capillaries with endothelial thickening, collagenous walls, and perivascular cuffing were observed. Nilson et al,[77] irradiating the basilar artery of the cat by narrow beams from the ^{60}Co gamma unit, observed a thickening of the intima as an expression of late vascular repair. Some of the small arteries in the surrounding brain parenchyma, but never the basilar artery, were more or less occluded. Dollinger et al[20] and Pearson[86] published cases of coronary occlusion after radiotherapy.

It has been mentioned that changes in the larger vessels are discrete and of a segmental pattern in the early postirradiation periods. This fact can lead to an underestimation of their frequency. However, lesions become more obvious at longer intervals after irradiation, and they increase progressively. Although the precise mechanism of damage to the large vessels is unclear, there is physiologic and pathologic evidence suggesting that progressive sclerosis with subsequent occlusion of the vasa vasorum after irradiation interferes with nutrition of the vessel wall and leads to features reminiscent of an endarteritis obliterans.

Historical Sketch

Before total surgical excision was established as the treatment of choice for AVM by the work of Olivecrona[82,83,84] and Norlén at the Karolinska Hospital[81] decompression, carotid ligation, ligation of the feeders, and conventional x-ray therapy had been used. In 1921 V. Magnus[69] published a case where an AVM was operated on and irradiated with radium in Oslo as early as 1914 and noted a decrease in the frequency and the cessation of the epileptical seizures of the patient.

Cushing had in the 1920s and early 1930s advocated x-ray therapy following decompression. In "Tumors Arising From the Blood Vessels of the Brain" published in 1928,[15] he gives the history of a case with AVM.

> On January 17, 1924, a left osteoplastic exploration which proved to be a most desperate procedure was made. The astonishing lesion consisted of a tangle of small thin-walled actively pulsating arterioles. The Sylvian vessels were greatly dilated and a large pulsating vein evidently containing arterial blood passed up around the posterior margin of the lesion. The tumor itself felt firm in consistency and was fairly well circumscribed, but it was inconceivable that it could be attacked without fatal hemorrhage.

After this exploration, a series of deep x-ray treatments was instituted. The patient was reoperated in 1927.

> "The reopening of the dura disclosed a most unexpected condition. The lesion proved to be of stony hardness. The tangle of pulsating vessels previously encountered was largely thrombosed and transformed into a multitude of small bloodless shreds. It was found that the central lesion could be easily separated from the adjacent normal-looking cortex. . . The experience of brushing the solidified tumor away from its surroundings was a most surprising one: the multitude of small vessels, most of them "dead" so they could be parted like deteriorated rubber bands and a few others "living" which were easily secured either by clips or by using a coagulating current, gave the impression of a lesion which had died out in consequence of the prolonged radiation.

Cushing then describes the microscopy of the specimen with the intima of these arteries usually greatly proliferated so that "the lumen was often completely occluded."

Ray,[91] McKissock,[68] and Olivecrona[82,83,84] concluded on the basis of their experience that irradiation was of little or no benefit. Many others agreed.[26,33,43,88,114] In two of Krayenbühl's 19 cases where irradiation had been used as a complement to ligation of the carotid artery, clipping of feeders or decompression, and studied by Wegmann (1969) the AVM did not fill on follow-up angiograms. However, in one of these cases the angiographic study was incomplete, and a subsequent rebleed indicated that the malformation was not obliterated and that an angiogram of the vertebral system, if performed, would probably have visualized it. Svien and Peserico[108] describe the decrease of one AVM after x-ray therapy.

In his Hunterian Lecture delivered at the Royal College of Surgeons of England in 1955, Potter[89] presented 10 cases of irradiated AVMs and was impressed that only one patient died and four of the ten had survived for more than 20 years after treatment. However, since no follow-up angiogram had been performed, there was no proof that the AVMs had been obliterated. Nevertheless, Potter made a plea for the reconsideration of radiotherapy. Johnsson[35] presented 20 AVMs treated with conventional radiotherapy. Follow-up angiography performed 2 to 20 years after treatment showed that 45% of the cases had been cured, 25% had improved, and 25% were unchanged. Kjellberg et al[39] mention in a paper on Bragg peak the partial disappearance on the angiogram of an AVM previously irradiated with proton beams. In 1977 they reported 33 cases of AVM treated by the stereotactic Bragg peak proton beam method.[40] The angiography follow-up in 27 cases demonstrated that every treated case showed a marked reduction in the small-vessel component of the malformation and in two cases total obliteration had occurred.

In conclusion, radiotherapy was often used as a last resort, and despite some occasional successes, until 1970 it had been considered ineffective and had been abandoned. Olivecrona expressed a general feeling when saying: "The choice lies between removing the lesion or leaving it alone. In the latter case roentgen treatment may be tried, even if not much is to be expected from such therapy."[84]

However, the establishment and development of a method of treatment is often dependent on the rate of technologic innovation and research. During the last three decades a wealth of radiobiologic evidence concerning the sensitivity of vessels to irradiation accumulated. Furthermore, attempts to supplant instruments used in neurosurgery with stereotactically directed narrow beams of ionizing radiation were made.* The ^{60}Co gamma unit I was constructed in 1968 and installed in the Department of Neurosurgery, Karolinska Institute, Stockholm.

In 1970 I used the narrow ionizing beams from the ^{60}Co gamma unit I to irradiate an AVM for the first time. Thus, in the same department where 30 years earlier Olivecrona pronounced radiation therapy as useless, a project for the reassessment of this method started. The first results were published a few years later,[105,106] and further reports on the study in progress followed.

Stereotaxic Radiosurgery for Cerebral AVMs

Radiotherapy Versus Radiosurgery in AVM

In the publications on radiotherapy for AVM hitherto published (Table 6.1), the details of treatment were often lacking, the fields of irradiation approximate, and accuracy in dosimetry usually absent. Furthermore, doses were often low and given over a long period. Evaluation of results, usually based on clinical criteria and follow-up with angiography, if done at all, was unsystematic. Although inspired by early radiotherapy, radiosurgery in AVM differs from radiotherapy in principle and technique. Generally speaking, radiotherapy is based on the biologic difference in radiosensitivity between the cells of the pathologic and surrounding tissue. In radiosurgery accurate stereotactic localization combined with fields of radiation with steep gradients makes the biologic differentiation less critical, and the physically determined concentration of the radiation on the target becomes one of the important factors of treatment. Thus, a high single dose with a sharp gradient can be focused on a well-delineated tissue volume with little effect on the surrounding brain substance.

Method and Material

The ^{60}Co Unit

The main components of the stereotaxic gamma unit are the beam sources, the collima-

* References 1, 38, 49, 50, 53, 55, 56, 60, 70, 92.

Table 6.1. Publications on conventional x-ray therapy in arteriovenous malformations.

Ref.	Author	Year (19—)	Cases	Radiation type[a]	Dose (krad)	Time[b]	Follow-up Years	Follow-up Angiography
69	Magnus V	'21	1	R	2	F Rep	7	0
See 103	Marque AM	'27	2	X	2	F Rep	?	0
15	Cushing H Bailey P	'28	8	X	2	F Rep	>3	0
See 103	Cade	'31		R		F	?	0
91	Ray BS	'41	3	X	3–13	F Rep	>3	0
33	Jefferson G	'48	2	X	?	F	?	0
See 103	Krayenbühl HA	'54	4	X	?	F Rep	3	+
89	Potter JM	'55	10	X R	?	F Rep	Up to 22	0
See 103	Tönnis Schiefer	'55		X		F	?	+
85	Peterson JH McKissock W	'56	11	X R	?	F Rep	Up to 14	0
See 103	Olivecrona H Riives I	'58	?	X R	?	F Rep	10	+
105	Svien HJ Peserico I	'60	1	X R	3.7	F Rep	8	+
45	Krenchel NJ	'61	5	X	3	F	?	0
88	Pool JL	'65	?	X	?	F Rep	?	0
See 103	Johnson RT	'69	20	X	4.5	F Rep	2–20	+
26	French LA Chou SN	'69	<6	X R	?	F Rep	2	+
112	Wegmann HY	'69	17	X	?	F	Up to 19	+

[a] R, radium; X, x-ray.
[b] F, fraction; Rep, repeated.
[c] C, clinical; O, Operative; A, angiography.

tors, the operating table, and the instrument panel. The beam source consists of a number of ^{60}Co rods, 20-mm long and 1-mm in diameter, orientated radially and enclosed in a heavily shielded hemisphere. The distance from them to the focal point is 38 cm (Figs. 6.1, 6.2).

The collimator system, made from heavy alloy cylinders, consists of an outer helmet fixed to the bottom of the central hemispherical body and an inner helmet—the collimator helmet—attached to the operating table and provided with two adjustable axis rods for supporting the patient's head. The cross-section of the beams can be varied by changing the inner part of the collimator helmet. Beam cross-sections with a diameter of 3 mm in the anteroposterior and 5 or 7 mm in the transverse direction at the focal point with unit I can be obtained. With unit II, the cross-section of the beam is circular and can be adjusted to 8 or 14 mm in diameter. In unit II any of the 179 cobalt sources can be obliterated as required by plugging its respective collimator channel. Opening and closing the heavy radiation shield of the apparatus, as well as the

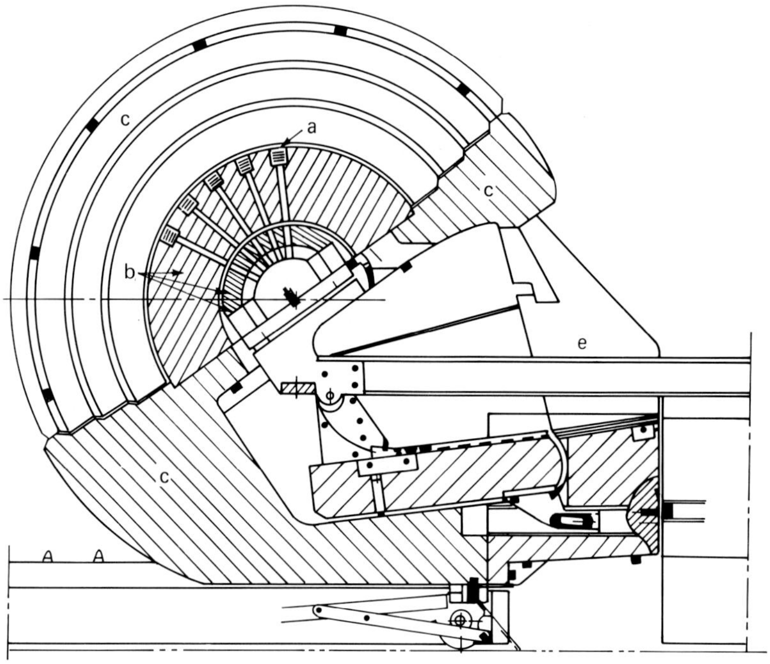

A

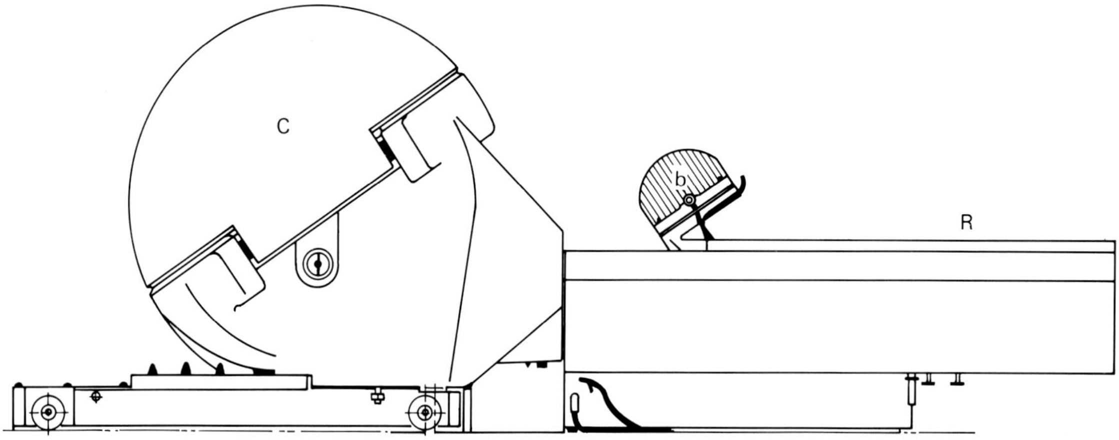

B

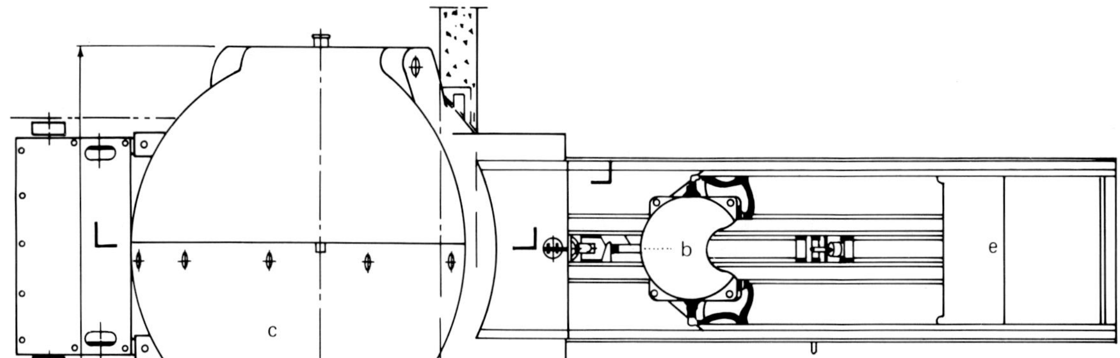
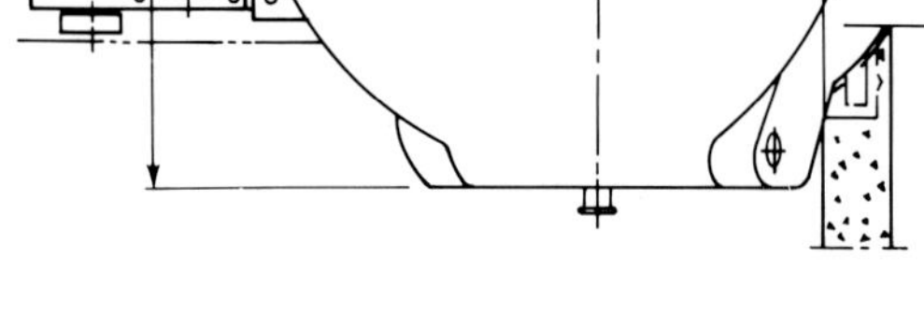

C

Fig. 16.1 A–C. Schematic of the stereotactic ^{60}Co gamma unit. *Key:* ^{60}Co source, (*a*) collimator helmets, (*b*) shielding material, (*c*) central beam (*d*), movable operating table (*c*).

Fig. 6.2. Stereotactic ^{60}Co gamma unit.

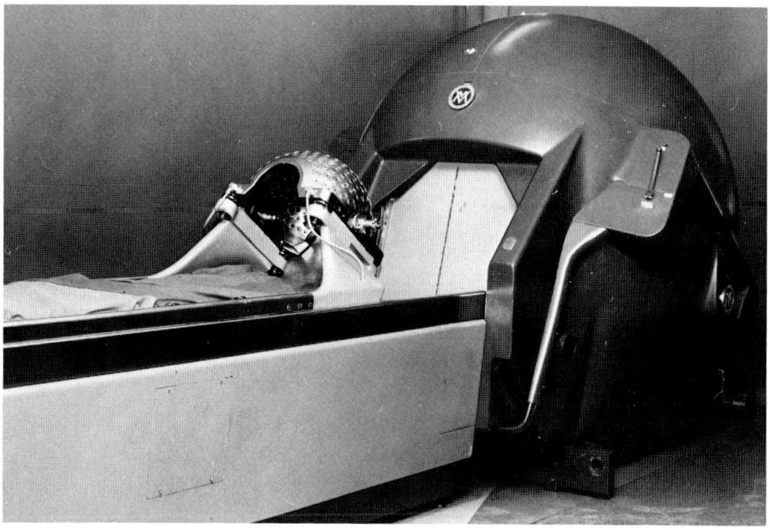

movement of the table in and out of the unit, is effected by means of a remote-controlled hydraulic system.

The Target for Radiation

Although the cluster of pathologic shunting vessels represented the logical target for radiation, the cross-section of the radiation beam available initially was too small and the first AVM to be treated too large to be covered by the radiation field. Therefore, only the feeding arteries were included in the 50% isodose distribution curve.

Case 1, E.B. The first patient, a 69-year-old man with hypertension and chronic nephritis, was admitted to our department in December 1969 after a subarachnoid hemorrhage. He had no neurologic deficits apart from a transient superior homonymous quadrantic hemianopsia. Angiography revealed a large AVM in the medial part of the left occipital lobe fed by a dilated posterior cerebral artery. The malformation and the feeding artery filled only from the vertebrobasilar system (Fig. 6.3). Radiosurgery was performed in March 1970 and the target point located so that the two terminal branches of the feeding artery were included in a single radiation field (Fig. 6.3); 5 krads were given over a period of about half an hour. The angiograms repeated in November 1971 no longer visualized the malformation, and the feeding vessels were obliterated (Fig. 6.3).

The following second case was small enough to be completely covered by the radiation field.

Case 2, S.E. Angiography following a subarachnoid hemorrhage in a 10-year-old girl revealed a small AVM in the right basal ganglia (Fig. 6.4). At radiosurgery in April 1972 a single dose of 5 krads was delivered so that the cluster of pathologic vessels was almost completely covered. Subsequent angiography after 1 year showed no filling of the malformation.

In 1975 the ^{60}Co unit II was installed at the Karolinska enabling spherical fields of up to 25 mm in diameter to be covered by the field of irradiation.

The Patients

Our first two cases treated revealed the value, limitations, and most of the problems of radiosurgery in AVM, and they shaped the clinical management and research in this field.

On the basis of management, the patients have been grouped according to the following (Fig. 6.5): Group A includes those in whom the radiation field completely covered the cluster of pathologic vessels. Group B includes those in whom the cluster of pathologic vessels could be only partially covered by the radiation field. Group C comprises those cases where all feeding arteries were included in the 50% isodose configuration. Group D comprises those cases where the radiation field included only some of several feeding vessels. The total number of pa-

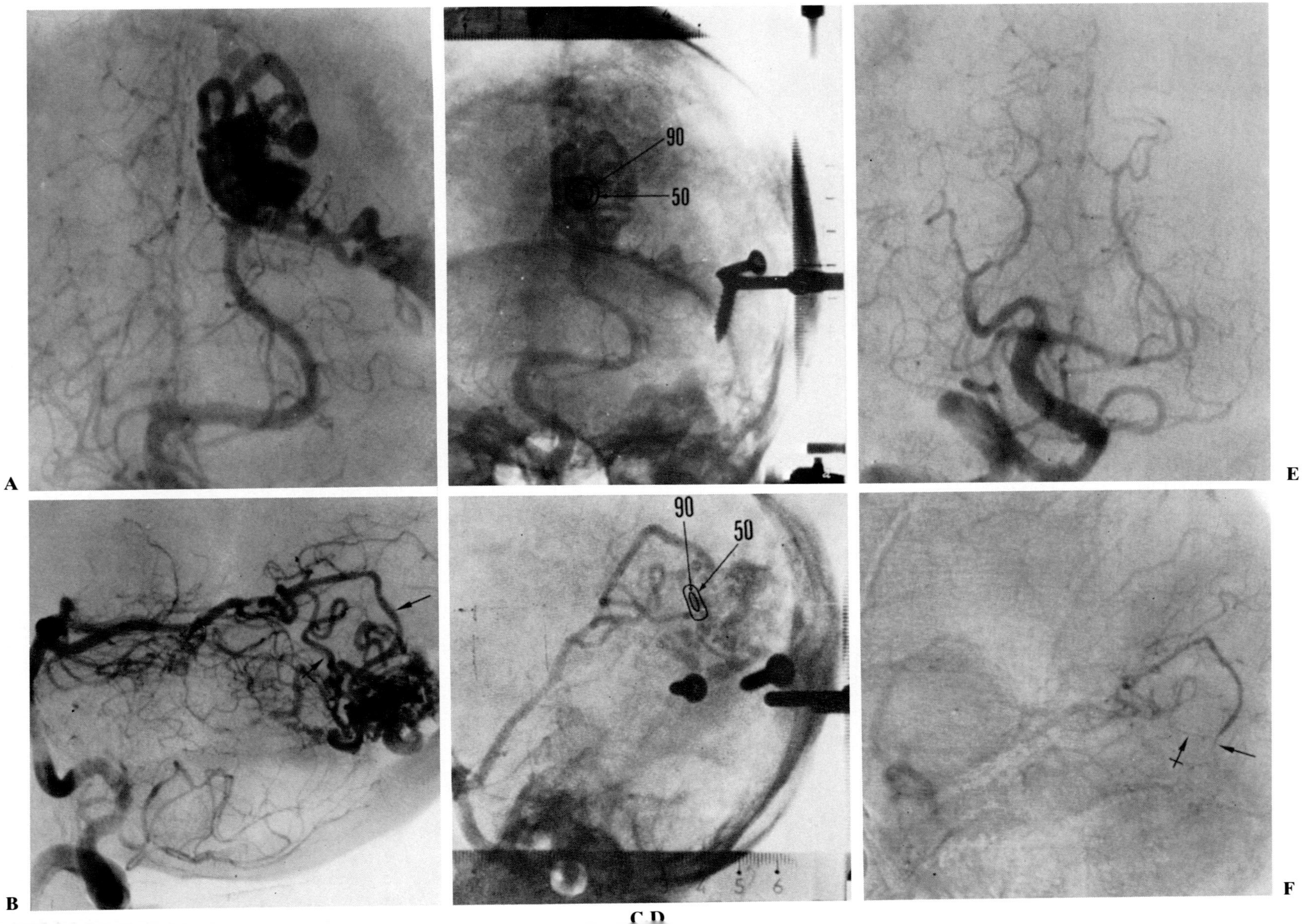
A
90
50
E
B
90
50
F
C D

Fig. 6.3. Vertebral angiograms, frontal and lateral views. **A** and **B.** AVM fed by two branches (*arrows*) of the psterior cerebral artery (reproduced by courtesy of Acta Chir Scand). **C** and **D.** On day of radiosurgery; two feeding arteries included in 50% isodose distribution. **E** and **F.** Angiography 19 months later showing no filling of AVM, decrease to normal of the posterior cerebral artery and local constriction in lumen of two feeding arteries (*arrows*). This constriction corresponds to course of vessels through target area.

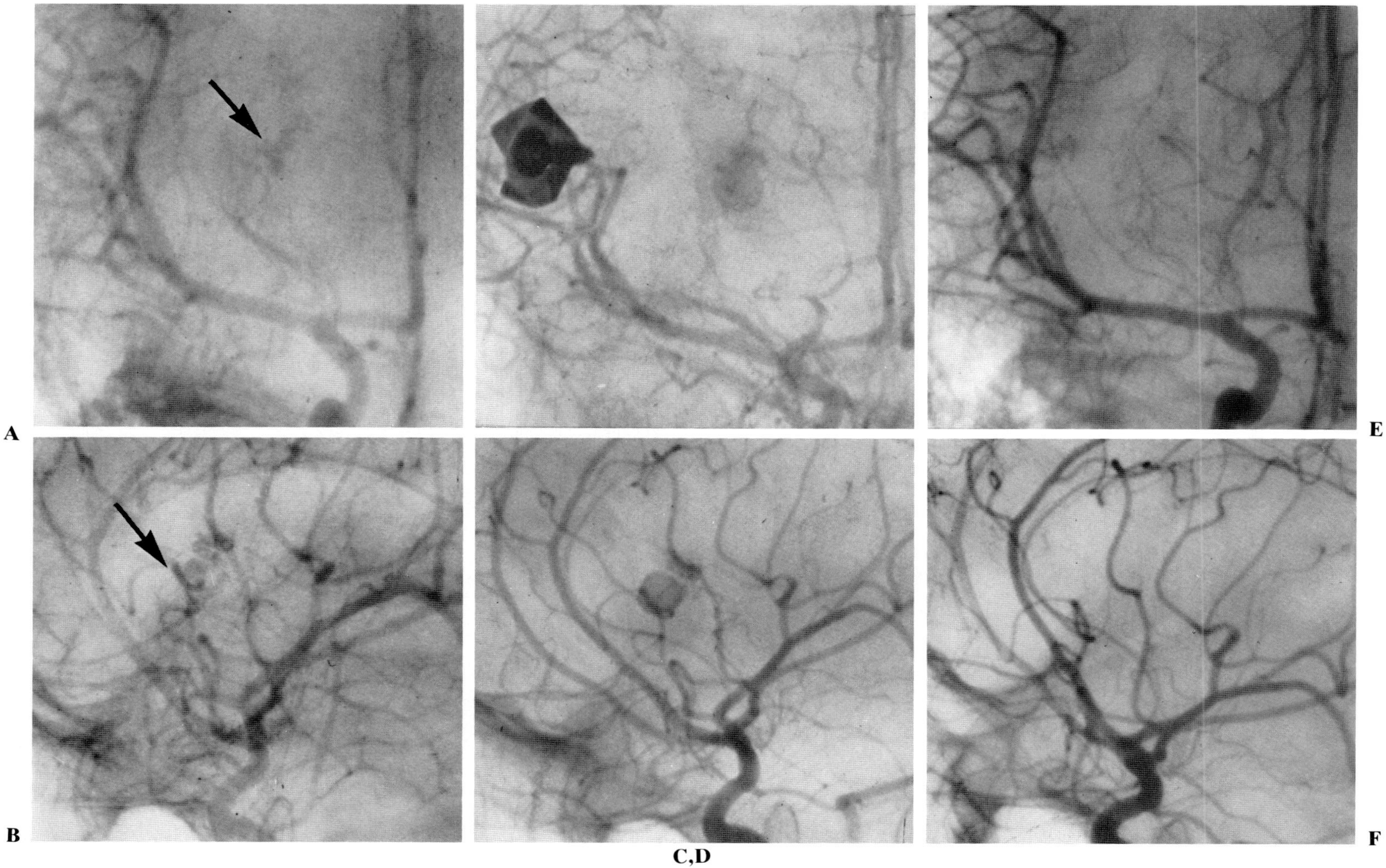

Fig. 6.4. Angiograms, frontal and lateral views, demonstrating **A** and **B**, small AVM fed by hypertrophied striothalamic artery immediate after subarachnoid bleed (*arrows*). **C** and **D**. Time of radiosurgery. **E** and **F**. One year after treatment with no filling of the AVM.

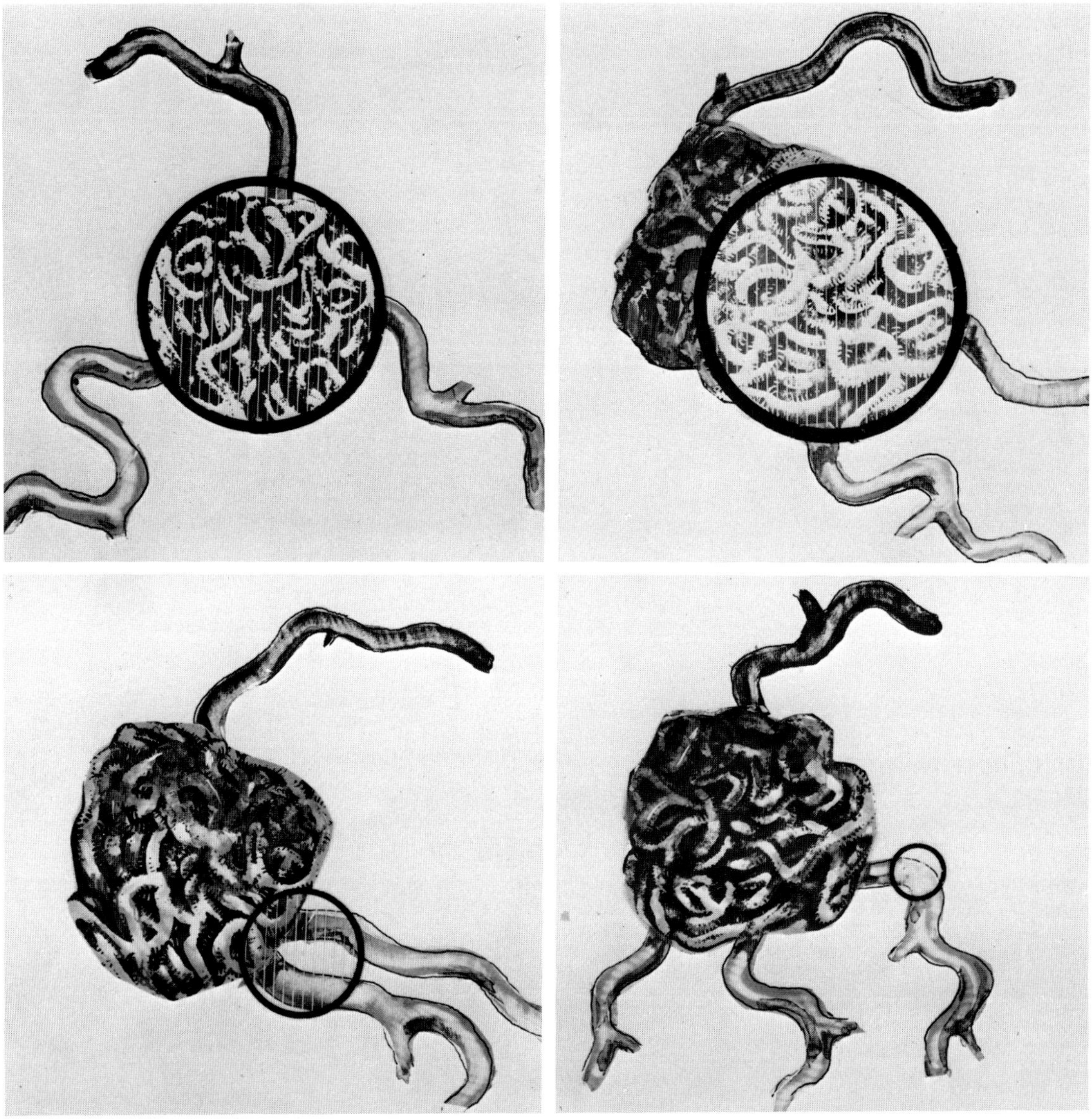

A C B D

Fig. 6.5. Relationship of AVM and radiation field. According to this relationship, patients treated were grouped in those in whom **(A)** AVM was totally covered by optimum radiation dose, **(B)** all feeding arteries were included, **(C)** only part of AVM was irradiated and **(D)** only part of multiple feeders were irradiated.

tients treated was 300; 162 females and 138 males. Their mean age was 29 years; the range was 4 to 70 years. Irradiation was repeated in nine cases where no results were obtained and the initial treatment was considered technically unsatisfactory.

Follow-up

Angiography, brain scanning, computerized tomography (CT), EEG, and clinical asessment were carried out postoperatively at 3-, 6-, 12-, 36-, and 60-month intervals. One of the foreign patients could not be traced, two refused follow-up angiography. This assessment is based on a total of 300 cases. In two patients the feeding arteries were irradiated without satisfactory results; when the treatment was ultimately repeated, the whole cluster of pathologic vessels was covered by the radiation field. These two cases are included in group C as well as in

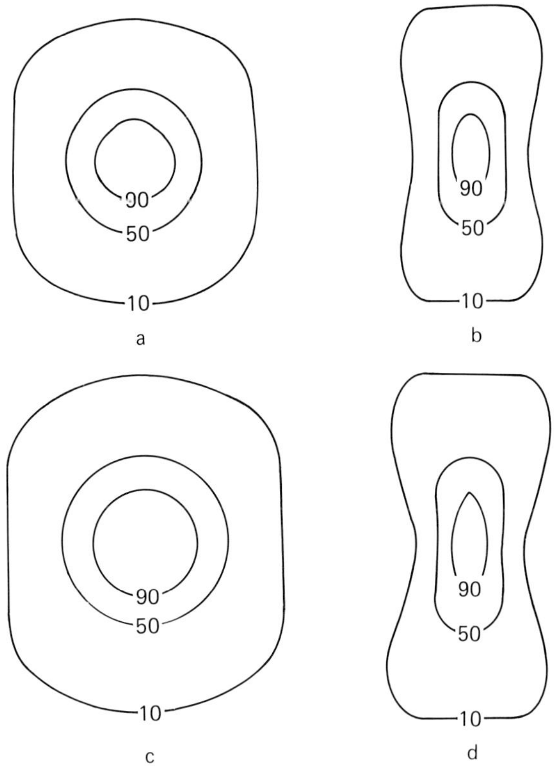

Fig. 6.6. Dose distribution in unit I. **A** and **B.** frontal, **C** and **D** lateral views. ▷

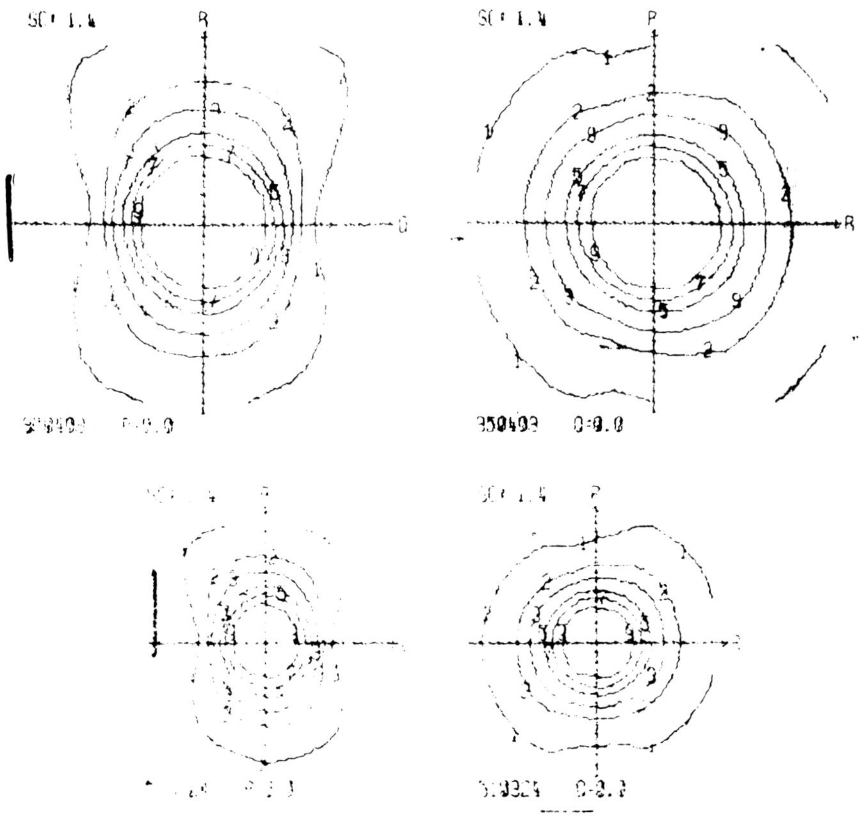

Fig. 6.7. Dose distribution in unit II. **A** and **B.** lateral, **C** and **D** frontal views. ▽

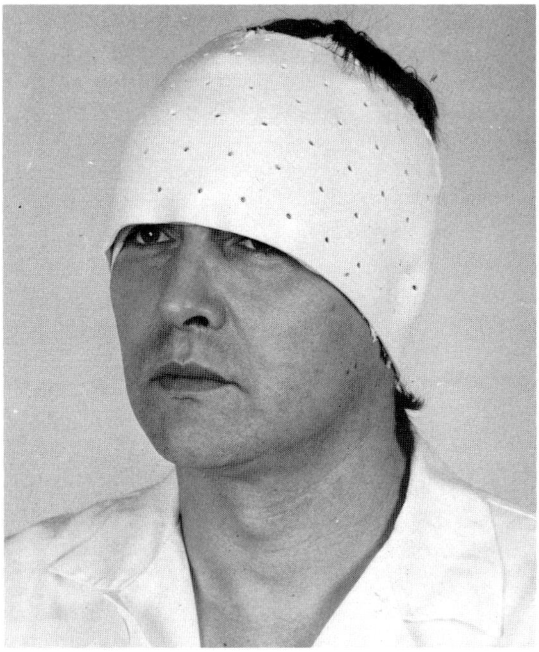

Fig. 6.8. Patient with thermoplast molded around his head.

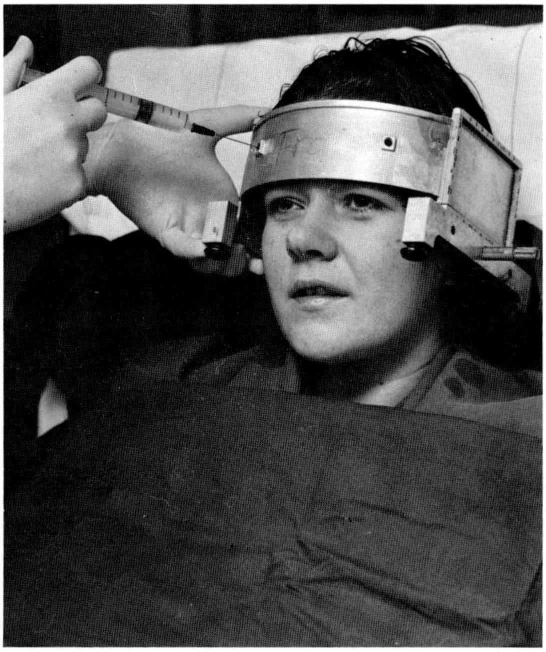

Fig. 6.10. Instead of thermoplast, metal frame with built-in coordinate scales is fixed to patient's skull.

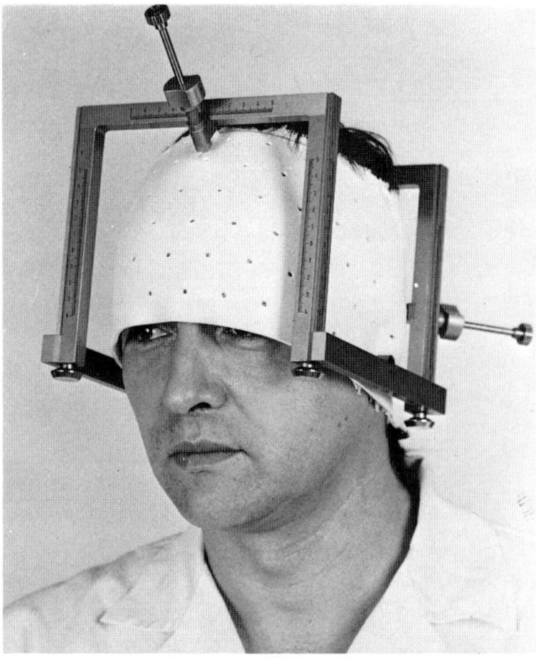

Fig. 6.9. Neurosurgical stereotactic frame fixed to plastic shell.

group A. All patients entering the study had one to five follow-up examinations during a period varying from three months to 7 years. A final follow-up angiography was carried out 5 years after total obliteration.

Procedure

Four-vessel rapid serial angiography and CT scans were carried out in every case of AVM. Every effort was made to identify all the feeding arteries on the lateral and anteroposterior films. The location and size of the malformation, as well as the pattern of feeding vessels, determine whether conventional surgery or radiosurgery will be performed. If radiosurgery is chosen, the place and size of the AVM are transposed on lateral and anteroposterior plain x-ray films of the skull, which are used for dose planning.

Dose plans are calculated with the PCP 11 minicomputer in a three-dimensional matrix,[3] taking into consideration the individual parameters. Size of the skull, position and size of the target volume are fed into the computer via a

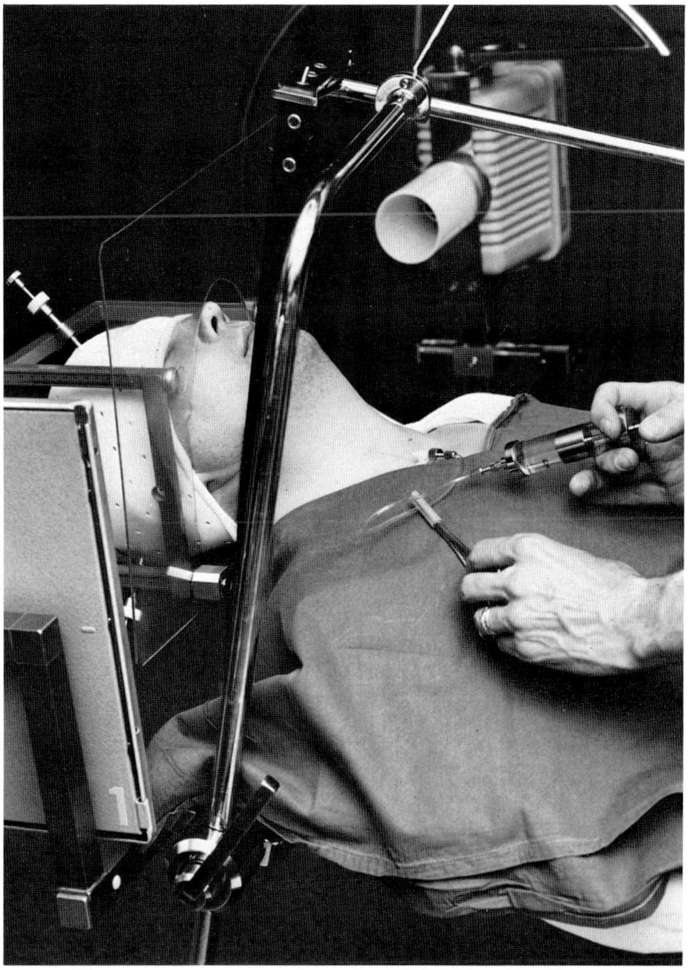

Fig. 6.11. Patient in position for stereotactic angiography.

keyboard and a curve digitizer. Maximum, minimum, average, and integral doses and isodose plans are displayed on a graphic screen and on an incremental plotter. The dose planning by computer may define a radiation field that matches spatially to the tangle of vessels to be irradiated. Examples of dose-distribution curves used in the first cases treated are reproduced in Fig. 6.6, and computer-calculated individual dose distributions for the collimators 14 and 8 mm are reproduced in Fig. 6.7.

The patient's hair is washed but not cut on the evening before the operation. Except in children and cases with altered state of consciousness, the operation can usually be performed with the patient awake. However, premedication is necessary because of the angiography. The procedure includes the following steps: The coordinate frame is afixed. In the first cases the stereotactic frame was fixed to a cap of plaster applied to the patient's head. The plaster has since been supplanted by the following alternatives: (1) A thermoplast (Orthoplast) is moulded around the patient's head and hooked on four small metal screws previously fixed into the outer table of the skull (Fig. 6.8). The stereotactic coordinate frame is then fixed to the plastic shell (Fig. 6.9). As the use of metal screws fits badly to "a bloodless procedure," one may omit them provided the moulded plastic fits firmly to such skull prominences as the orbital ridge, preventing any movement during radiation. (2) A circular metal frame with built-in coordinate scales is fixed directly to the skull by four screws after local anesthetic is injected at the fixation points. The coordinate frame is aligned on the patient's head corresponding to the location of the AVM

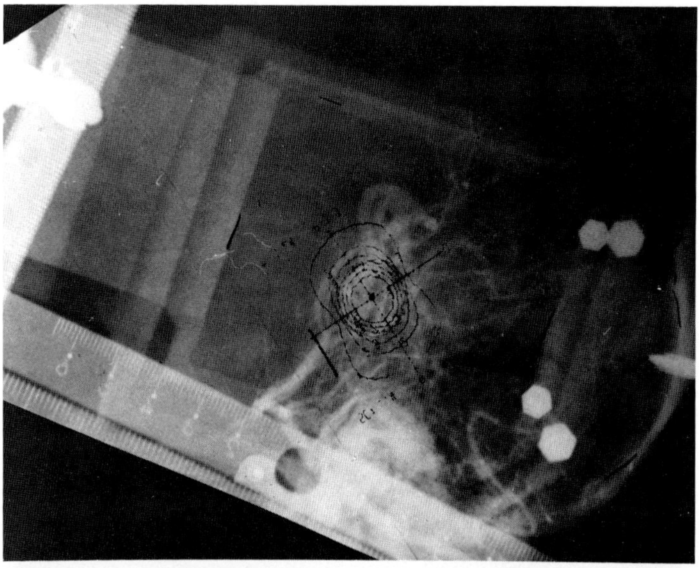

A

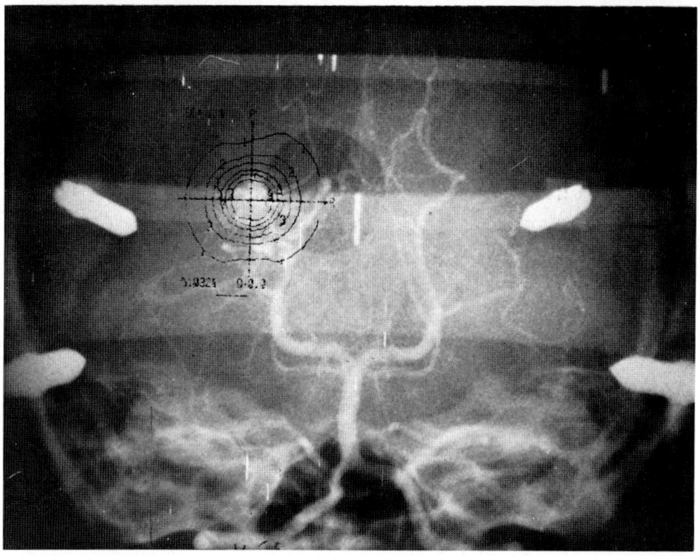

B

Fig. 6.12. Individual dose plane superimposed on stereotactic angiogram in **A** lateral and **B** frontal views.

(Fig. 6.10). Stereotaxic angiography of the vessels harboring the malformation is performed in both lateral and anteroposterior projections by direct injection or catheterization of the vessels via the femoral artery (Fig. 6.11). If the malformation presents two areas of vascularity, both are visualized, and by superimposing the angiograms, the composite picture of the pathologic vessels is drawn on the film to be used for determining instrument coordinates of the target. The stereotactic films are compared with the preoperative angiograms and the target area determined. The x and y coordinates for the midpoint of this area are calculated.

Bergström, Greitz and Steiner,[11] worked out a method of coordinate determination by computer without using a given geometric relationship between the patient (the sterotactic frame fixed on the head of the patient) and the x-ray focus and film. The point of intersection between one horizontal and two vertical planes can be determined by feeding into the computer the coordinates of these three planes, defined by verticals passing through the target and the scales. The dose distribution is then superimposed on the AVM on the stereotactic film so that the tangle of pathologic vessels is optimally covered by a sufficient dose and minor adjust-

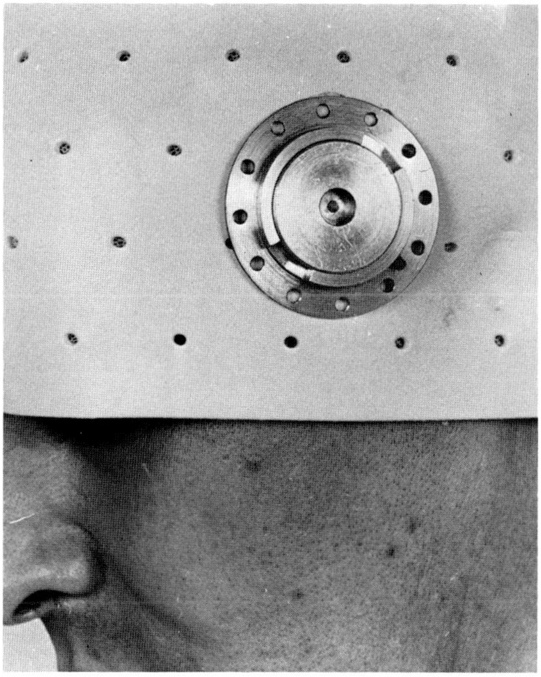

Fig. 6.13

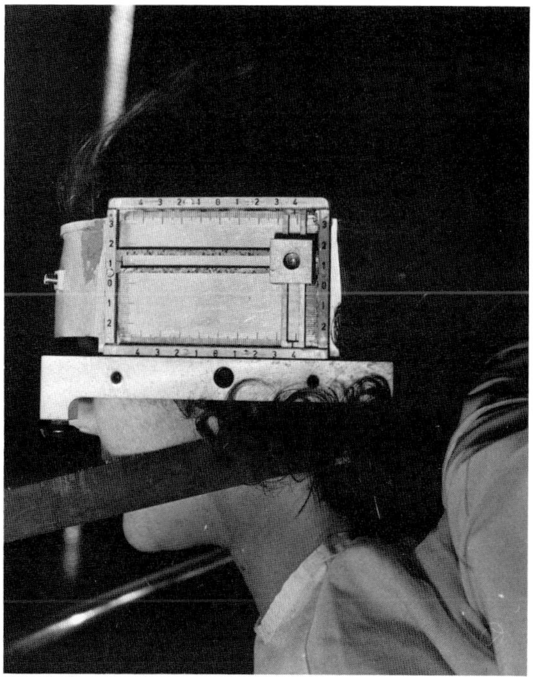

Fig. 6.14

Fig. 6.13. Metal bearings glued in orthoplast.

Fig. 6.14. Metal bearings attached to metal frame according to coordinates.

Fig. 6.15. Patient on operating-room table with head placed in the collimator helmet supported by axis rods inserted in bearings.

Fig. 6.16. Instrument panel. Intercommunication system and TV monitor to communicate with and observe patient during treatment.

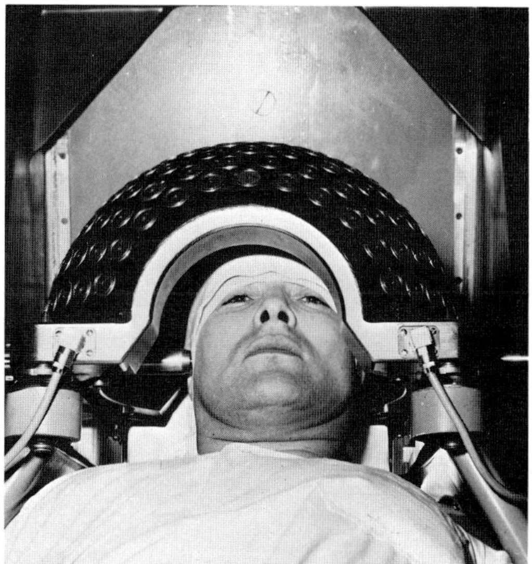

Fig. 6.15

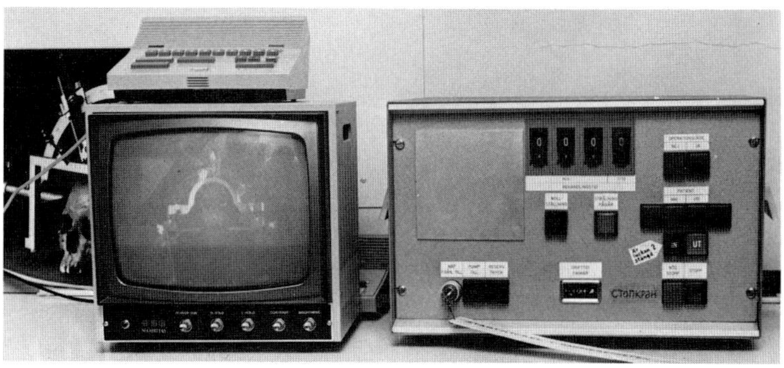

Fig. 6.16

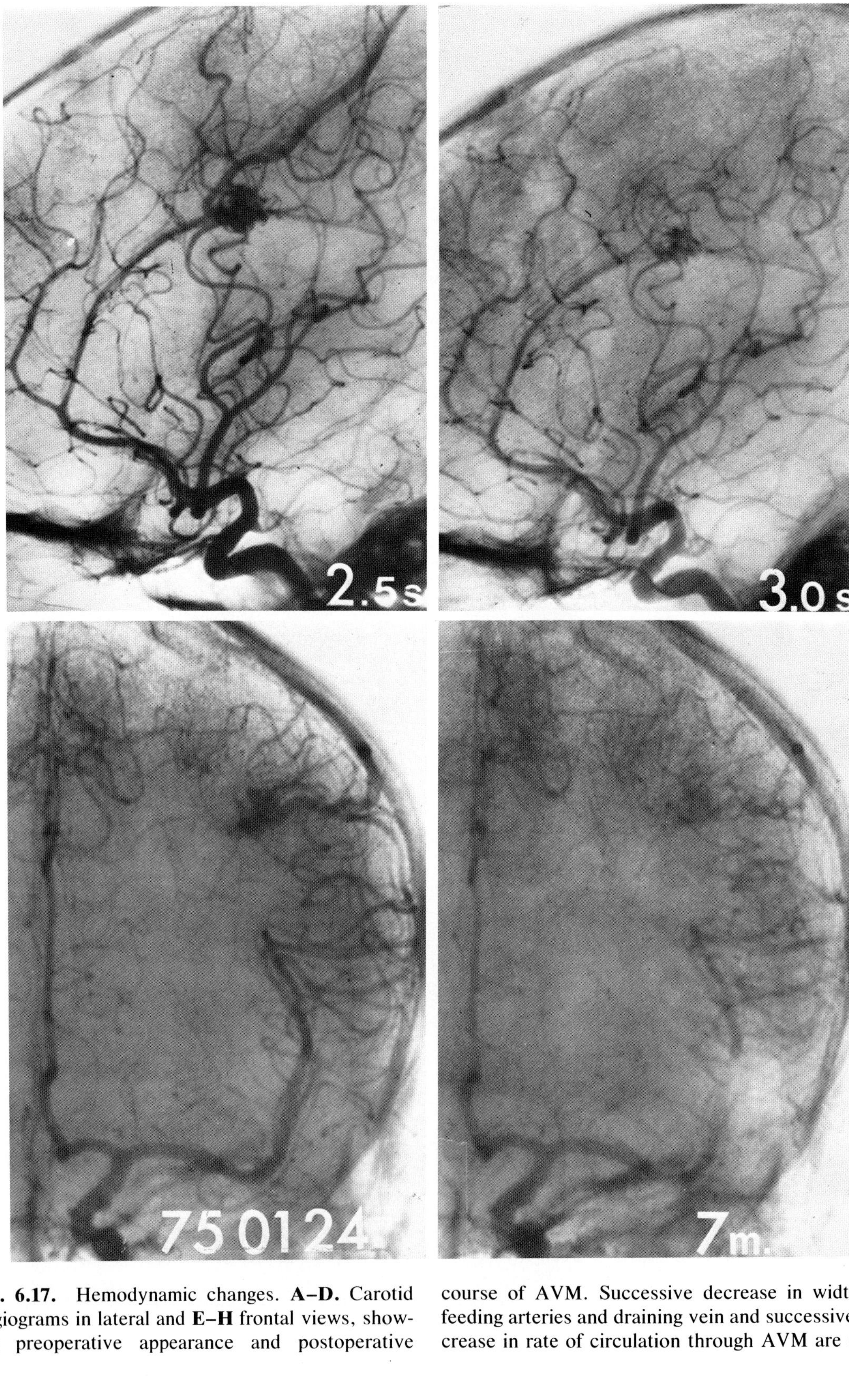

A B E F

Fig. 6.17. Hemodynamic changes. **A–D.** Carotid angiograms in lateral and **E–H** frontal views, showing preoperative appearance and postoperative course of AVM. Successive decrease in width of feeding arteries and draining vein and successive decrease in rate of circulation through AVM are seen

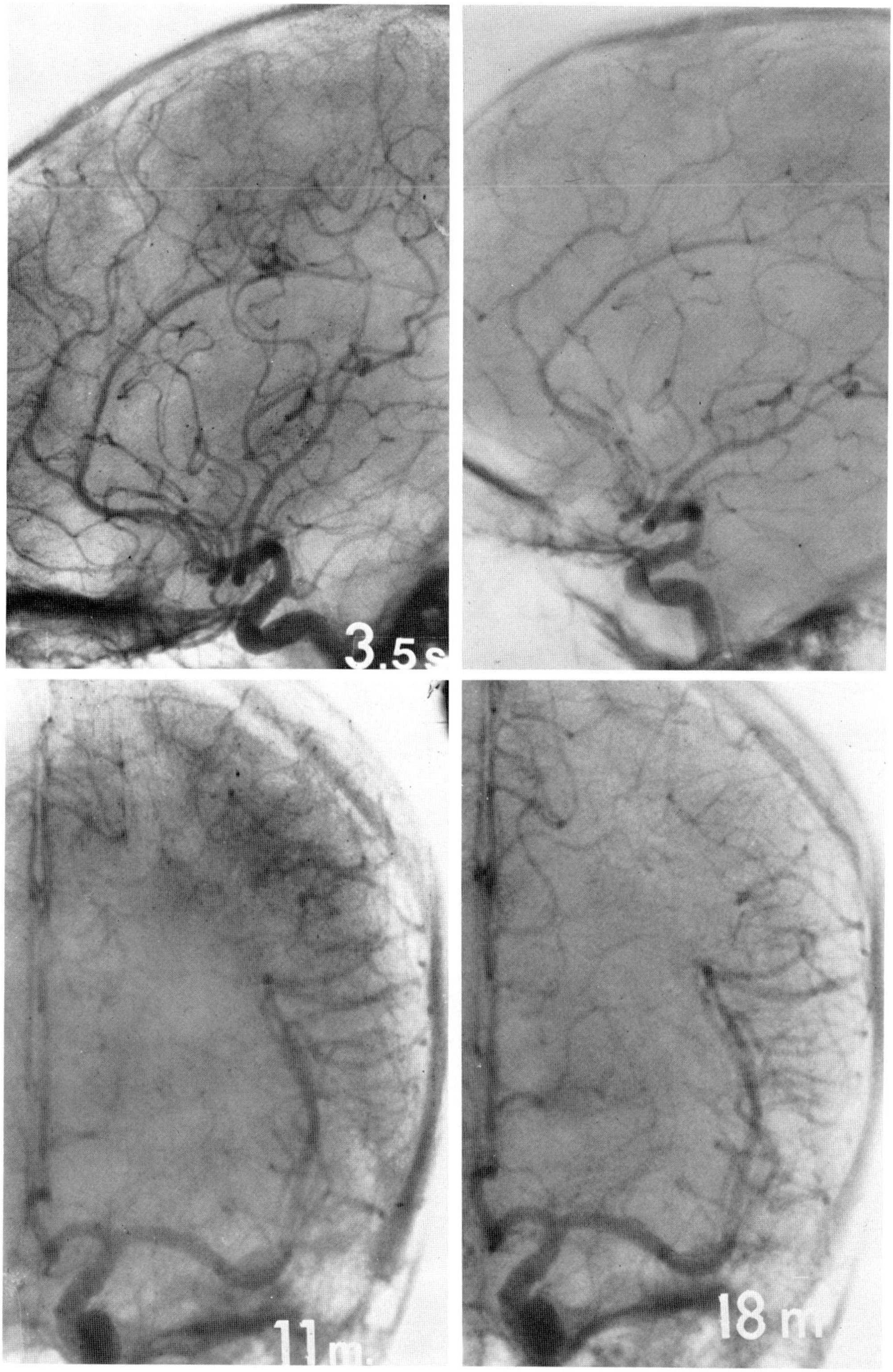

C D G H

from delayed appearance time of draining vein **(A–C).** Time after start of injection shown in **A–D.** Follow-up carried out 7, 11, and 18 months after treatment. On last occasions **(D** and **H)** AVM is no longer filled.

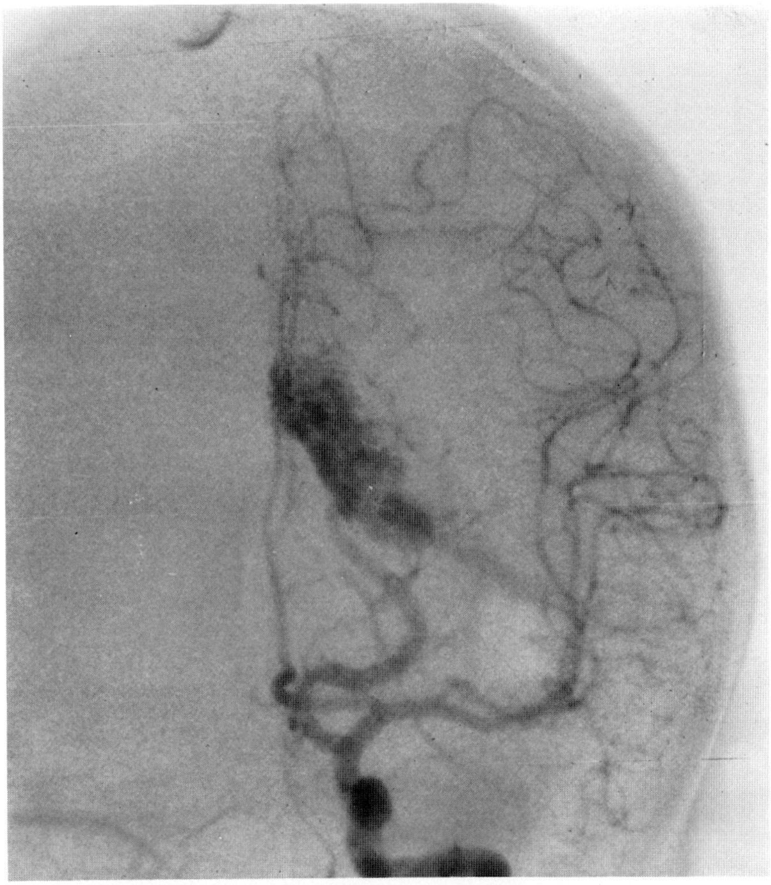

A

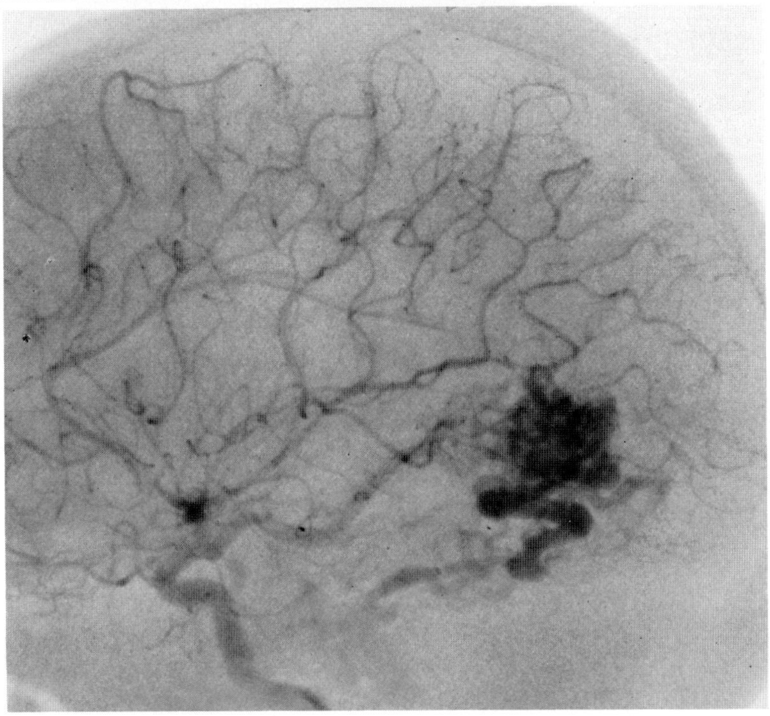

C

Fig. 6.18. Carotid angiography. **A.** Frontal and **C** lateral views of AVM fed by branches from posterior cerebral artery draining to transverse sinus. One year after treatment subtotal obliteration of AVM has been achieved. **B** and **D.** Posterior cerebral artery and drawing vein decreased in size.

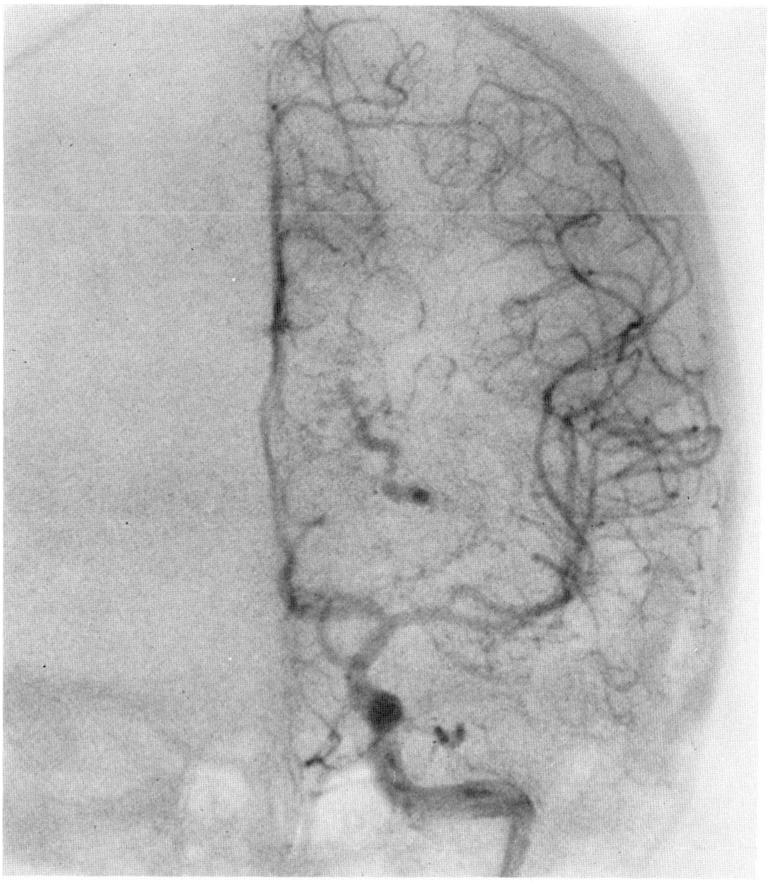

B

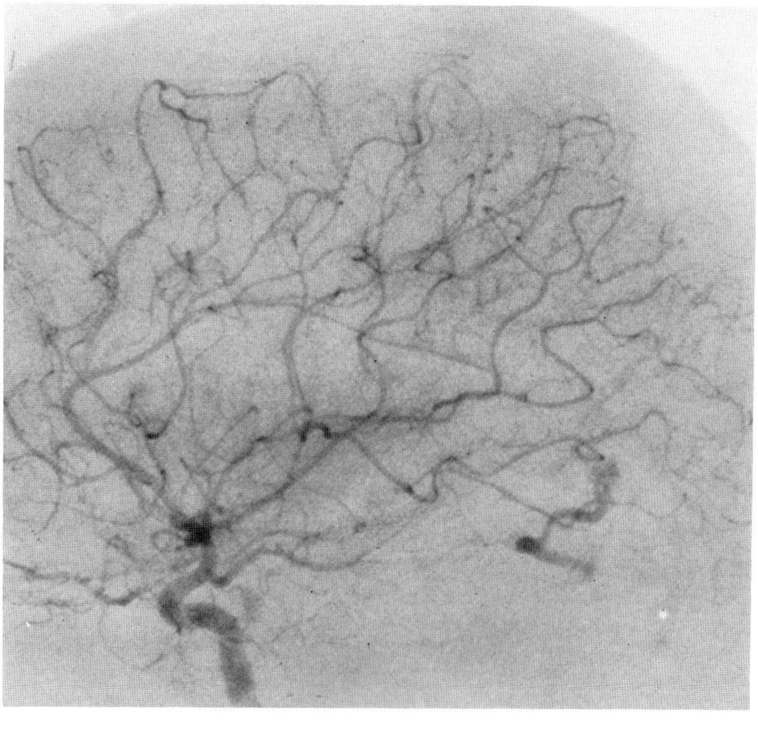

D

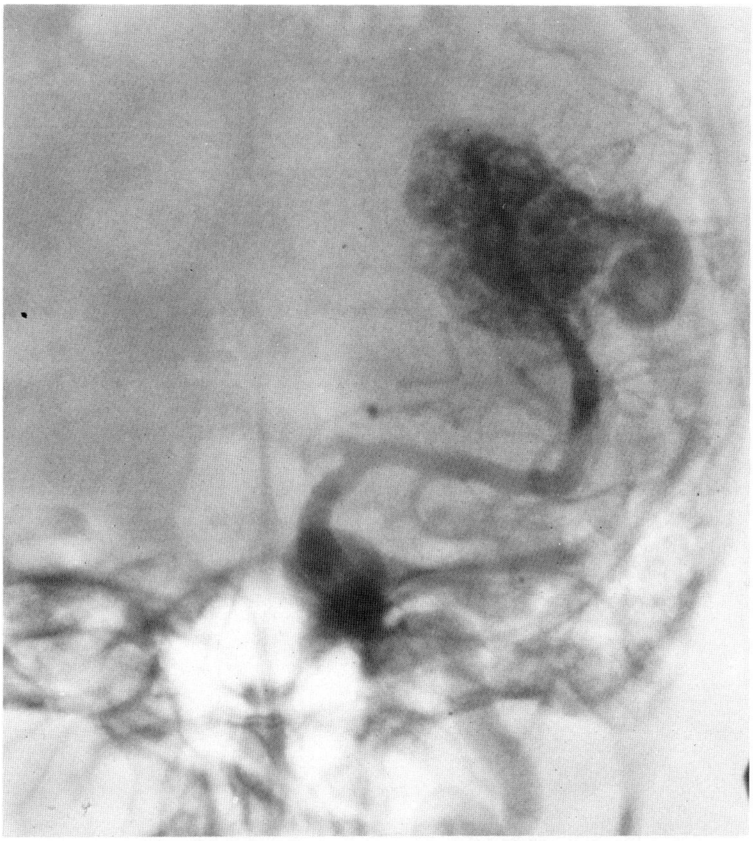

A

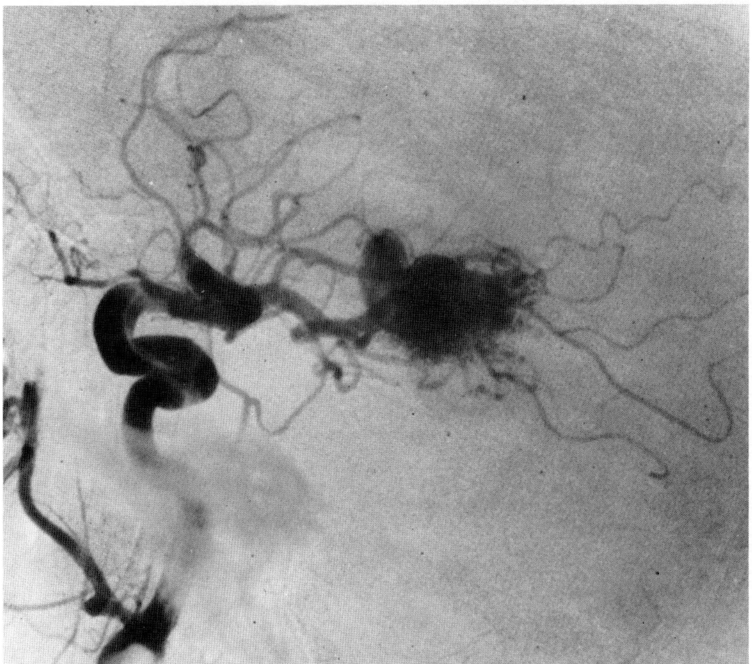

C

Fig. 6.19. Carotid angiography. **A.** Frontal and **C** lateral views of AVM fed by branches of left middle cerebral and anterior choroidal arteries draining to superior anastomic vein left transverse sinus and sagittal and cavernous sinuses. **B**, **D**, and **E**. Sixteen months after treatment subtotal obliteration of the malformation (examination carried out in Department of Neurosurgery, Sheffield).

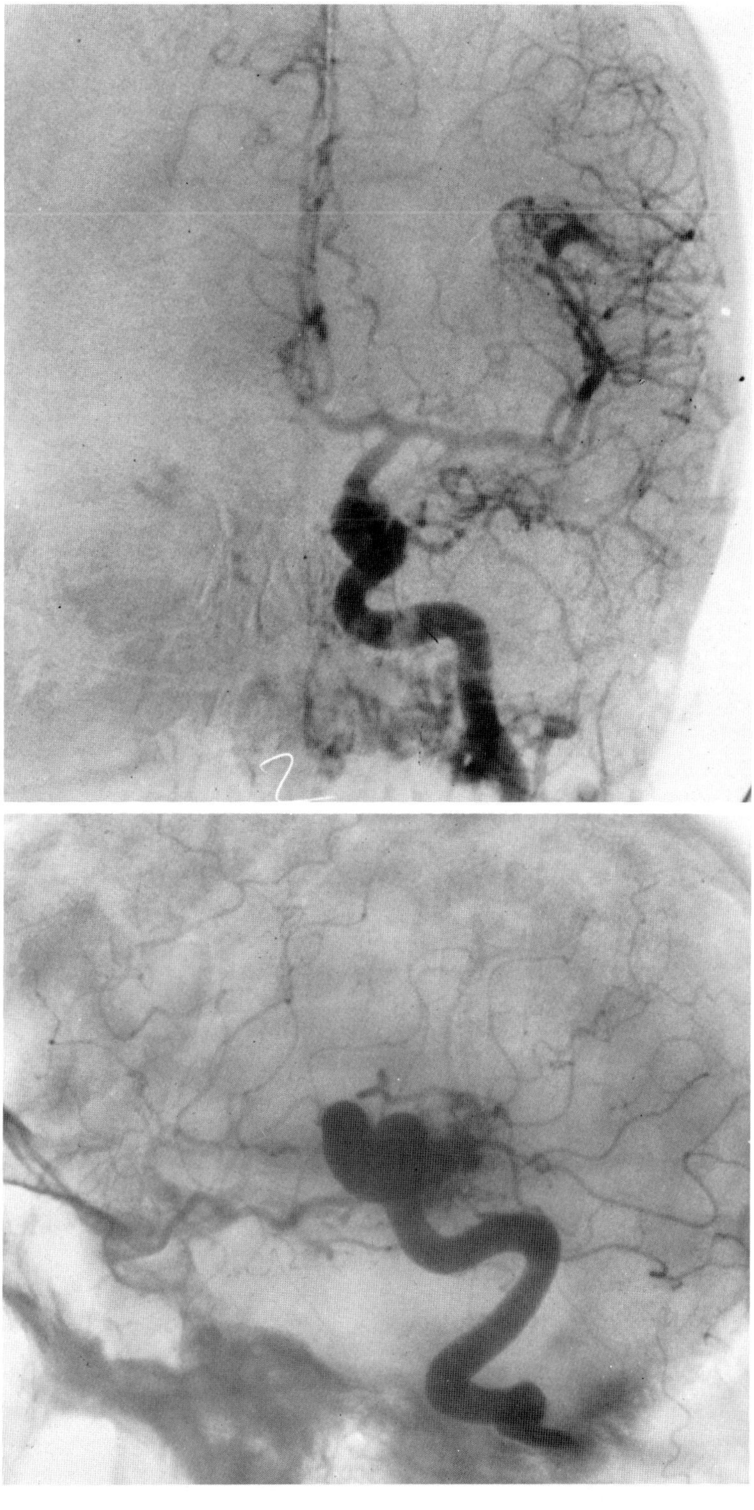

B

D

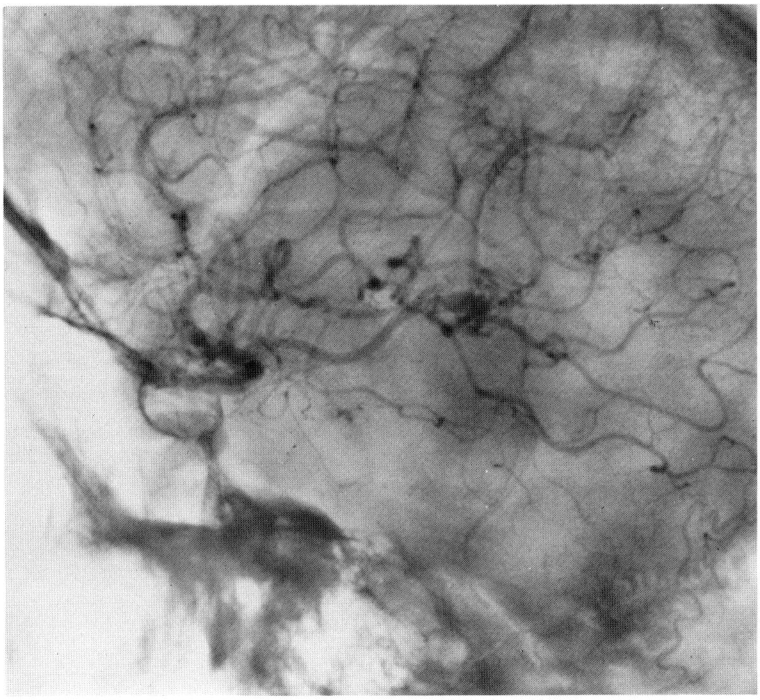

Fig. 6.19E

ments of the coordinates are made as required (Fig. 6.12).

The *x* and *y* coordinates of the target determine the position of two metal bearings for the axis rods of the collimator helmet, the bearings being glued in the plastic shell (Fig. 6.13). In the case of the metal frame, the bearings are attached to the scales and adjusted according to the coordinates (Fig. 6.14). New anteroposterior x-ray view is taken and the *Z* coordinate, which determines the lateral position of the head in the apparatus, is calculated. At this stage, when plaster or plastic is used, the stereotactic frame is removed. During this time the required inner collimator helmet is placed in position. The patient is moved to the operating table. The axis rods are inserted in the bearings, and the patient's head is positioned according to the *Z* coordinate (Fig. 6.15). The radiation time corresponding to the decided dose and the dose rate of the gamma unit at the specific time of the operation is calculated and the timer on the instrument panel programmed. After a final check of the axis readings and the position of the head, the irradiation shield of the unit is opened, and the operating table with the patient is moved into position. The inner and outer collimators marry and the target is cross-fired with the narrow ionizing gamma beams. The patient is observed by the operator on a TV screen, and they communicate by an intercom (Fig. 6.16). When the timer signals that the required dose of irradiation has been given, the operating table is taken out again and the radiation shield is closed. The axis rods of the collimator helmet are disconnected and the plaster or the metal frame is removed. Sterile dressings are placed on the four screw wounds. The patient may eat normally immediately after the procedure. Following the treatment the patient remains in bed for 12 to 24 hours as a routine precaution observed after cerebral angiography. Single radiation doses varying between 3 and 12.5 krads to a target point at the center of the vascular cluster have been used. In two small series, fresh plasma or the antifibrinolytic drug ε-aminocaproic acid (EACA) have been used as adjuvants.

Follow-up includes angiographic studies; however, if repeated too often, they may yield total radiation doses above permitted levels. CT scans may be carried out instead of control angiographies. However, CT is of use only if it reveals that the malformation was not obliterated. If, on the contrary, the malformation is not visualized, angiography has to be performed. In certain cases even on an angiogram an early filling of a draining vein is the only evidence that the pathologic shunt is still not completely sealed.

Results and Discussion

Angiographic Studies

The changes observed on postoperative angiograms may be summarized as follows:

1. No visible changes. Some of these cases may respond later to the treatment.
2. Hemodynamic changes consisting of a decrease in the flow rate through the malformation reflected in a decrease in the size of the feeding arteries (Fig. 6.17). Hemodynamic changes, if they occurred, were usually observed before gross morphologic changes occurred in the AVM.
3. Partial obliteration of the AVM.

Case 3., R.M. A 32-year-old housewife was admitted to the department of neurosurgery following a subarachnoid hemorrhage. On admission she had a superior homonymous quadrantic hemianopsia. Angiography revealed a large AVM fed by two branches of the right posterior cerebral artery and drained by a dilated vein to the transverse sinus (Fig. 6.18). Irradiation of the feeding arteries by 5 krad induced only a slight reduction of the malformation, and 3 years later the entire tangle of pathologic vessels was covered by 8.5 krad. One year later a subtotal obliteration of the AVM could be confirmed (Fig. 6.18).

Case 4, M.M. The patient was a 23-year-old student who had suffered from migraine for 10 years. Angiography following a subarachnoid hemorrhage visualized in the posterior part of the left Sylvian fissure a 3.5 by 2.5 by 2.5 cm large AVM fed by hypertrophied branches of the left middle cerebral and anterior choroidal arteries and draining into the vena Labbé, to the left transverse sinus and through superficial cortical veins to the sagittal and cavernous sinuses. The pathologic vessels could be covered by a single radiation field of 10 krad. On an angiogram performed 16 months later, the remaining abnormality appeared to be a short region of dilatation on a branch of the left middle cerebral artery and a few suspicious small vessels in the immediate neighborhood of the dilated segment. Therefore, some residual malformation could not be excluded completely (Fig. 6.19).

4. Total obliteration of the AVM.

Case 5, L.M. A 20-year-old student had transient aphasia and right hemiparesis following subarachnoid hemorrhage. The AVM was localized on the medial aspect of the left hemisphere close to the tentorial notch, fed by branches from the posterior cerebral and pericallosal arteries and draining into the straight sinus via the great vein of Galen. Ten krad were given, the whole malformation being included in the isodose configuration. The malformation became successively smaller and did not fill on angiogram 1 year later. (Fig. 6.20). The neurologic deficiencies improved and she continues her studies.

Case 6, K.M. A 16-year-old girl presented with a subarachnoid hemorrhage from an AVM situated at the level of the left ambient cistern behind the pulvinar thalami, fed by branches from the posterior choroidal arteries and drained by superficial veins on the inferior surface of the temporal and occipital lobes to the lateral aspect of the transverse sinus. The tangle of pathologic vessels was irradiated by a single dose of 10 krad and did not fill when angiography was performed 9 months later. There was a narrowing of the posterior cerebral artery within the target area (Fig. 6.21). The patient is now free of symptoms.

Case 7, E.Ö. A 4-year-old boy presented with a subarachnoid bleed from an AVM on the medial aspect of the left occipitotemporal region, fed by branches from the posterior cerebral artery and drained via the great vein of Galen to the straight sinus. Radiosurgery was performed, the whole malformation was covered by the irradiation field, and a single dose of 10 krad was given. One year later the malformation was found to be obliterated (Fig. 6.22). The boy is developing normally.

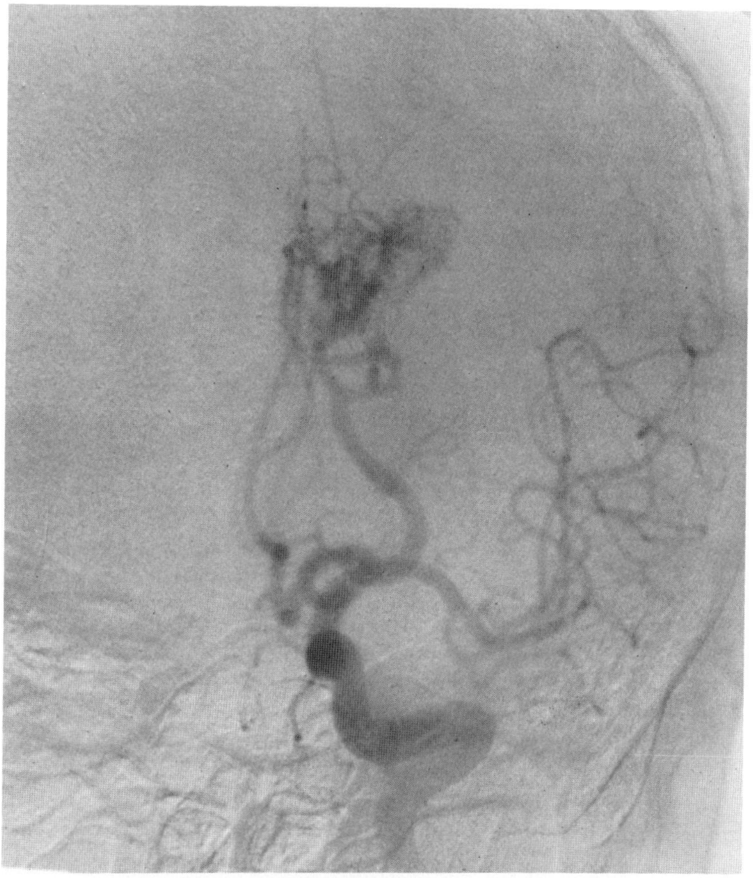

A

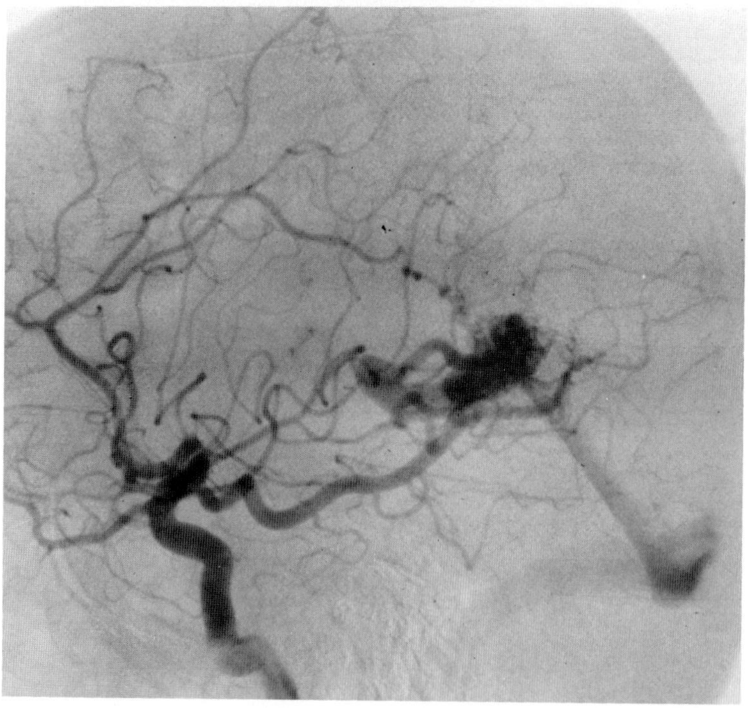

C

Fig. 6.20. Carotid angiography. **A.** Frontal and **C** lateral views of AVM fed by branches from posterior cerebral and pericallosal arteries draining to straight sinus. **B** and **D.** After 1 year AVM disappeared, size of posterior cerebral artery decreased and feeding arteries became occluded.

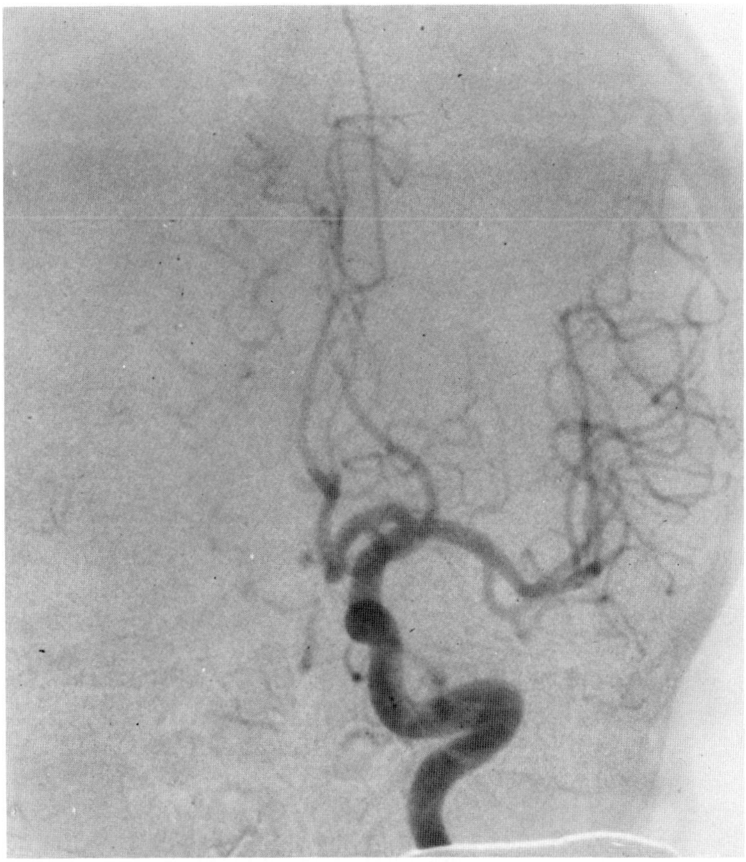

B

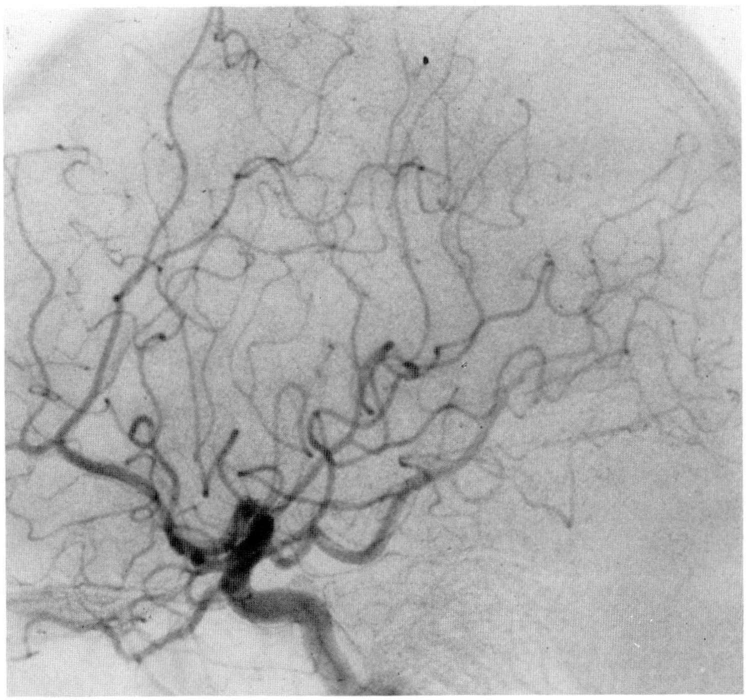

D

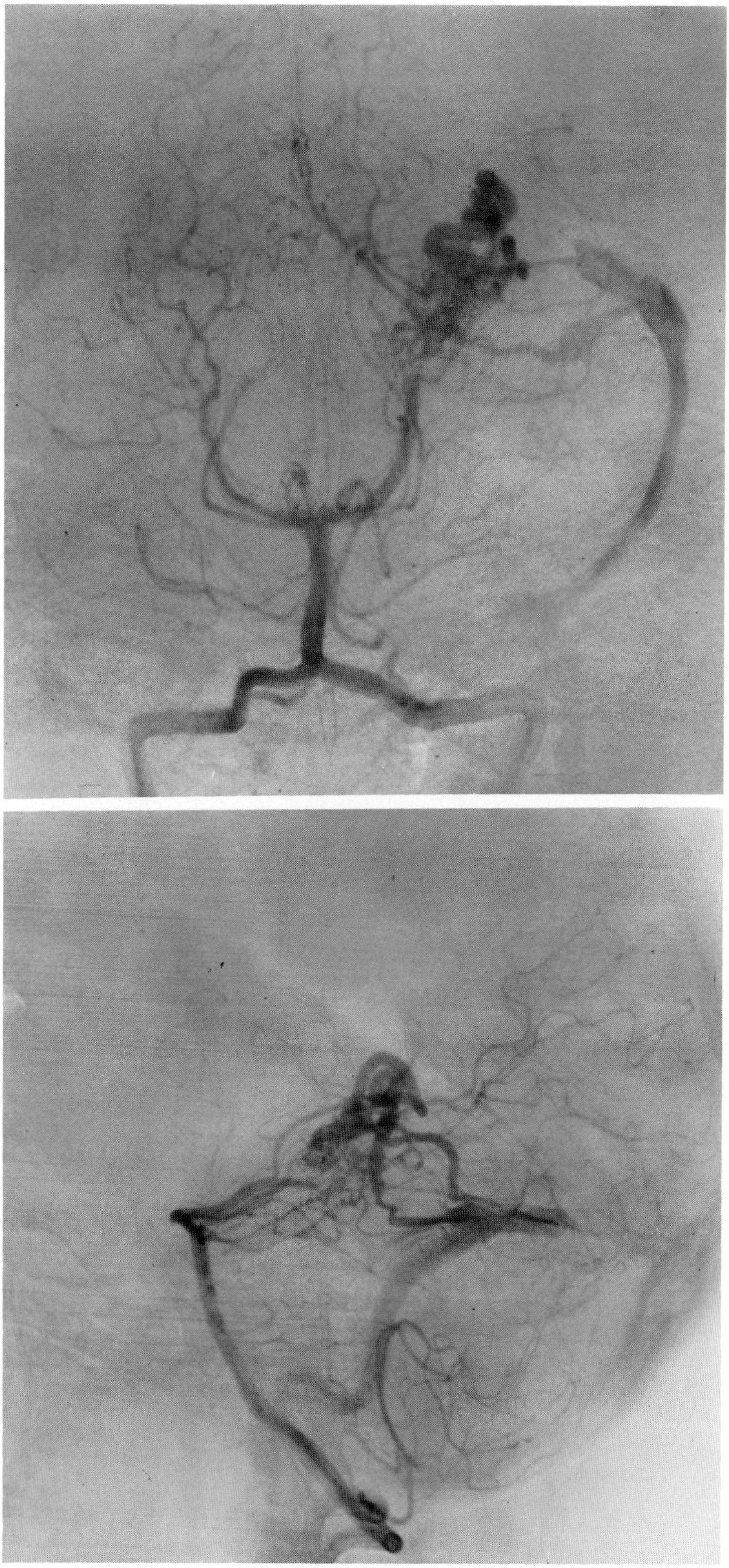

A

C

Fig. 6.21. Vertebral angiography. **A**. Frontal and **C**, lateral views of AVM in wing of ambient cistern behind pulvinar thalami draining to transverse sinus; 9 months after treatment, no filling of malformation is seen; **B** and **D**, narrowing of posterior cerebral artery within the target area.

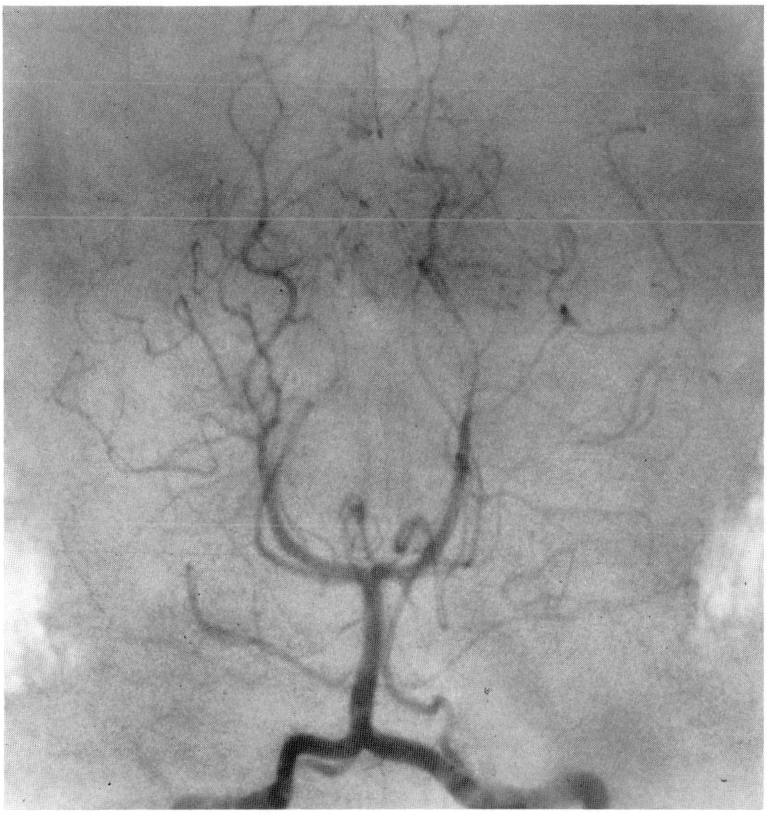

B

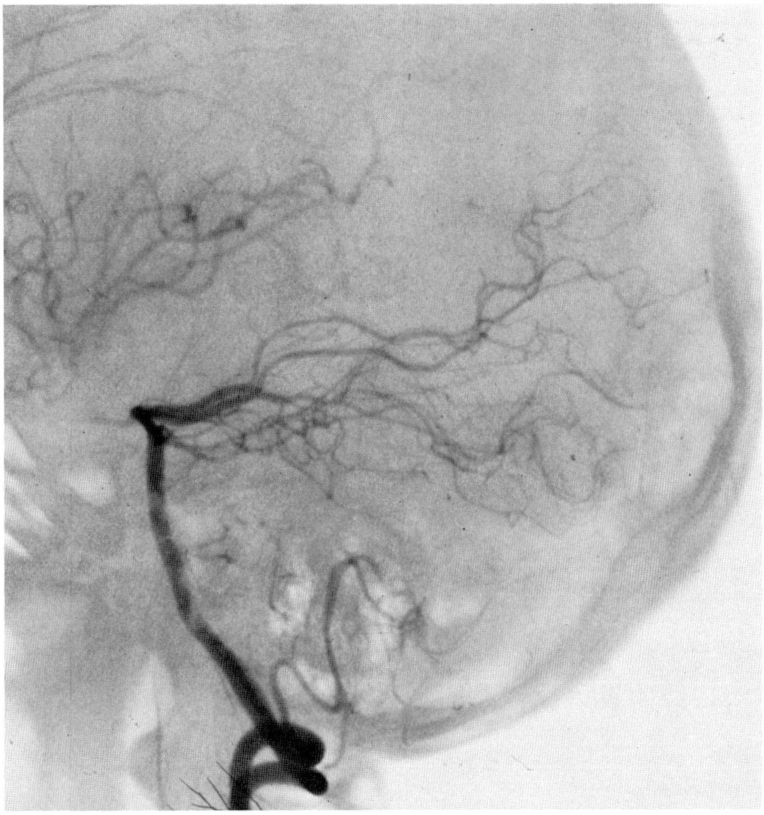

D

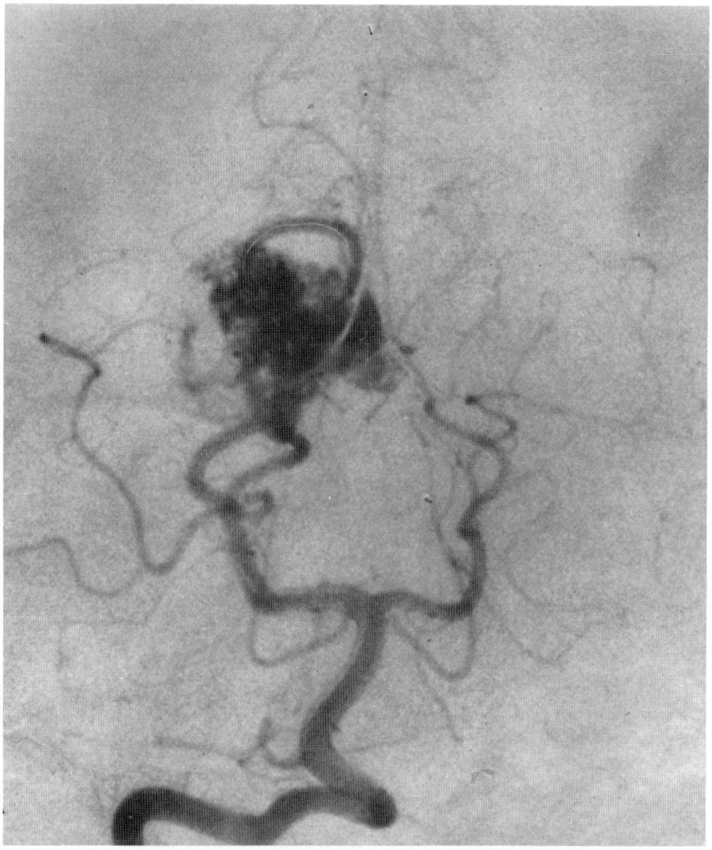

A

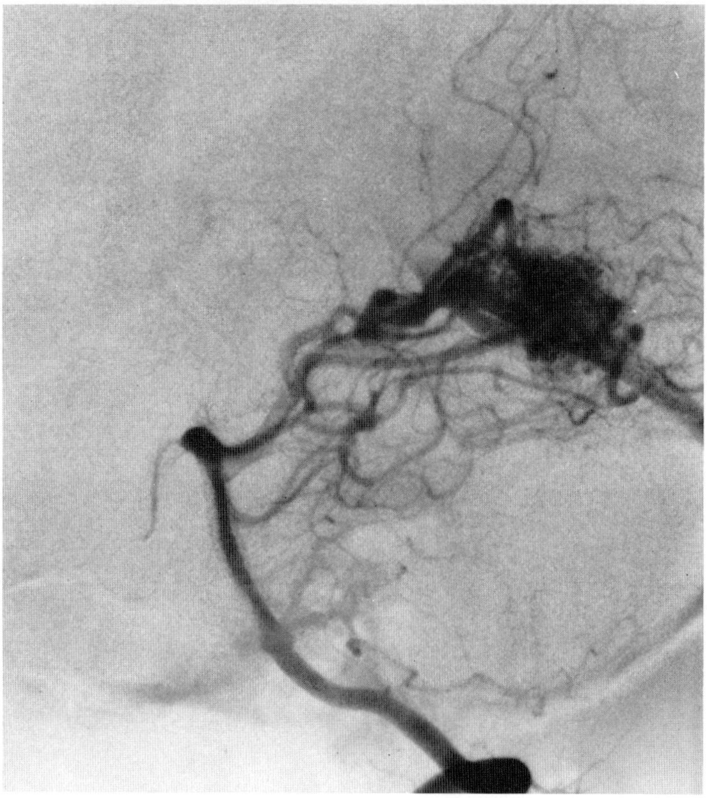

C

Fig. 6.22. Vertebral angiography. **A.** Frontal and **C,** lateral views of AVM adjacent to falx cerebri and tentorium, close to notch. Malformation is fed by branches from posterior cerebral artery and is drained by great vein of Galen to straight sinus. **B** and **D**. One year after treatment, AVM is no longer filled.

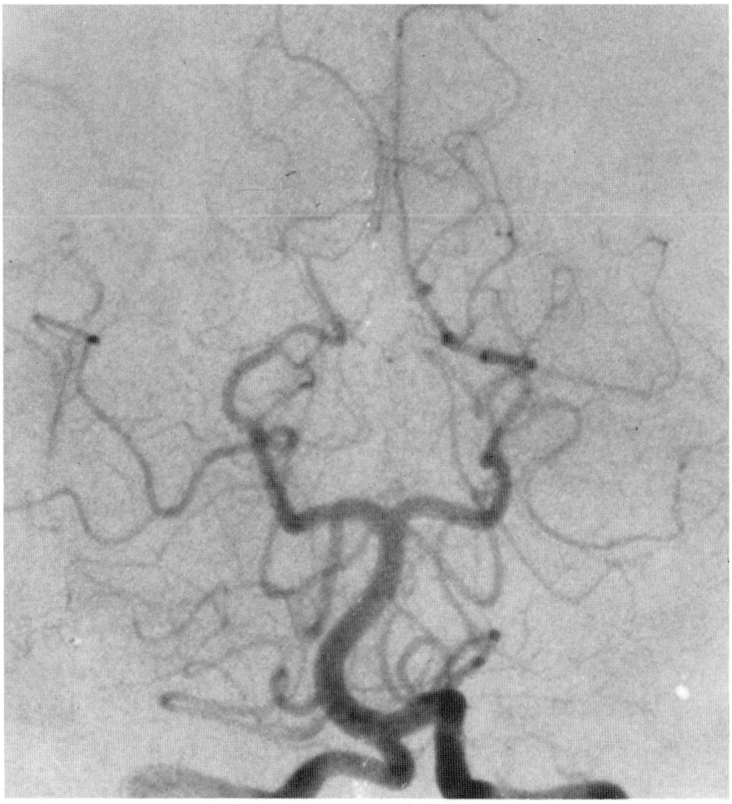

B

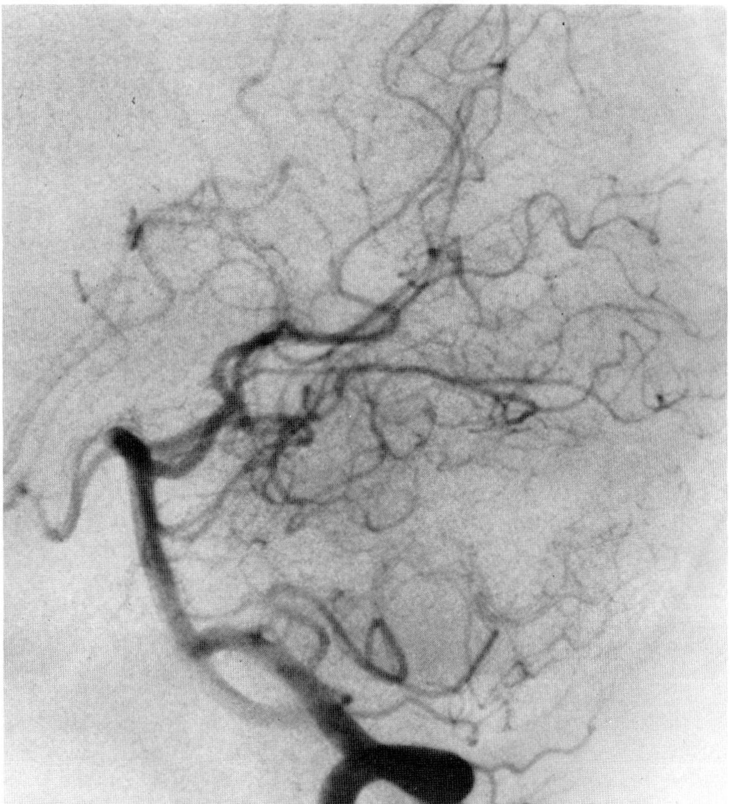

D

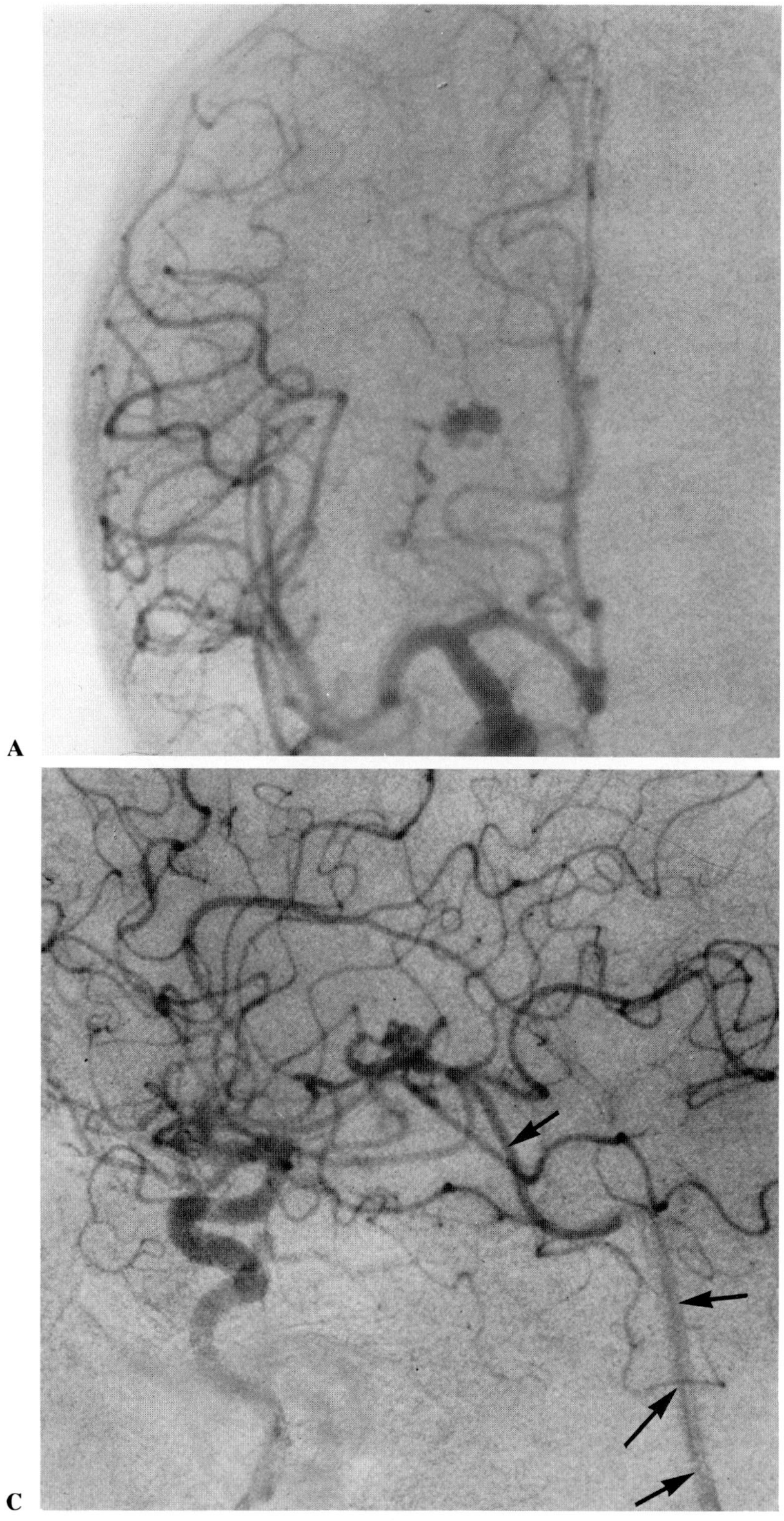

Fig. 6.23. Carotid angiography. A. Frontal and C, lateral view of an AVM adjacent to the ventricular system fed by thalamostriate branches and obliterated after radiosurgical treatment. Postoperative angiography shows disappearance of the AVM on B, frontal and D, lateral projections.

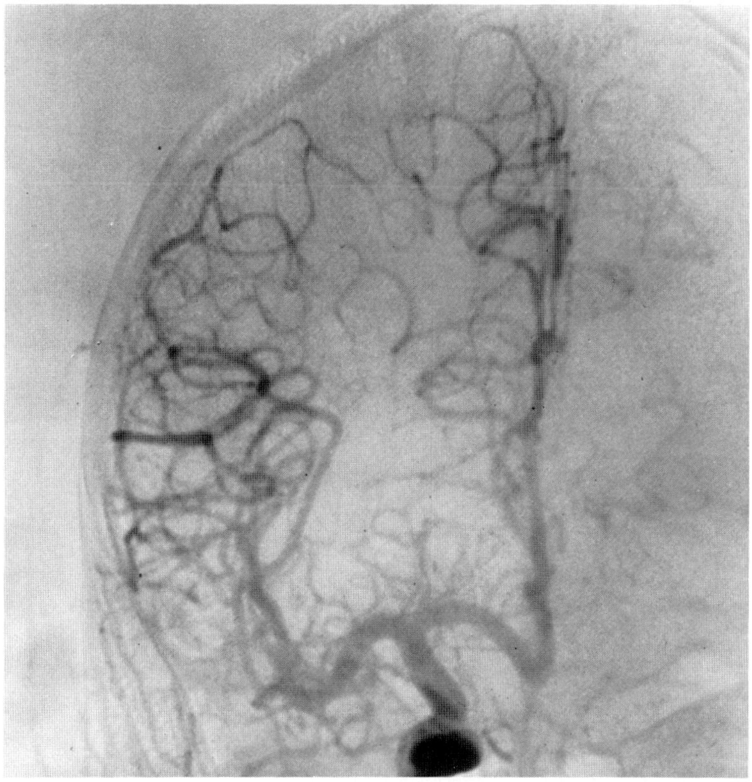

B

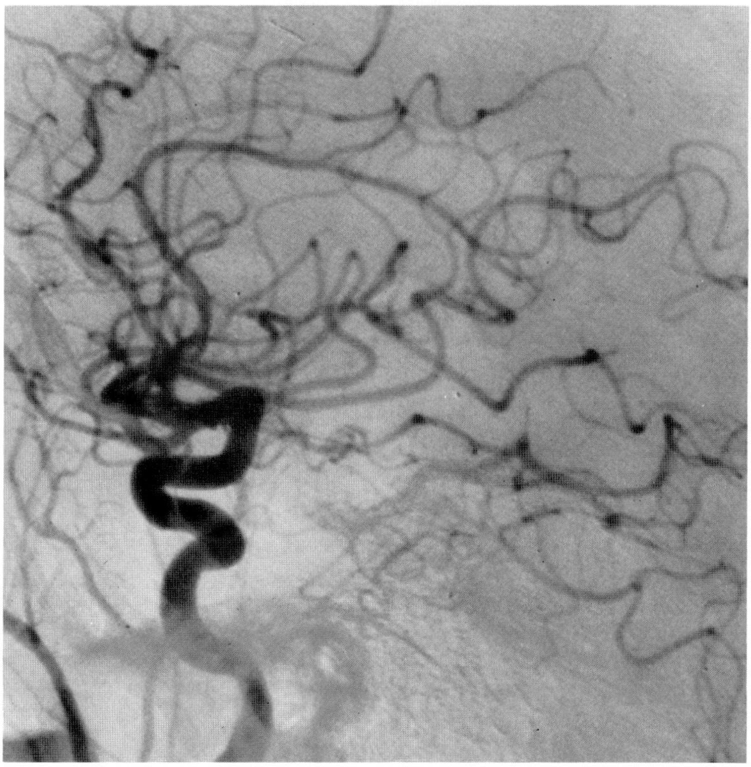

D

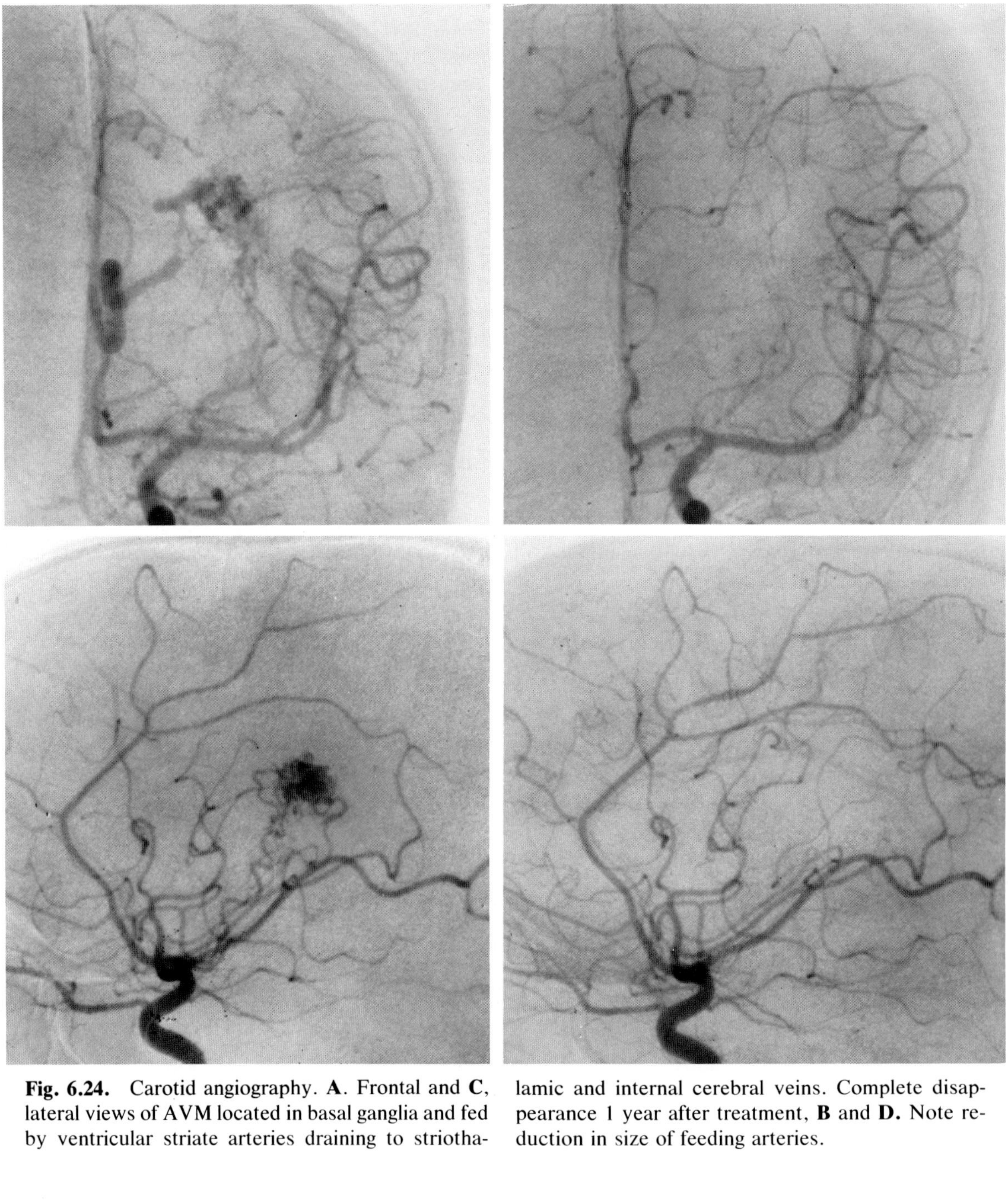

Fig. 6.24. Carotid angiography. **A**. Frontal and **C**, lateral views of AVM located in basal ganglia and fed by ventricular striate arteries draining to striothalamic and internal cerebral veins. Complete disappearance 1 year after treatment, **B** and **D.** Note reduction in size of feeding arteries.

Case 8, J.H. A 14-year-old boy was admitted to the referring hospital after a subarachnoid bleed. He was drowsy and had a left-sided hemiparesis. Angiography revealed a small AVM in the right basal ganglia fed by a hypertrophied lenticulostriate artery and draining directly into the vena cerebri interna (Fig. 6.23). At the time of the admission to our department, the left hemiparesis had disappeared. A single dose of 5 krad was delivered, the radiation field covering the entire malformation, and it did not fill on an angiogram 1 year after treatment (Fig. 6.23).

Case 9, E.J. A 16-year-old girl was admitted to our department with aphasia and right hemiparesis following a subarachnoid and intracerebral hemorrhage from an AVM in the midthalamic region adjacent to the lateral ventricle, fed by dilated ventricular striate arteries and drained into the striothalamic and internal cerebral veins (Fig. 6.24). Only a slight decrease in the size of the malformation occurred 2 years after the feeding arteries had been irradiated with a single dose of 5 krad. The treatment was repeated, and a single dose of 10 krad was given so that the cluster of pathologic vessels was completely covered by the radiation field. The malformation progressively decreased in size and became obliterated 1 year later (Fig. 6.24). Her aphasia and hemiparesis disappeared almost completely.

Table 6.2 summarizes the results of the angiographic follow-up. In group A (248 patients) in 166 cases a one year and in 104 cases a two years follow-up is available. Within 1 year partial obliteration was seen in 96 cases (57.9%) total obliteration in 56 cases (33.7%) and no changes in 14 cases (8.4%). Within 2 years partial obliteration occurred in 12 cases (11.4%), total obliteration in 90 cases (86.5%) and no change in 2 cases (1.9%). It may be assumed that subsequent follow-up will reveal further cases of total obliteration. To date no definite pattern concerning the duration of the latency from the time of the treatment to the time of occlusion of the malformation or concerning the optimal dose required for total obliteration could be established.

In group B (32 patients) follow-up angiographies (1–5 years) in 19 patients were carried out. Hemodynamic changes occurred in two and reduction in the size of the malformation occurred in seven cases.

In group C (16 patients) with follow-up in three cases the obliteration was total in one case (Fig. 6.3), partial in another, and no reduction was observed in a third case.

In group D (4 patients) marked decrease in the size of the malformation could be observed

Table 6.2. Angiographic follow-up in 192 of 300 irradiated cerebral AVMs.

Group A,	Follow-up	1year (166 cases)	Follow-up	2 years (104 cases)
(248 treated cases)	No	%	No	%
Hemodynamic changes	0	0	0	0
Partial obliteration	96	57.9	12	11.4
Total obliteration	56	33.7	90	86.5
No result so far	14	8.4	2	1.9
Group B,	Follow up	(19 cases)	Follow-up	(19 cases)
(32 treated cases)				
Hemodynamic changes	2		2	
Partial obliteration	7		7	
Total obliteration	0		0	
No result	10		10	
Group C,	Follow-up	(3 cases)	Follow-up	(3 cases)
(16 treated cases)				
Hemodynamic changes	0		0	
Partial obliteration	1		1	
Total obliteration	0		1	
No result	2		1	
Group D,	Follow-up	(4 cases)	Follow-up	(4 cases)
(4 treated cases)				
Partial obliteration	0		1[×]	
No result	4		3	

[×] Five years following radiosurgical treatment.

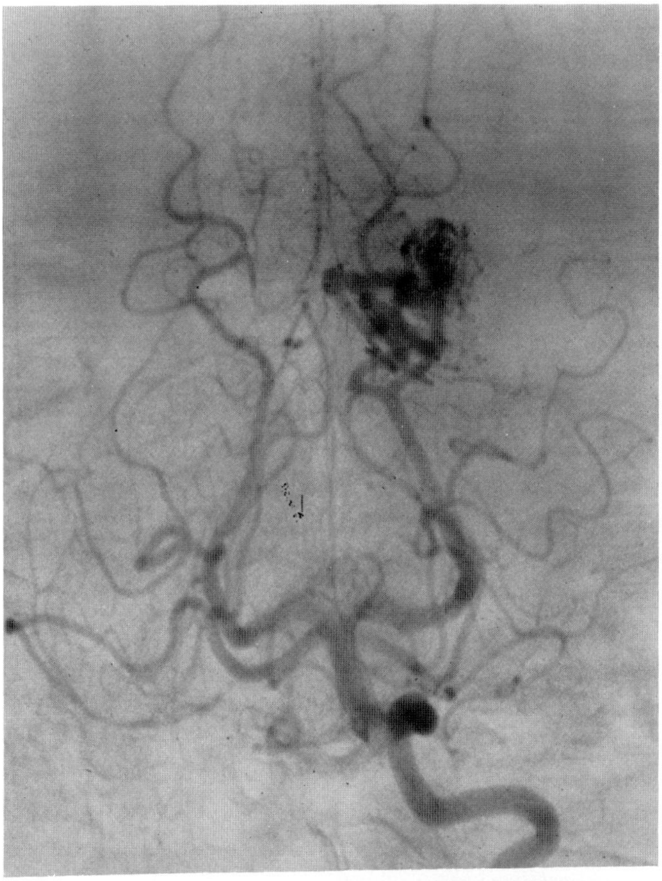

A

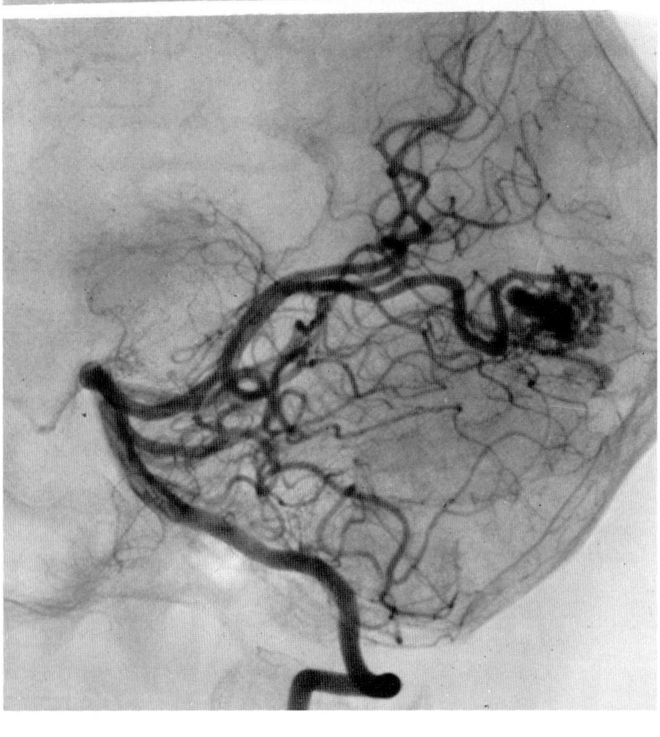

C

Fig. 6.25. Vertebral angiography. **A.** Frontal and **C** lateral views of AVM on medial aspect of occipital lobe, fed by branch from dilated calcarine artery draining to transverse sinus close to torcular herophili. Seven months after treatment, AVM has disappeared and size of feeding artery is decreased considerably. **B** and **D**. Delayed and incomplete filling of peripheral branches supplying medial portion of occipital lobe.

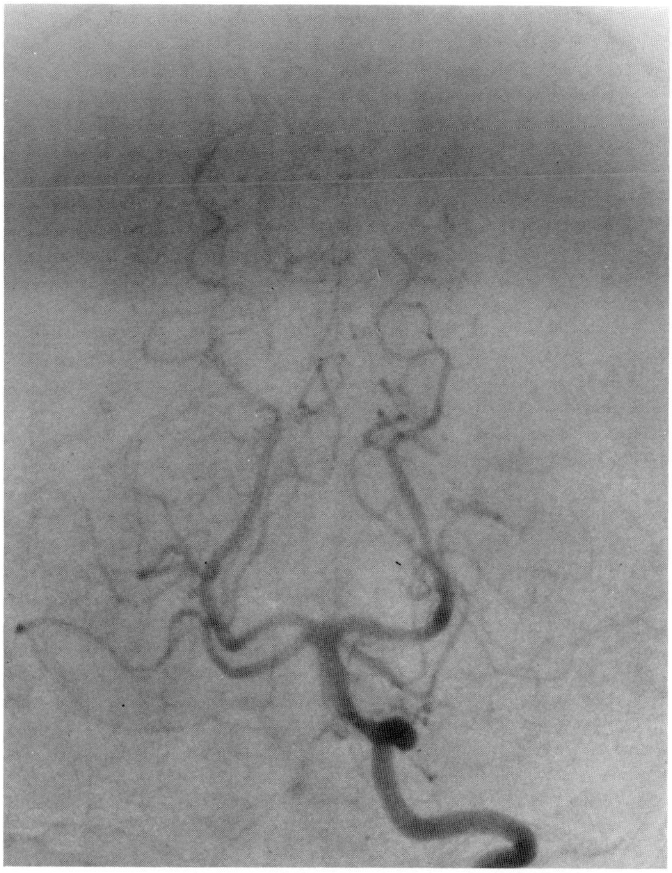

B

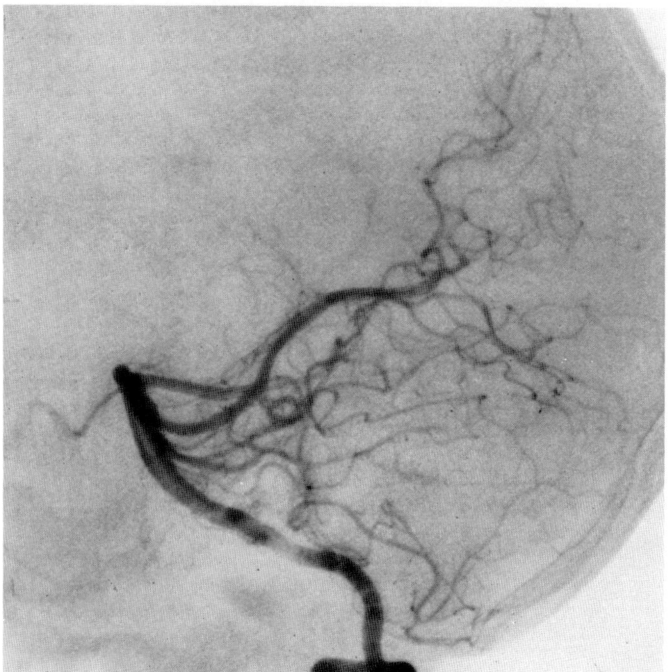

D

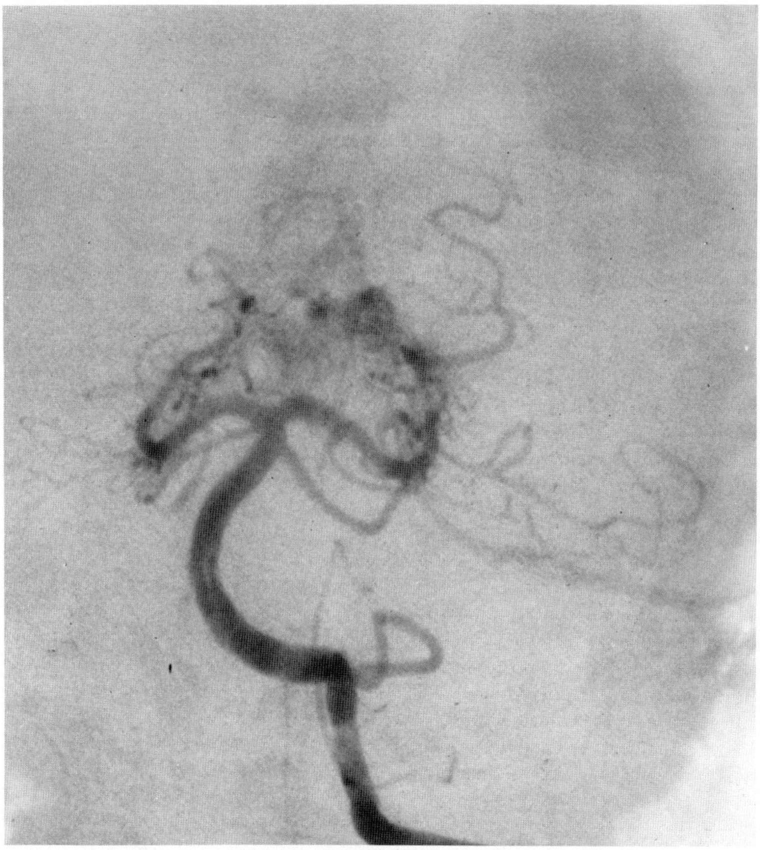

A

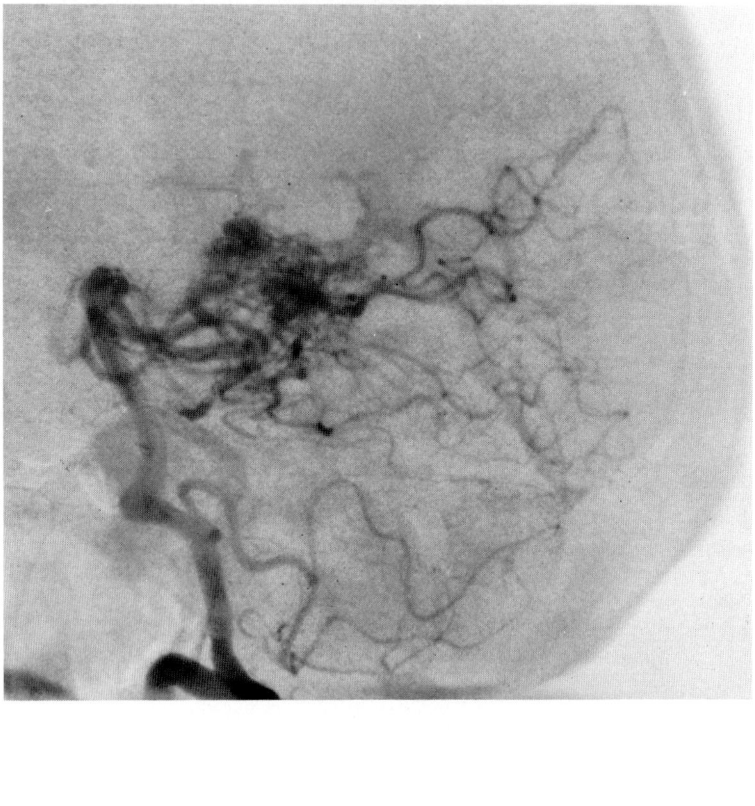

C

Fig. 6.26. Vertebral angiography of AVM located in posterior part of left thalamus. **A** and **C**. Before and **B** and **D**, after irradiation. Marked decrease in the size of malformations seen (examination carried out in the Department of Neuroradiology, Umeå).

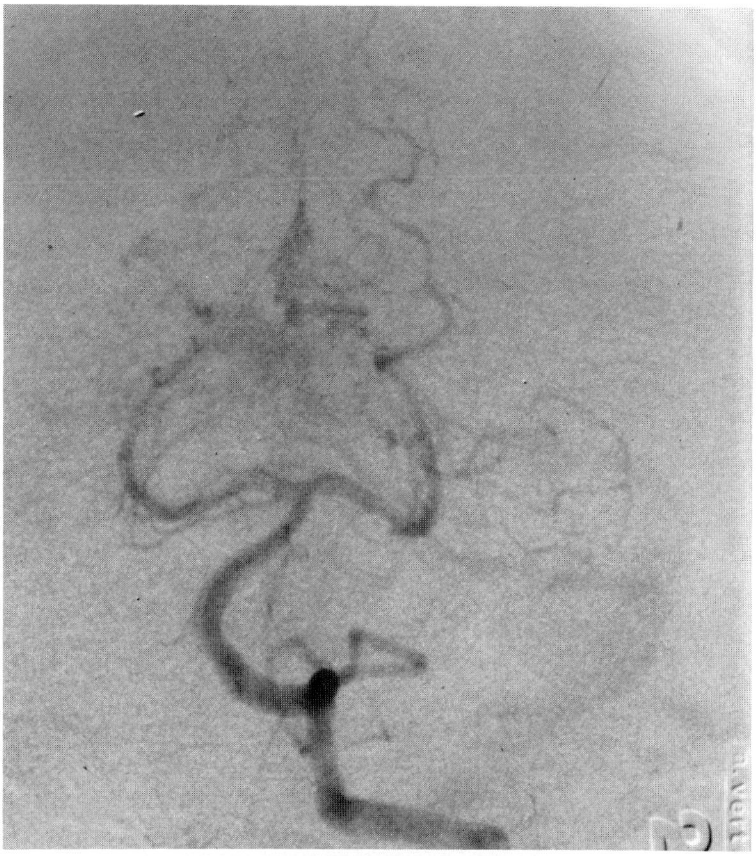

B

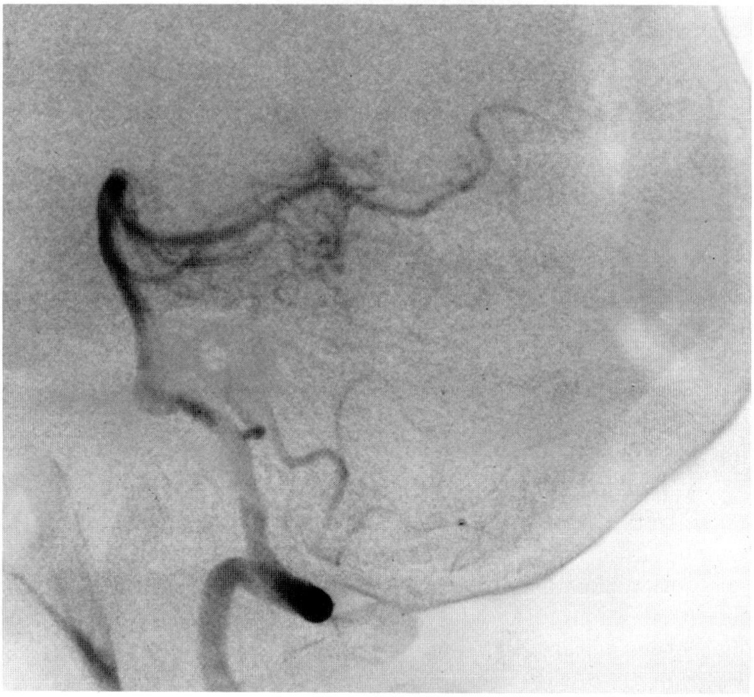

D

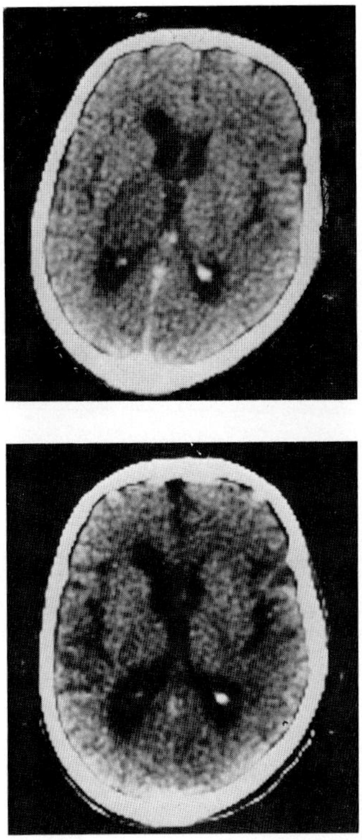

A

B

Fig. 6.27. CT scan of patient whose AVM is shown in Fig. 6.26 revealed a lesion of low attenuation corresponding to **A**, irradiated area; **B**, this area of radionecrosis was smaller on CT scan carried out two years later (examination carried out in Department of Neuroradiology, Umeå).

5 years after the radiation in one case. Whether this change was caused by the treatment or was spontaneous is impossible to determine.

In group D selective radiation of one or more but not all of multiple feeders resulted in therapeutic failure, as anticipated. In group B despite the fact that hemodynamic changes and reduction in the size of the malformation could be seen in those cases in which only part of the cluster of pathologic vessels could be covered by the irradiation field, the results have to be considered unsatisfactory. It remains to be determined whether the treatment made some of the inoperable lesions in this group surgically accessible. In group C, cases where all the feeding arteries were included in the radiation field, there are too few patients to allow valid conclusions to be drawn. Nevertheless, this group does stimulate an old discussion concerning the therapeutic value of the ligation of the feeding vessels.

Radiation of the Tangle of Pathologic Vessels vs Radiation of the Feeding Arteries

In AVM the logical target of surgery—conventional or radiosurgery—is the site of the pathologic shunt. The rationale for that is the peculiar flow pattern in the malformation as determined by the multiform character of its blood supply. The malformation is built up of a number of vascular units or "vascular modules," each unit consisting of a cluster of pathologic arteriovenous shunts and their feeders. Total resection or obliteration of the system of abnormal arteriovenous shunts secures a permanent cure. Holman[31] and Potter[89] among others, discussed suggestively how the remaining shunting mechanism after ligation of the feeding arteries could invite arterial blood from somewhere else on the basis of flow toward "low resistance." Nevertheless, ligation of the main feeding arteries has been used with success by many investigators.[26,27,29,30,46,68,93] Many others occluded the afferent vessels by embolization,[5,65,67,98] by the catheter-balloon,[96] and by using cryotherapy.[112]

A 5-year follow-up study of one of the early cases in our series treated by irradiation of the feeding arteries (Fig. 6.3) indicates that total and presumably permanent angiographic disappearance of an AVM after radiation of all the feeding arteries is possible. The many failures observed after occlusion of afferent vessels by open surgery may be explained by the fact that the deep-seated feeders were left untouched. The narrow ionizing gamma beams can be directed on feeding vessels, independently of their location in the skull. In this way, if all feeding arteries are occluded, a permanent cure is possible. However, it may be difficult sometimes to identify the vessels and to include them in the isodose distribution on the lateral and anteroposterior films. A stereophotogrammetric evaluation of angiograms worked out by Ederyd and Östman[21] in the department of neuroradiology, Karolinska, may improve identification of vessels on the lateral and anteroposterior x-ray views and avoid errors that may account for some of the therapeutic failures after radiation aimed to occlude the feeding arteries.

Latency

The main drawback of radiosurgery in AVM is the long latent period before the effect can be assessed. Hemodynamic changes, if they occur, can be seen already three months after treatment. The latency between time of treatment and complete angiographic disappearance of the malformation varies from 6 to 22 months. The long latency corresponds presumably to the slow development of the reparative histologic changes in the wall of the irradiated vessels. They are scarce and spotty in the early postirradiation phase, the obliterative endothelial damage being a late event.

The present material is too small and the scatter of the parameters too great to allow relevant evaluation of possible factors influencing the length of the latency. The shortest latencies observed were 6 months after 7 krad, 7 months after 7.5 krad, and 8 months after 5 krad. But similar doses were related also to longer latencies. The large doses used in this series reflect an attempt at shortening the latency. But it is uncertain whether increased doses correlate with an earlier radiobiologic response. The mechanism of occlusion of small blood vessels by edema and later by the increase in the number of the endothelial cells may be inhibited when the dose rate and size exceed a critical level.[77,94] In theory, antifibrinolytic drugs given additionally or activation of the coagulation mechanism could promote thrombosis and shorten the latent period.

Two pilot studies using ε-aminocaproic acid or fresh plasma after the radiation are concluded. Since the follow up is still in progress no definite results are yet available. Further experimental studies may show whether the latency and final extent of the obliterative process can be controlled by other pharmacologic or physical adjuvants. Animal studies in progress aim to enhance the radiation effect by additionally inducing hyperpyrexia[106] or deep hypotension,[105] the adversive effect on radiation being counteracted by increasing the O_2 saturation in the blood of the animal.

Neurologic Condition

The patients in this series were admitted with one or more of the following clinical conditions: subarachnoid and/or intracerebral hemorrhage in 240 cases, neurologic deficits in 60 cases, headache in 93 cases, and epilepsy in 18 cases. Changes in the intracerebral hemodynamic state following treatment of the AVM may theoretically result in a decrease of neurologic deficits, subjective complaints, or in the frequency of seizures. Nevertheless, the natural course of the disease or the placebo effect may also account for improvements. Changes in the anticonvulsant medication may furthermore be responsible for changes in seizure frequency. Therefore we have not drawn any conclusions from any single observation where improvement of neurologic signs or in the frequency of seizures occurred. New neurologic deficits occurred in six cases.

Case 10, T.S. A 52-year-old woman with a history of epileptic seizures had no neurologic signs on admission. Angiography visualized small AVM on the medial aspect of the occipital lobe, fed by a branch of the dilated calcarine artery and drained into the transverse sinus close to the torcular herophili (Fig. 6.25). Radiosurgery was performed with a single dose of 7.5 krad. Seven months after treatment the malformation had disappeared, and the feeding artery had decreased considerably in size. There was a delayed and incomplete filling of the peripheral branches supplying the medial portion of the occipital lobe. Eight months after treatment the patient observed a right homonymous hemianopsia, which presumably may be explained by the vascular changes seen on the angiogram.

The neurologic deficits in the five remaining cases were due to delayed radiation necrosis.

Delayed Radiation Necrosis

Case 11, R.E. A 61-year-old patient in group B had an AVM located in the posterior part of the left thalamus (Fig. 6.26). It was partially obliterated after radiation with a single dose of 7.5 krad using the widest collimator. A right-sided hemianaesthesia appeared 11 months after treatment. A CT scan at the time of the neurologic deterioration revealed a lesion of low attenuation corresponding to the irradiated area (Fig. 6.27). The hemianaesthesia slowly improved, but the regress of the symptoms was incomplete. Marked decrease of the low attenuation area could be seen on a CT scan repeated 20 months after treatment (Fig. 6.27).

Case 12, E.G. This patient was a 25-year-old female with Addison's disease who had had two subarachnoid hemorrhages in the past 10 years.

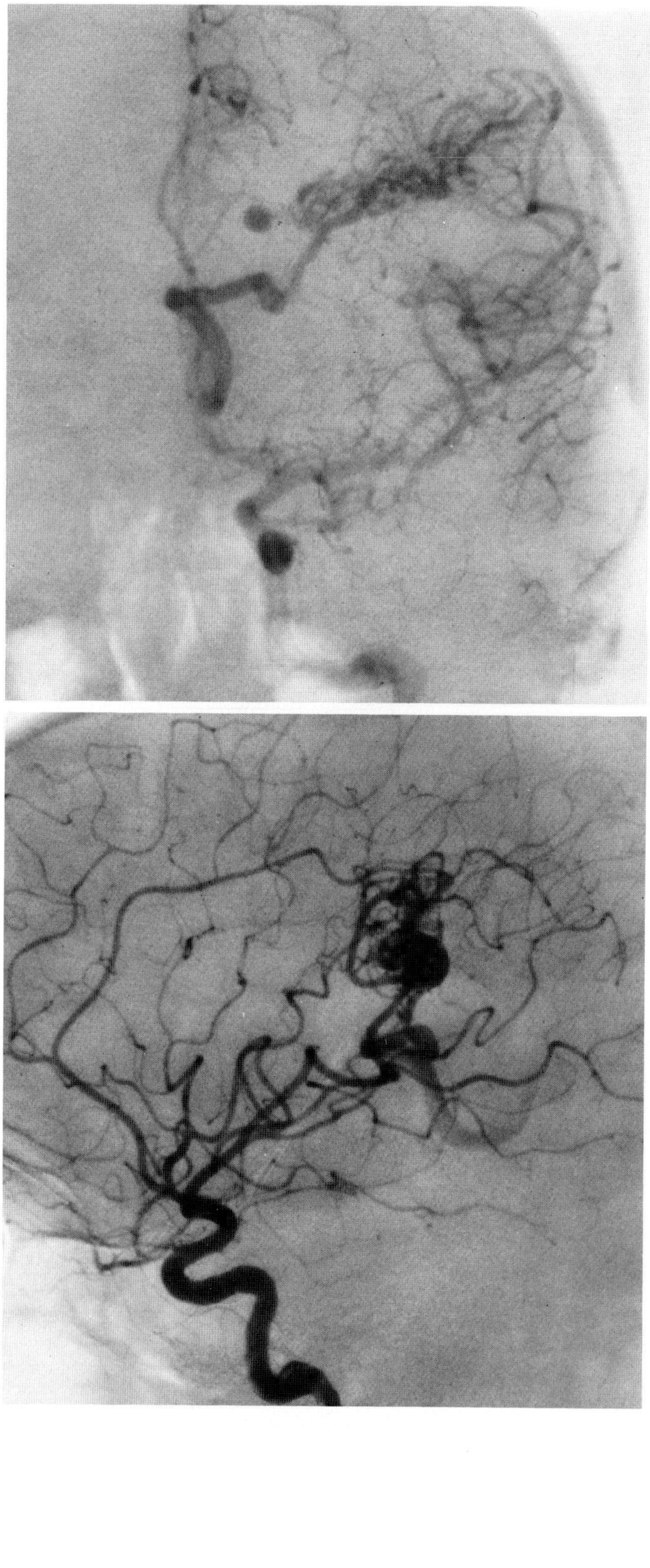

A

C

Fig. 6.28. Carotid angiography. A. Frontal and C lateral views of AVM fed by hypertrophied left posterior parietal artery draining to internal cerebral vein. B and D, eleven months after treatment, AVM did not fill.

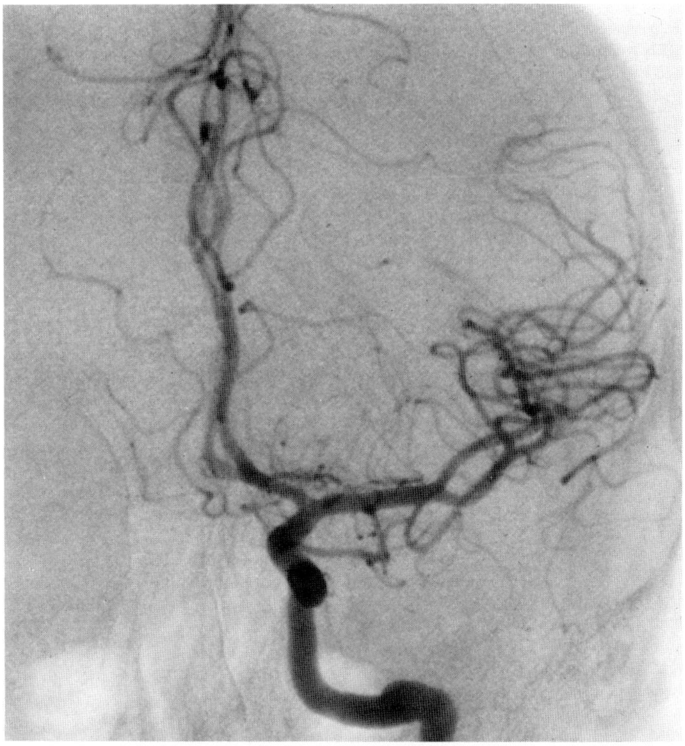

B

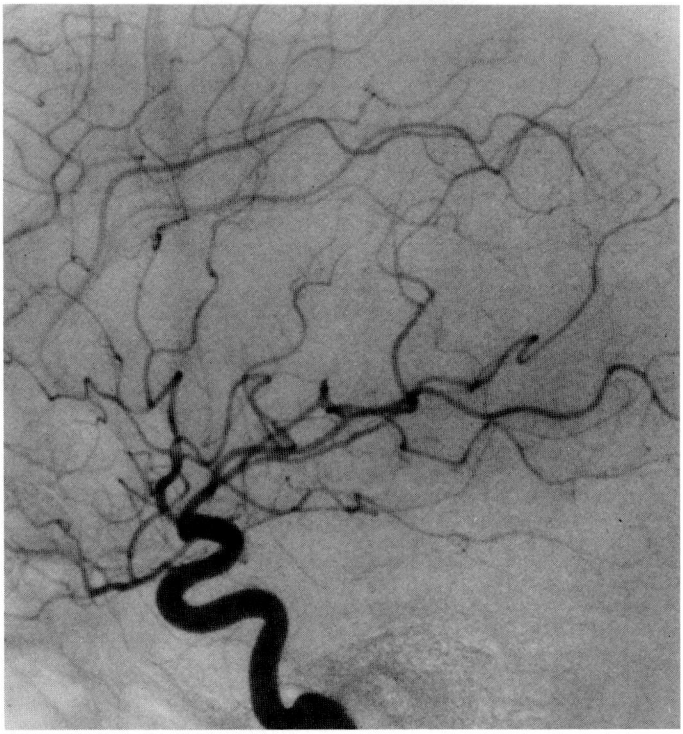

D

An AVM fed by a hypertrophied left posterior parietal artery and drained through a parietal and ventricular vein to the internal cerebral vein was revealed by angiography (Fig. 6.28). Two targets within the malformation separated by 17 mm were crossfired with 5 krad × 2 using the widest collimator of gamma unit II to obtain the maximum radiation field. Three months after treatment, the patient complained of headaches and vomiting, slight dysarthria, and right hemianaesthesia. There were only hemodynamic changes to be seen on the angiogram. The unilateral symptoms successively increased, and 6 months after irradiation the patient had a slight aphasia, moderate right-sided hemianaesthesia, and a spastic hemiparesis. Angiography revealed partial decrease in the size of the malformation and a CT scan showed the presence of a slightly expansive lesion of low attenuation (Fig. 6.29). Angiography performed 11 months after treatment showed complete obliteration of the AVM (Fig. 6.28). The patient was treated with large doses of dexamethasone. Repeated CT scans showed progressive decrease of the lesion of low attenuation, and 22 months after irradiation the CT scan was completely normal (Fig. 6-29). The neurologic deficiencies improved progressively but the hemiparesis is still present. Nevertheless, she fulfills her duties well as a secretary in a research institute.

Case 13, B.A. A 20-year-old female suffered a right-sided hemiparesis 6 months after radiosurgery for an AVM in the region of the left trigonum. One field of radiation (collimator 8 of the gamma unit II) was used and 10 krad given. A CT scan at the time of the occurrence of the neurologic deterioration revealed an expansive lesion with low and high attenuation areas in the

A B C D

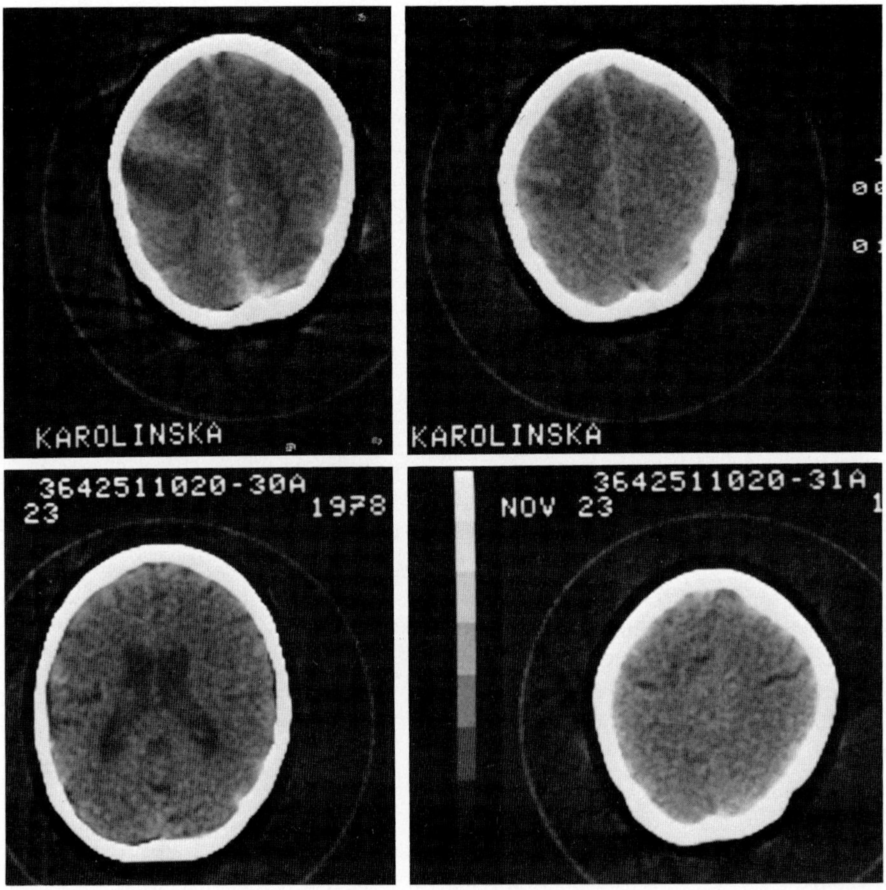

Fig. 6.29. CT scan of patient whose AVM is shown in Fig. 6.28, **A–B,** expansive lesion of low attenuation 6 months after irradiation; **C–D,** 22 months after irradiation, CT scan tomography became normal.

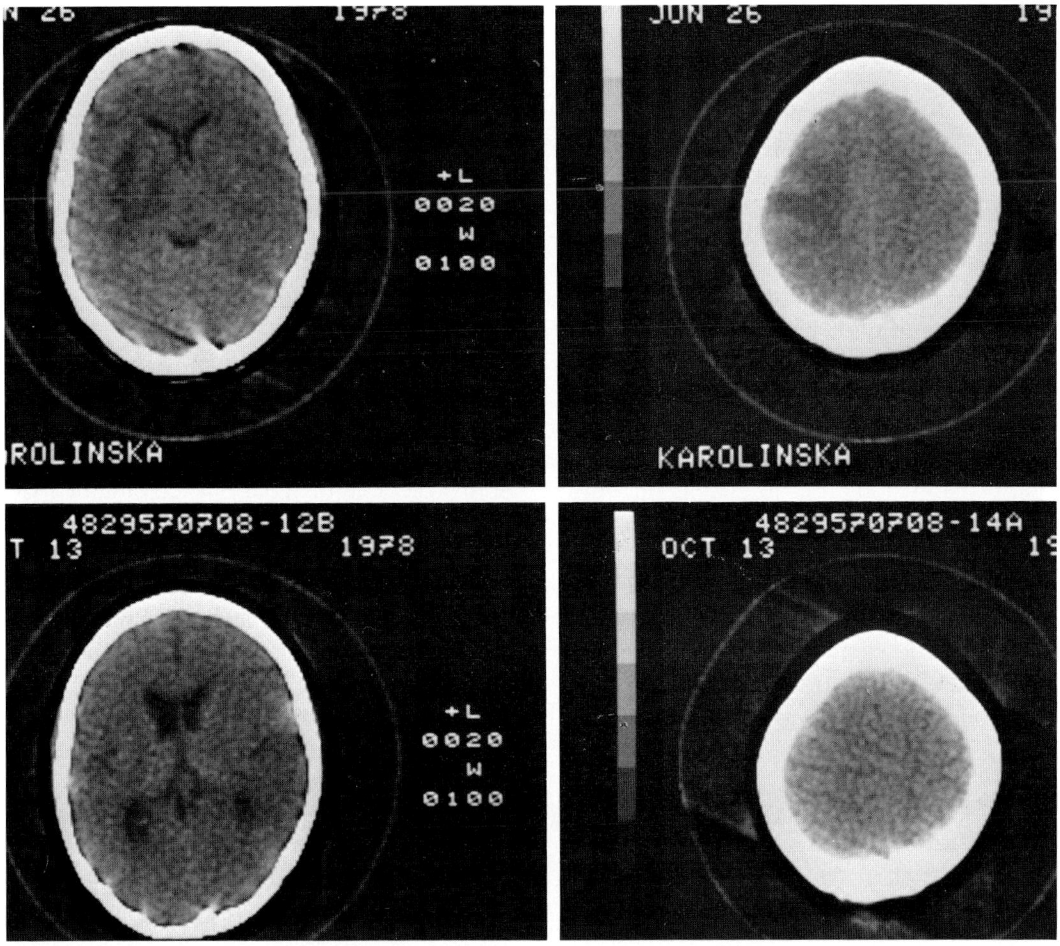

A B C D

Fig. 6.30. CT scan showing **A–B,** radionecrosis 6 months after irradiation; **C–D,** decrease of expansive low-attenuation area 11 months after treatment.

left thalamic region, extending into the parietal lobe (Fig. 6-30). The patient was given dexamethasone, starting with doses of 16 mg daily and rapidly tailing off to 1 mg/day. Six months after the occurrence of the neurologic picture, there has been a progressive improvement of the hemiparesis, and the patient continues her previous work as a secretary. The AVM no longer filled on the follow-up angiogram 2 years after treatment. Repeated CT studies showed a successive decrease of the postradiation lesion (Fig. 6-30). There were two additional cases of radionecrosis in non eloquent brain revealed by the routine follow-up CT scan.

In summary, 7 of 300 patients who underwent radiosurgery for AVM had delayed radionecrosis of brain parenchyma. The doses inducing the necrosis ranged from 5 krad, given in 2 fields to 7.5 or 10 krad given in 1 field or radiation. Clinical signs and symptoms were first observed 3 to 11 months after treatment.

Since there is a certain volume of brain parenchyma within the tangle of pathologic vessels covered by the radiation field, the steep radiation field gradient and the accurate localization of the radiosurgery are only of limited value. Brain tissue included in the radiation field will absorb the dose directed on the target, and the degree of histopathologic damage will depend on the dose size and rate, volume of tissue involved, and time factor. Actually, it is easier to understand the occurrence of radionecrosis in the 7 cases than the absence of lesions consistent with radionecrosis in the remaining cases, despite the high doses used and the extreme temporal concentration of radiation exposure.

Since Fisher and Halfelder described for the

first time radiation necrosis of brain,[22] a wealth of controversial clinical and experimental data has been accumulated. Diengdoh and Booth[19] described these changes after fast neutron therapy with doses of 7 krads; Martins et al,[72] and Michael[73] after doses of 6 to 7 krad in fractions of about 200 rads/day. Nakagaki et al[76] demonstrated that the critical dose of radiation for monkeys ranges between 5 and 6 krads, fractionated at 200 rads/day. However, Brownson et al[12] reported brain damage induced by low dosage x-irradiation, and Foltz et al[23] reported late morphologic changes at doses of 1.3 to 3.5 krads—much lower than those thought to be tolerated by the central nervous system. On the other hand, radiation in excess of 6 krads used in craniopharyngiomas seldom gave undue effects.[41,42] No definite conclusion concerning the role of dose or the size of the radiation field can be drawn in our material. Although radionecrosis occurred in a number of cases where single doses ranging from 7.5-10 krads were given using a collimator of 14 mm diameter there were more cases treated in the same way and within subsequent radionecrosis. Radionecrosis occurred in one case with 50 krad only and using small collimator.

The basic mechanism in the pathogenesis of delayed radiation necrosis of the brain may be a direct effect of radiation on the parenchyma,[18] or of vascular changes, e.g., obliteration of small vessels with consequent necrosis of dependent tissue[72,94] or an alteration in the antigenic structure of the brain, leading to an autoimmune vasculitis.[14] It seems pertinent to assume that individual parameters could play also some role.

Rebleed

In 300 irradiated AVMs rebleed occurred in 11 cases.

In Group A with 248 cases there were 6 rebleeds. One patient bled 6 months after irradiation of the AVM with 12 krads. An angiography prior to the hemorrhage had shown partial obliteration of the AVM localized in the region of the right motor cortex. The patient was operated on in his home country, an intracerebral hematoma was evacuated, and the malformation extirpated. In the operative specimen, vessels with organized or fresh thrombi were seen together with patent vessels. One other patient rebled 3 weeks after the treatment. Six months later the AVM no longer filled on the follow-up angiogram

In Group C with 16 cases no rebleed occurred.

In Group B with 32 cases and Group D with 4 cases there were 5 rebleeds.

One patient in this group had a rebleed 22 months after treatment. In this case only part of several feeding arteries were radiated, and they received 10 krads. A second patient had additionally to the AVM 2 arterial aneurysms on the left pericallosal artery and an AVM occipitally on the left side, fed by four arteries from the left pericallosal and posterior cerebral arteries. Only part of the tangle of pathologic vessels could be included in the radiation field and 5 krads were given. Subsequent follow-up showed only a slight decrease in the size of malformation, and a fatal rebleed occurred 33 months following treatment. The histologic study of the postmortem specimen showed completely obliterated small vessels along with patent arteries. Another AVM that rebled was more than 4 cm × 3 cm × 4 cm large and was located in the left thalamus. The patient died following the hemorrhage 40 months after the AVM was radiated with a single dose of 10 krads, only part of the malformation being covered by the radiation field. The vessels of the AVM seemed patent at macroscopic examination. The histologic study is not available.

Little information is currently available about the potential risk of vascular rupture after large single-dose irradiation. Berdjis[9] states with some reservations that the large- and medium-sized arteries can tolerate radiation doses of 5 to 6 krads when given over 5 to 6 weeks. Eleven cases of ruptured large elastic arteries (aorta and carotid) after irradiation for neoplastic disease (dose, 5 krads over 41–47 days) were reported by Marcial-Rojas and Castro.[71] However, all their cases were complicated by infection and salivary fistulas. Spontaneous ruptures of the carotid artery and aorta have been reported in surgically treated patients with salivary fistula or infection even without radiotherapy.[94] Rojas has also seen a large group of patients treated with similar doses without any complications. No rupture has occurred in cats receiving single doses from 5 to 20 krads to the carotid artery[105] or the basilar artery,[77] nor in rats receiving 40 krads[105] to the aorta and inferior vena cava.

In this series of patients irradiated by single doses ranging from 3 to 12.5 krads, the rebleed rate of 6.7% does not exceed the rebleed in the natural history of the AVM given as 21.6% by Mingrino.[75] Nevertheless, the long latency between the radiation and the obliteration of the malformation with the risk of rebleed during this period remains the main drawback of radiosurgery in AVM and a serious argument against radiation of operable malformations.

The Mechanism of Obliteration of AVM Induced by Radiation

It is still too early to do more than speculate about the exact mechanism that leads to the occlusion of an irradiated AVM. Nevertheless, some facts support the assumption that proliferation of the endothelial lining, as well as thrombosis, is the main factor. The fact suggesting the role of endothelial proliferation in the obliteration of the AVM are as follows:

1. Extensive experimental and clinical evidence of progressive and proliferative changes in the vessel wall induced by ionizing radiation (see Radiobiology in this Chapter).
2. In our case 1, the two feeding arteries showed a local constriction corresponding to their course through the target area (Fig. 6.3).
3. Rather impressive changes were observed in an arterial aneurysm. In case 14, A.A., a 61-year-old woman was stuporous for several weeks from the ischemic effects of vasospasm following a subarachnoid hemorrhage. An arterial aneurysm on her left posterior communicating artery was irradiated in two overlapping fields with a single dose of 5 krads given in each field. The aneurysm progressively diminished in size and was completely obliterated after 11 months. The calibre of the posterior cerebral artery adjacent to the aneurysm had successively narrowed and was finally occluded (Fig. 6.31). It needs to be emphasized that radiosurgery is an inadequate treatment for aneurysms that have recently bled, and it remains to be determined whether it has any place in the treatment of aneurysms that have not bled.
4. In irradiated cases some of the feeding arteries occasionally underwent progressive narrowing until total occlusion occurred (Fig. 6.32).

It is possible that in addition to proliferation of the endothelial cells, thrombosis also has a role in the occlusion of the pathological vessels. Jörgensen,[36] in discussing thrombogenesis, reformulated Virchow's triad.[118] Factors promoting thrombosis are vascular injury; deviation of blood flow from a laminar pattern or flow at increased or reduced rates of shear; and increased platelet reactivity, increased activation of coagulation, or decreased fibrinolytic activity. At least two of the preceding set of factors, namely, an abnormal blood flow and endothelial damage, are present in irradiated vessels. Whether early radiation-induced changes in endothelial cells—including degeneration, swelling, and necrosis—increased platelet reactivity has still to be proved. Thrombus formation in irradiated vessels was observed in clinical cases as well as under experimental conditions. On the other hand, Nilsson et al[77] did not find vascular thrombosis in the irradiated basilar artery and surrounding small arteries in the cat. That there was a complete absence of platelet adhesions or aggregations leads to the assumption that the mechanisms for the initiation of this activity—e.g., liberation of adenosinediphosphate, formation of pro-collagen by endothelial cells, and electrical potentials of the endothelium—may have been seriously disturbed by too high doses of irradiation in these experiments.

Little is known about the role of age, repeated small hemorrhages, menses, previous use of oral contraceptive drugs, and the propensity of pathologic vessels for thrombosis in contributing to the occlusion of a malformation after radiation. The possibility of spontaneous thrombosis[13,32,81,85] must also be mentioned. However, in the present series the fact that the obstructed segments of the feeding arteries (Fig. 6.3) or the obliterated tangles of pathologic vessels coincided precisely with the preoperatively determined target area and that the

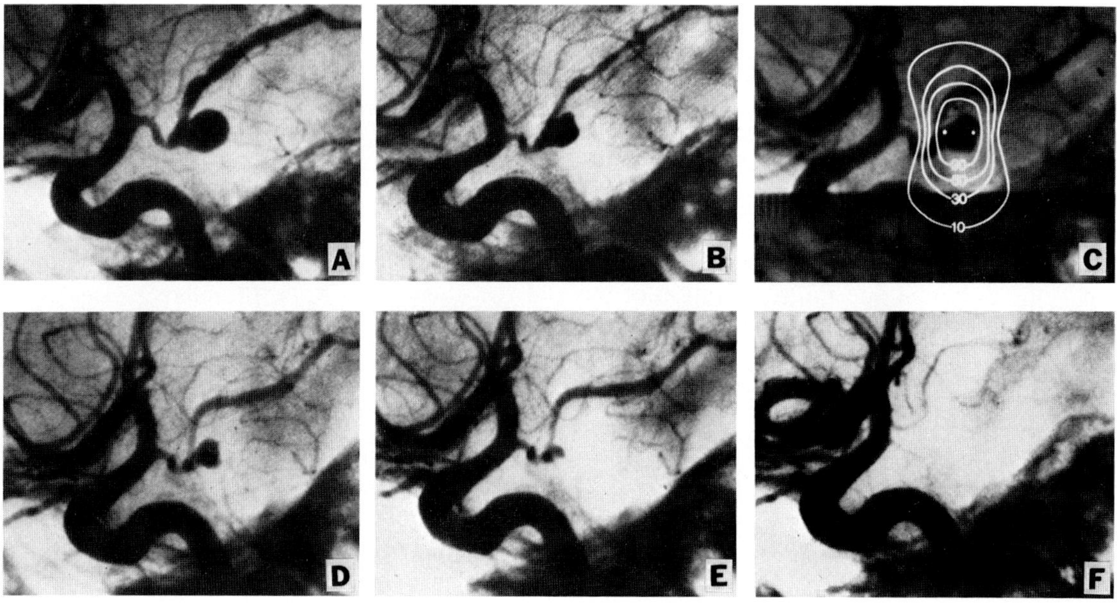

Fig. 6.31. Angiography. **A**. Lateral views two days after subarachnoid hemorrhage; **B**, one week later, showing spasm of posterior communicating and posterior cerebral arteries; **C**, at time of radiosurgery, showing that no spasm is present; **D**, 6 months later showing that aneurysm has become smaller; **E**, the caliber of segment of the posterior cerebral artery (→) adjacent to the aneurysm has diminished; **F**, further decrease in size of aneurysm and persistent narrowing of adjacent arteries.

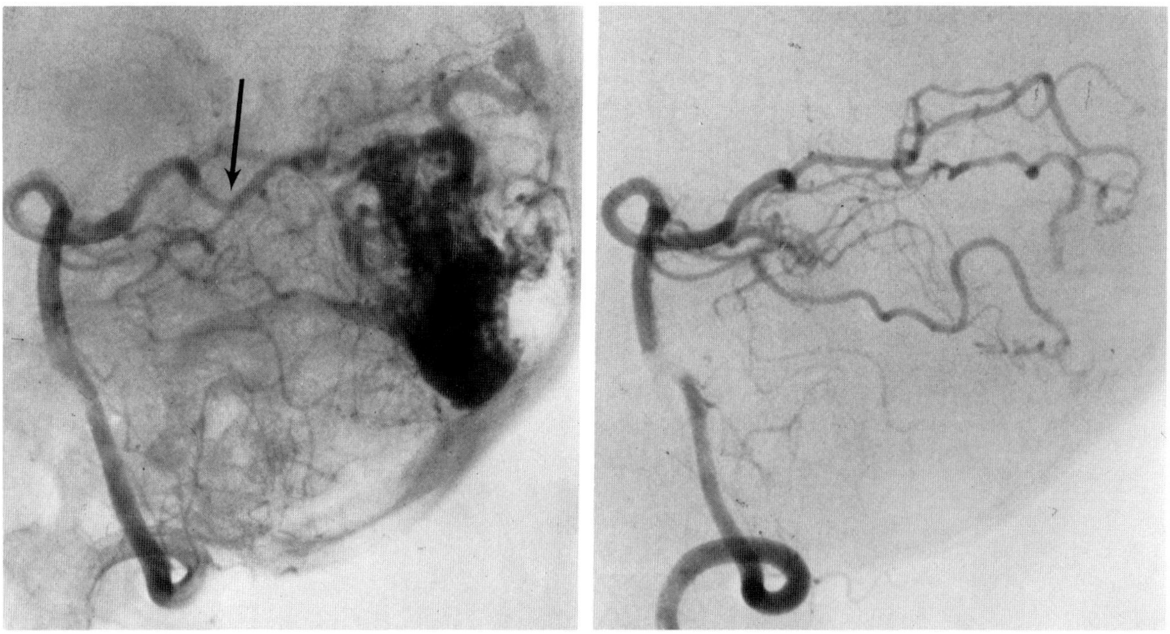

A

Fig. 6.32. Vertebral angiography, lateral views before and after radiosurgery. Arteriovenous malformation in the posterior part of the occipital lobe, close to the tentorium, fed from the a. calcarina, the occipital and temporal branches of the arteria cerebri posterior **(A)**. The patient had radiosurgery and fifteen months later there is a total obliteration of one of the large feeding arteries **(B)**.

results were reproducible make a spontaneous obliteration independent of the radiosurgical procedure extremely improbable.

Conclusion

For the purpose of occluding AVM the ^{60}Co unit in the Department of Neurosurgery at the Karolinska Hospital, Stockholm, proved to be an efficient tool. However, Kjellberg et al[40] also reported successes using proton beams. Although the method of stereotactically directing beams on the pathologic vessels as used in Stockholm and Boston have obvious advantages compared with nonstereotactical radiation, the results in the treatment of AVM with conventional radiotherapy without stereotactic localization obtained by Johnson[35] are noteworthy.

Technical development in the field of particle accelerators may result in equipment that will surpass the possibilities offered by those currently available and may prevail in the radiosurgery of the future. Larsson et al contends that the electron accelerator for super-voltage x-ray production would seem an attractive alternative, provided further improvement of the currently employed systems of acceleration and beam transport, as well as of the mechanical precision, are achieved. Larsson et al[51] also recommends ^{192}Iridium for further testing, "especially when higher neutron flux densities will be available." They contend that the disadvantageous short half-life may be compensated for by designing convenient source exchange. And, finally, they believe that ^{45}Scandium might also be a possible future alternative. It appears that obliteration of AVM by ionizing radiation is feasible. In correctly selected cases obliteration occurred in 86% within a period of 2 years. It may be assumed that further obliteration will be demonstrated with subsequent follow-up angiographies.

In addition to the permanent cure achieved by total obliteration of the malformation partial occlusion may prove to be useful in the management of some inoperable AVMs converting them into lesions accessible to open surgery.

The incidence of undue effects is low and there is no mortality. The rebleed rate during the long latency between the time of the treatment and the time when total obliteration of the AVM occur is not higher than that seen in the natural history of the disease.

References

1. Andersson B, Larsson B, Leksell L, Mair W, Rexed B, Sourander J, Wennerstrand J: Histopathology of late radiolesions in the goat brain. Acta Radiol 9:385–394, 1940
2. Arndt J, Backlund E-O, Larsson B, Leksell L, Norén G, Rosander K, Rähn T, Sarby B, Steiner L, Wennerstrand J: Stereotactic irradiation of intracranial structures: physical and biological considerations. INSERM Symposium No 12, Ed: Gabor Szikla, pp. 81–92, Elsevier/North-Holland Biomedical Press, 1979.
3. Arndt J, Backlund E-O, Dahlin H, Ekström P: A computer controlled dose planning system for irradiation of small volumes of the brain with a multicobalt unit. Proc 3rd Congr Soc Radiol Europ, Edinburg, 1975
4. Arnold A, Bailey P, Harvey RA: Intolerance of the primate brain stem and hypothalamus to conventional and high energy radiations. Neurology 4:575, 1954
5. Ausman JI, Gold LH, Tadavarthy SM, Amplatz K, Chou SN: Intraparenchymal embolization: a new technique for obliteration of an intramedullary arteriovenous malformation of the spinal cord. Neurochirurgie, 1977, in press
6. Backlund E-O, Johansson L, Sarby B: Studies on craniopharyngiomas. II: Treatment by stereotaxis and radiosurgery. Acta Chir Scand 138:749–759, 1972
7. Backlund E-O, Rähn T, Sarby B: Treatment of pinealomas by stereotaxic radiation surgery. Acta Radiol (Ther Phys Biol) 13:368–376, 1974
8. Backlund E-O, Arndt J, Dahlin H, Grietz T, Leksell L, Steiner L: Radiosurgery in intracranial arteriovenous malformations. International Congr Series No 433. Neurol Surg. Carrea R (ed.) Le Vay D (co-ed.). Excerpta Medica, Amsterdam-Oxford, 1977
9. Berdjis CC, et al: Cardiovascular system and radiation: —late effects of x-rays on the arteries of the adult. Strahlentherapie 112:595–602, 1960
10. Bergstrand H, Olivecrona H, Tönnis W: Gefässmissbildungen und Gefässgeschwülste des Gehirns. G Thieme, Leipzig, 1936
11. Bergström M, Greitz T, Steiner L: An approach to stereotaxic radiography. Acta Neurochir 54:157–165, 1980.
12. Brownson RH, Suter DB, Diller DA: Acute

brain damage induced by low dosage x-irradiation. Neurology 13:181–191, 1963
13. Conforti P: Spontaneous disappearance of cerebral arteriovenous angioma. J Neurosurg 34:432–434, 1971
14. Crompton MR, Layton DD: Delayed radionecrosis of the brain following therapeutic x-radiation of the pituitary. Brain 84:85–101, 1961
15. Cushing H, Bailey P: Tumours arising from the blood vessels of the brain. CC Thomas, Springfield, Ill, 1928
16. Dahlin H, Sarby B: Destruction of small intracranial tumours with 60 Co gamma radiation. Physical and technical considerations. Acta Radiol (Ther Phys Biol) 14:209–227, 1975
17. Dandy WE: Arteriovenous aneurysms of the brain. Arch Surg 17:190–243, 1945. Surgery of the brain. Hagerstown, 1928
18. Davidoff LM, Dyke CG, Elsberg CA, Tablov IM: The effect of irradiation applied directly to the brain and spinal cord. 1. Experimental investigations of Macacus rhesus monkeys. Radiology 32:451–463, 1938
19. Diengdoh JV, Booth AR: Postirradiation necrosis of the temporal lobe presenting as a glioma. Case report. J Neurosurg 44:732–734, 1976
20. Dollinger MR, Lavine DM, Foye LV Jr: Myocardial infarction due to postirradiation fibrosis of the coronary arteries. Case of successfully treated Hodgkin's disease with lower esophageal involvement. JAMA 195:316–319, 1966
21. Ederyd J, Östman A: Stereofotogrammetrisk angiografi. Institutionen för Fotogrammetri, KTH, Stockholm, 1978
22. Fisher AW, Holfelder H: Lokales Amyloid im Genirn: eine Spätfolge von Röntgenbestrahlung. Dtsch Z Chir 227;475, 1930
23. Foltz EL, Holyoke JB, Heyl HL: Brain necrosis following x-ray therapy. J Neurosurg 10:423, 1953
24. Forster DMC, Leksell L, Meyerson BA, Steiner L: Gammathalamotomy in intractable pain. Pain 194–198. Georg Thieme Publishers, Stuttgart, 1972
25. Forster DMC, Steiner L, Håkansson S: Arteriovenous malformation of the brain. A long-term clinical study. J Neurosurg 37:562–570, 1972
26. French LA, Chou SN: Conventional methods of treating intracranial arterio-venous malformations. Prog Neurol Surg 3: 274–319. Karger, Basel, 1969
27. Frugoni P, Ruberti R: Observations sur 54 cas d'anévrysms artërio-veineux soustentoriels traités chirurgicalement. Neurochirurgie 9:377–389, 1963
28. Giombini S, Morello G: Cavernous angiomas of the brain. Account of fourteen personal cases and review of the literature. Acta Neurochir 40:61–82, 1978
29. Guiot G, Rougerie J, Sachs M, Hetzog E, Molina P: Repérage stéréotaxique de malformations vasculaires profondes intracérébrales. Paris, Sem Hop 36:1134–1143, 1960
30. Hayne RA, Kempe LG, Coxe W: The surgical treatment of arterio-venous malformations of the head. J Neurosurg 13:259–270, 1956
31. Holman E: Experimental studies in arteriovenous fistulas. I. Blood volume variations. Arch Surg Chicago, ix, 822–836, 1924. III. Cardiac dilation and blood vessel changes. Arch Surg Chicago, ix. 856–879, 1924.
32. Höök O, Johanson C: Intracranial arteriovenous aneurysms. A follow-up study with particular attention to their growth. Arch Neurol Psychiatry 80:39–54, 1958
33. Jefferson G: Les hemorrhagies sous-arachnoidiennes par angiomes et aneurysmes chez le jeune. Rev Neurol 80:413–432, 1948
34. Johns HE, Cunningham JR: The physics of radiology. Charles C Thomas, Springfield, Illinois, USA, 1978.
35. Johnson RT: Radiotherapy of cerebral angiomas. With a note on some problems in diagnosis. Cerebral angiomas—advances in diagnosis and therapy. Springer-Verlag, Berlin-Göttingen-Heidelberg, 1975, pp 256–258
36. Jörgensen L: Vessel wall and thrombogenesis: Vascular injury, arteriosclerosis. Thromb Diathes Haemorrh (Stuttg) Suppl 54:309–316, 1973
37. Kjellberg RN, Kliman B: A system for therapy of pituitary tumours. In Kohler PO, Ross GT (eds.): diagnosis and treatment of pituitary tumours. Excerpta Medica, Amsterdam, 1973, pp 234–252
38. Kjellberg RN, Koehler AM, Preston WM, Sweet WH: Intracranial Lesions Made by the Bragg Peak of a Proton Beam. In Haley TJ, Sinder RS (eds.): Response of the Nervous System to Ionizing Radiation. Little, Brown and Company, Boston, 1964, pp 36–53
39. Kjellberg RN, Nguyen NC, Kliman B: Le bragg peak protonique en neuro-chirurgie stéréotaxique. Neurochirurgie (Paris) 18,3:235–264, 1972
40. Kjellberg RN, Poletti CE, Roberson GD, Adams, RD: Bragg peak proton beam treatment of arteriovenous malformations of the brain. International Congress, Series No 433, Neurol Surg Editor: Carrea R, Co-editor: Le Vay D. Excerpta Medica, Amsterdam-Oxford, 1977
41. Kramer S, Southard M, Mansfield CM: Radiotherapy in the management of craniopharyngiomas. Amer J Roentgenol 103:44–52, 1968

42. Kramer S, Lee KF: Complications of radiation therapy: the central nervous system. Semin Roentgenol 9:75–83, 1974
43. Krayenbühl HA: Discussion des rapports sur "Les angiomes supratentoriels." Ier Congrès International de Neurochirurgie, rapports et discussions. Braxelles, 1957
44. Krayenbühl HA: Angiographic contribution to the problem of enlargement of cerebral arteriovenous malformations. Acta Neurochir 36:215–242, 1977
45. Krenchel NJ: Intracranial racemose angiomas: A clinical study. Universitetsforlaget, Aarhus, 1961
46. Laine E, Galibert P: Anévrysmes artério-veineux et circoides de la fosse postérieure. A propos de quarante observations. Rev Neurol (Paris) 115:276–288, 1966
47. Larsson B: Blood vessel changes following local irradiation of the brain with high-energy protons. Läk Fören Förh (Uppsala) 65:61, 1960
48. Larsson B, Andersson B, Rexed B, Sourander P, Mair W: Lesion in the depth of the brain produced by a beam of high energy protons. Acta Radiol 54:251, 1960
49. Larsson B, Leksell L, Rexed B, Sourander P, Mair W, Andersson B: The high-energy proton beam as a neurosurgical tool. Nature 182:1222, 1958
50. Larsson B, Leksell L, Rexed B: Use of high-energy protons for cerebral surgery in man. Acta Chir Scand 125:1–7, 1963
51. Larsson B, Lidén K, Sarby B: Irradiation of small structures through the intact skull. Acta Radiol (Ther Phys Biol) 13:513–534, 1974
52. Larsson B, Sarby B: Equipment for radiation surgery using narrow 185 MeV proton beams. The Gustaf Werner Institute, Uppsala University, Uppsala, 1974
53. Lawrence JH, Tobias CA, Born JL, Linfoot JA, D'Angio GJ: Heavy particles in experimental medicine and therapy. JAMA 196:166–170, 1966
54. Lawrence JH, Tobias CA, Linfoot JA, Born JL, Chong CY: Heavy particle therapy in acromegaly and Cushing's disease. JAMA 235: 2307–2310, 1976
55. Leksell L: The stereotaxic method and radiosurgery of the brain. Acta Chir Scand 102:316–319, 1951
56. Leksell L: Cerebral radiosurgery. Washington DC: 2nd Int Congr Neurol Surg Excerpta Medica Int Congr Series No 36, S5, 1961
57. Leksell L: A note on the treatment of acoustic tumours. Acta Chir Scand 137:763–765, 1971
58. Leksell L: Stereotaxic and Radiosurgery. An Operative System. Charles C Thomas, Springfield, Ill, 1971
59. Leksell L: Stereotaxic radiosurgery in trigeminal neuralgia. Acta Chir Scand 137:311–317, 1971
60. Leksell L, Larsson B, Andersson B, Rexed B, Sourander P, Mair W: Lesions in the depth of the brain produced by a beam of high energy protons. Acta Radiol 54:252–264, 1960
61. Lidén K: Physikalische Grundlagen für die Verwendung ionisierender Strahlung bei gezielter Hirnchirurgie. In Olivecrona H, Tönnis W (eds.): Handbuch der Neurochirurgie, Band VI. Springer, Heidelberg, 1957
62. Lindsay S, Entenman C, Ellis EE, Geraci CL: Aortic arteriosclerosis in the dog after localized aortic irradiation with electrons. Circ. Res. 10:61–67, 1962 A
63. Lindsay S, Kohn HI, Dakin RL, Jew J: Aortic arteriosclerosis in the dog after localized aortic x-irradiation. Circ Res 10:51–60, 1962 B
64. Luessenhop AJ: Artificial embolization for cerebral arteriovenous malformations. Year Book Publishers, Basel, Karger, and Chicago. Progr Neurol Surg 3:320–362, 1969
65. Luessenhop AJ: Artificial embolization of inoperable arteriovenous malformations. In Pia HV, Gleave JRW, Grote E, Zierski J (eds.): Cerebral Angiomas, Springer-Verlag, Berlin-Heidelberg-New York, 1975, pp 198–205
66. Luessenhop AJ, Kachman R Jr, Shevlin W, Ferraro AA: Clinical evaluation of arterial embolization in the management of large cerebral arterio-venous malformations. J Neurosurg 23:400–417, 1965
67. Luessenhop AJ, Spence WT: Artificial embolization of cerebral arteries. Report of use in a case of arteriovenous malformation. JAMA 172:1153–1155, 1960
68. McKissock W, Hankinson J: The surgical treatment of supratentorial angiomas. Rapports et discussions. 1er Congrès International de Neurochirurgie, Bruxelles, 1957
69. Magnus V: Bidrag till hjerchirurgiens klinik og resultater. Merkur, Kristiania, 1921
70. Mair W, Rexed B, Sourander P: Histology of the surgical radiolesion in the human brain as produced by high-energy protons. Radiat Res Suppl 7:384–389, 1967
71. Marcial-Rojas RA, Catro JR: Iradiation injury to elastic arteries in the course of treatment for neoplastic disease. Ann Otol Rhinol Laryngol 71:945, 1962
72. Martins AN, Johnston J, Henry JM, Stoffel TJ, Di Chiro G: Delayed radiation necrosis of the brain. J Neurosurg 47:336–345, 1977
73. Michael AM: Radiation necrosis of the brain:

Correlation between computed tomography, pathology, and dose distribution. J Comput Assist Tomogr 2:71–80, 1978
74. Minakova YI: 1977, Personal communication.
75. Mingrino S: Supratentorial Arteriovenous Malformations of the Brain. Advances and Technical Standards in Neurosurgery. Krayenbühl Zürich (ed.). Springer-Verlag, Wien, New York, 1978, pp 93–123
76. Nakagaki H, Brunhart G, Kemper TL, Caveness WF: Monkey brain damage from radiation in the therapeutic range. J Neurosurg 44:3–11, 1976
77. Nilsson A, Wennerstrand J, Leksell D, Backlund E-O: Stereotactic gamma irradiation of basilar artery in cat. A pilot study. Acta Radiol (Onocology) 17:150–160, 1978.
78. Nonne M: Ein Fall von Jacksonscher Epilepsie durch Trepanation geheilt. Münch Med Wochenschr 68:566, 1921
79. Norén G, Backlund E-O: Treatment of acoustic tumours by stereotactic radiosurgery. Proc 6th Congr Neurol Surg, Sao Paolo, 1977
80. Norén G, Grepe A, Backlund E-O, Leksell L: Stereotactic radiosurgery in acoustic neurinomas. (in press)
81. Norlén G: Arteriovenous aneurysms of the brain: Report of 10 cases of total removal of lesion. J Neurosurg 6:475–494, 1949
82. Olivecrona H, Ladenheim J: Congenital Arteriovenous Aneurysms of the Carotid and Vertebral Arterial Systems. Springer-Verlag Berlin-Göttingen-Heidelberg, 1957, p 91
83. Olivecrona H: Die arteriovenösen Aneurysmen des Gehirns. Deutsche Medizinische Wochenschrift, Nr. 36, 1950.
84. Olivecrona H, Riives J: Arteriovenous aneurysms of the brain. Their diagnosis and treatment. Arch Neurol Psychiatry 59:567–602, 1948
85. Peterson JH, McKissock W: A clinical survey of intracranial angiomas with special reference to their mode of progression and surgical treatment: A report of 110 cases. Brain 79:233–266, 1956
86. Pearson HES: Incidental dangers of x-ray therapy. Lancet 1:222, 1958
87. Pool JL: Treatment of arteriovenous malformations of the cerebral hemispheres. J Neurosurg 19:136–141, 1962
88. Pool JL: Aneurysms and arterio-venous anomalies of the brain. Diagnosis and treatment. Hoeber Medical Division, Harper and Row, New York, 1965
89. Potter JM: Angiomatous malformations of the brains; their nature and prognosis. Ann Roy Coll Surg (Engl) 16:227–243, 1955
90. Rähn T, Thorén M, Hall K, Backlund E-O: Stereotactic radiosurgery in Cushing's syndrome: Acute radiation effects. Surg Neurol, 14:85–92, 1980
91. Ray BS: Cerebral arterio-venous aneurysms. Surg Gynec Obstet 73:614–648, 1941
92. Rexed B, Mair, W, Sourander P, Larsson B, Leksell L: Effect of high-energy protons on the brain of the rabbit. Acta Radiol 53:289–299, 1960
93. Riechert T, Mundinger F: Combined stereotaxic operation for treatment of deep seated angiomas and aneurysms. J Neurosurg 21:358–363, 1964
94. Rubin Ph, Casarett W: Clinical radiation pathology, W.B. Saunders, Philadelphia, 1968, p 1057
95. Sarby B: Cerebral radiation surgery with narrow gamma beams. Acta Radiol (Ther Phys Biol) 13:425–444, 1974
96. Serbinenko FA: Balloon catheterization and occlusion of major cerebral vessels. J Neurosurg 41:125–145, 1974
97. Smith DJ: Effects of gamma radiation on isolated surviving arteries and their vasa-vasorum. Am J Physiol 201:901–904, 1961
98. Stein EM, Fraser RAR, Wolpert S: Embolization in the preparation for surgery of large cerebral arteriovenous malformations. J Neurol Neurosurg Psychiatry 38:407, 1975
99. Steiner L: Treatment of arteriovenous malformations by radiosurgery. In Intracranial arteriovenous malformations. Eds: Charles B Wilson, Benett Stein. Current Neurosurgical Practice, 1984.
100. Steiner L: Radiosurgery in intracranial tumour and arteriovenous malformations in children. In Tumours of the central nervous system in infancy and childhood, eds: Voth D, Gutjahr P, Langmaid C, Springer-Verlag Berlin Heidelberg 1982.
101. Steiner L, Greitz T, Backlund E-O, Leksell L, Norén G, Rähn T: Radiosurgery in arteriovenous malformations of the brain. In Stereotactic Cerebral Irradiation pp. 257–269. Ed. Szikla G, Elsevier, North-Holland Biomedical Press 1979.
102. Steiner L, Greitz T, Leksell L, Norén G, Rähn T, and Backlund E-O: Radiosurgery in intracranial arteriovenous malformations. II: A follow-up study. Proc 6th Int Congr Neurol Surg Excerpta Medica, Amsterdam, 1977, (in press)
103. Steiner L, Leksell L, Forster DMC, Greitz T, Backlund E-O: Stereotactic radiosurgery in intracranial arteriovenous malformations. Acta Neurochir (Suppl) 21:195–209, 1974
104. Steiner L, Leksell L, Greitz T, Forster DMC,

Backlund E-O: Stereotaxic radiosurgery for cerebral arteriovenous malformations. Report of a case. Acta Chir Scand 138:459–464, 1972
105. Steiner L, Lindquist C von Holst H: The effect on vessels of gamma-radiation combined with induced deep hypotension in cat. 1978, Unpublished
106. Steiner L, von Holst H, Lindquist C: The effect on vessels of the gamma-radiation combined with induced hyperpyrexia in cat. 1978, Unpublished
107. Svien HJ, McRae JA: Arteriovenous anomalies of the brain: fate of patients not having definite surgery. J Neurosurg 23:23–38, 1965
108. Svien HJ, Perserico J: Regression in size of arteriovenous anomaly. J Neurosurg 17:493–496, 1960
109. Thomas E, Forbus W: Irradiation injury to the aorta and the lung. Arch Path 67:256–263, 1959
110. Thorén M, Rähn T, Hall K, Backlund E-O: Treatment of pituitary dependent Cushing's syndrome with closed stereotactic radiosurgery by means of 60 Co gamma radiation. Acta Endocrinol 1978, in press
111. Walder HA: Application of cryotherapy in arterio-venous aneurysms. An experimental and clinical study. J Neurol Neurosurg Psychiatry 34:105, 1971
112. Walder HA, Jaspar HHJ, Meijer E: Application of cryotherapy in cerebrovascular anomalies. J Psychiatr Neurol Neurochir 73:471–486, 1970
113. Tobias CA, Anger HO, Lawrence JH: Radiologic use of high energy deuterons and alpha particles. American Journal of Roentgenology, Radium Therapy and Nuclear Medicine, 67:1–27, 1952
114. Wegmann H-J: Das Schicksal operierter Patienten mit arteriovenösem Aneurysma des Gehirns. Juris Druck and Verlag, Zürich, 1969
115. Wennerstrand J, Ungerstedt U: Cerebral radiosurgery. Acta Chir Scand 136:133–137, 1970
116. Wilson RR: Radiological use of fast protons. Radiology 49:487–491, 1946
117. Windholz F: Zur Kenntnis der Blutgefaessveraenderungen in Roentgenbestrahlten Gewebe. Strahlentherapie 59:662–670, 1937
118. Virchow R: Phlogose und thrombose im Gefassystem. In: Gesammelte Abhandlungen zur Wissenschaftlichen Medizin. Meidinger Sohn and Co, Frankfurt 1856, p 458
119. Wolbach SB: The pathologic history of chronic x-ray dermatitis and early x-ray carcinoma. J Med Res 21:415–449, 1909
120. Young MEJ: Radiological physics. London H.K. Lewis & Co. Ltd, 1957

7

Spinal Cord Arteriovenous Malformations

Ayub Khan Ommaya

Introduction

Surgical treatment of neural disorders are inevitably associated with improvements in diagnostic techniques, which lead to greater understanding of such diseases. The contributions of Egas Moniz (carotid angiography), Walter Dandy (pneumoencephalography), and G.N. Hounsfield (computerized tomography), all within the past 50 years, have created a virtual revolution in the diagnostic basis of modern neurosurgery. Application of such advances in diagnostic technique, as a general rule, has always been much slower for diseases of the spinal cord as compared with those of the brain. Vascular diseases of the spinal cord are no exception. Thus, it is not until 1969 that the first monograph on this subject, "Selective Arteriography of the Spinal Cord," describing our earliest experiences with arteriovenous malformations (AVMs) of the spinal cord, was published.[5] Although the pioneering work of R. Djindjian on the vascular radiology of the spinal cord began in the early '60s, it was not until the '70s that the diagnostic and therapeutic aspects of vascular diseases of the spinal cord, with special emphasis on the angiomas, became well understood. These developments are well summarized in a number of publications, the most notable being the excellent studies by Djindjian,[4] Aminoff,[1] and, most recently, the text edited by Pia and Djindian.[14] The intention of this chapter, therefore, is not to provide an exhaustive and comparative description of all that is known of spinal cord AVMs. Rather, we will seek to summarize our personal experience in the diagnosis and treatment of 104 cases of such lesions culled from more than 200 cases of nontraumatic myelopathy. These cases were referred as suspected AVMs of the spinal cord and were studied between 1961 and 1981 at the Clinical Center of the National Institutes of Health and the affiliated hospitals of the George Washington University. All 104 cases in this series were studied with selective spinal angiography (Fig. 7.1).

Terminology and Classification

AVMs or angiomas of the spinal cord are congenital abnormal clusters of blood vessels formed as a developmental anomaly of the spinal circulation. Turnbull described four stages in the development of the spinal vascular system, and it is at the end of the second or "initial" stage (third to sixth weeks) that maldevelopment leads to persistence of thin-walled tortuous vessels with poorly developed media and elastica, primitive capillary and precapillary channels, and abnormal arteriovenous shunts, all typically seen in AVM. These le-

1. Spinal Arteriovenous Malformations 104
2. Non-Traumatic Myelopathy of Unknown Origin 34
3. Tumors of the Spinal Cord (Primary) 24

   (a) Astrocytoma 12
   (b) Ependymoma 4
   (c) Hemangioblastoma 4
   (d) Neurofibroma 4

4. Cervical and Lumbar Spondylosis 20
   (Including Herniated Intervertebral Discs)
5. Syringomyelia 12
6. Motor Neuron Disease 2
7. Multiple Sclerosis 2
8. Chronic Arachnoiditis 2
9. Cholesteatoma of Posterior Fossa 1

Fig. 7.1. Discharge diagnosis of 200 patients referred as suspected cases of spinal cord AVMs, (1965 to 1981).

sions were first described in reports by Hebold in 1885 and by Gaupp in 1888, who picturesquely called them "hemorrhoids of the pia mater" and recognized them as a source for subarachnoid hemorrhage.[8,9]

AVMs are usually classified according to their regional localization by selective spinal angiography into three groups: cervical, thoracic, and thoracolumbar-sacral. Based on an angiographically analyzed series of 150 cases, Michael Djindjian gave overall regional percentages of 14% for cervical (Cl-Tl), 22% for thoracic (T2-T6), and 64% for the largest group of thoracolumbar-sacral AVM (T7 to cauda equina).[3] These figures are in rough agreement with our own series of 104 cases in which we have also observed an equivalent contribution of blood supply to the AVM from posterior arteries in 48% and from both anterior and posterior vessels in 52%. Our data also confirm the observation that more rostral AVMs have more anterior blood supply whereas the caudally placed AVMs have more posteriorly derived vascular inputs. Micheal Djindjian's observations at the Lariboisiere Hospital in Paris with A. Rey and R. Houdart on the classification of intramedullary AVM is an important contribution with great surgical significance, and the reader is referred to this work for further details.[3,4]

Our first radiologic classification of AVM recognized three basic types: the single-coiled, unbranched type 1 lesion, commonly seen in adults; the less common plexus of "glomus" type 2 lesion; and the variable rapid flow type 3 lesion with multiple feeding arteries often seen in younger patients and hence termed the "juvenile" type.[5] From the surgeon's point of view, a division of all spinal cord AVMs into low-flow and high-flow lesions is a simple rubric to separate the surgically easy, mainly extramedullary low-flow cases from the surgically difficult and often intramedullary, high-flow lesions.[12] High-flow AVMs are completely visualized by selective angiography in less than 5 seconds whereas low-flow AVMs require much longer times for dye clearance (Figs. 7.2, 7.3).

Incidence

In neurosurgical series, the incidence of spinal AVM ranges from a low of 3.3% in the preangiography era to a figure of 40% of all CNS vascular malformations after the introduction of selective angiography.[14] These figures certainly show that spinal AVMs are not rare lesions, but, in the absence of adequate epidemiologic data, the true incidence is not known. However, it is reasonable to expect that at least 10% of vascular space-occupying lesions of the spinal cord will be AVMs.[11] Incidence for sex showed males to be preponderant in our series (79%) whereas incidence for age was approximately equal from the second to the sixth decade. The incidence of high-flow AVM in adults was approximately one-fourth that of the low-flow type, which clearly emerged only in adults over 18.

Pathogenesis of AVM Effects on the Spinal Cord

In an earlier publication we discussed the pathogenesis of AVM signs and symptoms, considering particularly the factors of mechanical compression by the venous bulk of the lesion and vascular diversion ("steal").[10] These and other factors, including bleeding and progressive thromboses, are further discussed in the contributions of M. & R. Djindian.[14] The consensus points to a variable contribution of four major factors causing ischemia due to "steal," "compression" subarachnoid hemorrhage, and thrombotic phenomena. It is the variable contribution of these factors that may ex-

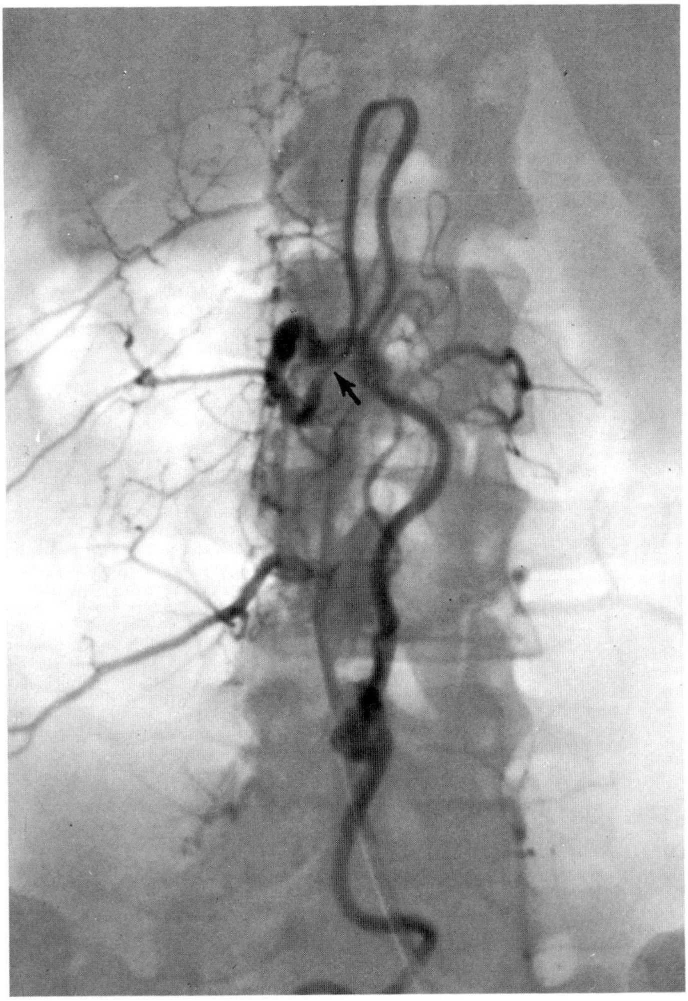

Fig. 7.2. Selective spinal angiogram of high-flow AVM. Note filling of part of venous drainage of lesion.

plain the often unpredictable response to embolization of feeders which cures the steal without relieving the compression as well as the genesis of so-called Foix-Aiajonanine disease as a thrombotic end-stage in the life of an untreated AVM as first suggested by Pia and Vogelsang.[15,17] The etiology of thrombosis in the AVM is unknown but that it occurs is unequivocally certain. The role of increased extramedullary venous pressure has been hypothesized by Aminoff, Barnard, and Logue.[2] These authors postulate a sequence of high venous back pressure causing reduced intramedullary AV pressure gradients which in turn cause reduced blood flow leading to spinal cord ischemia either directly or indirectly via intravascular thromboses. This mechanism is supported by our own work.[12]

Clinical Diagnosis

The most striking clinical fact about AVM of the spinal cord is the protean nature of its natural history, making early diagnosis (within 6 months of the first symptom) very difficult. Thus, in 60% of our 104 cases two years or more had elapsed. Figure 7.4 illustrates the extent of this delay in clinical recognition in the first 45 of the 104 patients referred to us. Note that only 17 of 45 were recognized as AVM cases within 1 year of symptom onset and that 19 of 45 were not properly diagnosed until 3 to 15 years after the original symptoms appeared. This difficulty of early diagnosis is often related to the insidious character of the onset of initial symptoms and signs. The most common deficits to appear first were either motor and sensory or

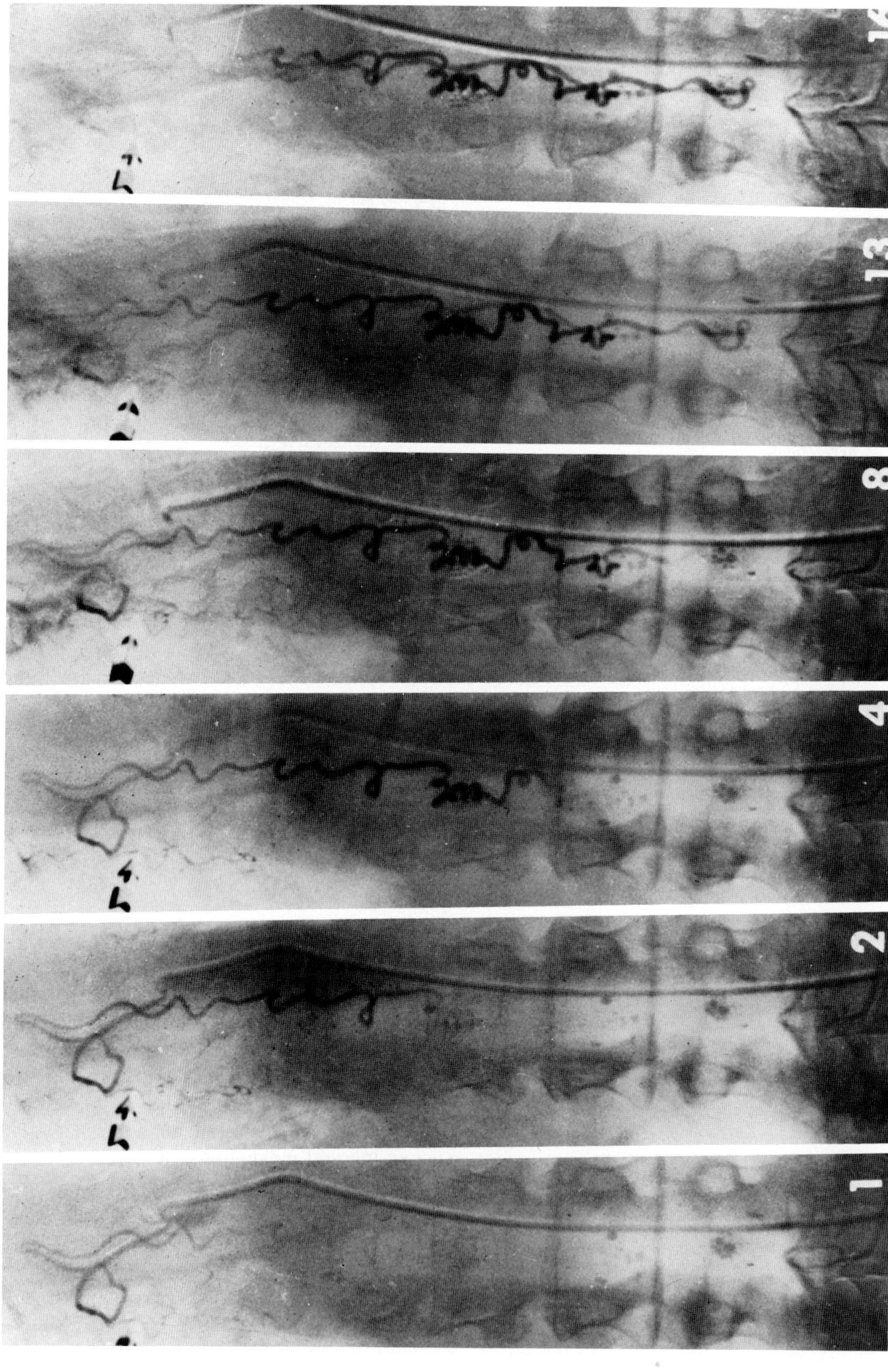

Fig. 7.3. Selective spinal angiogram of low-flow AVM. Note persistance of contrast medium within AVM for time shown.

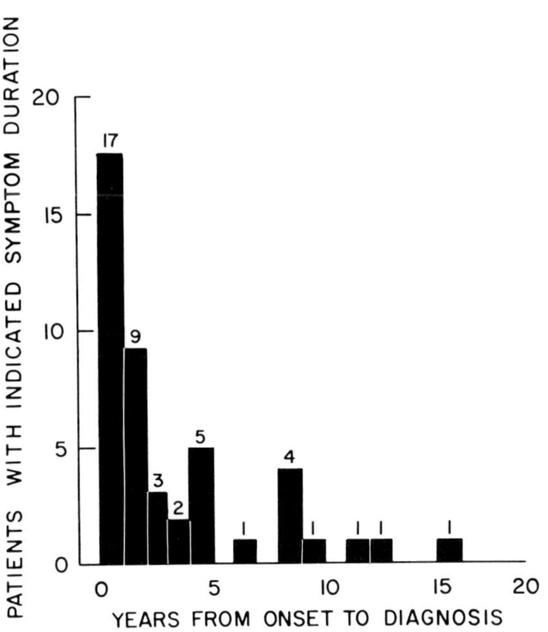

Fig. 7.4. Tabulation of duration of symptoms before recognition of presence of AVM in 45 patients. Note that majority of patients were not correctly diagnosed until at least 1 year had elapsed from onset of symptoms. (This group of patients were the first 45 cases in our series of 104 patients.)

	Incidence
Subarachnoid Hemorrhage*	11%
Fluctuating Course	32%
Progressive†	100%

* Bloody cerebrospinal fluid on lumbar puncture performed after an episode of neurological deterioration.
† Length of the final progressive episode varied from 1 week to 13 years.

Fig. 7.5. Incidence of three major features in the clinical course of spinal cord AVM.

both in 80%, with pain as a frequent component in nearly half the cases. Disturbances of sphincteral and sexual functions as initial signs were less common (9%), and acute onset of any or all of these symptoms and signs, usually due to subarachnoid hemorrhage, occurred in only 11% of our cases. The clinical course is almost invariably progressive, but in 32% of our cases the progression displayed a fluctuating intensity, a characteristic feature described by many

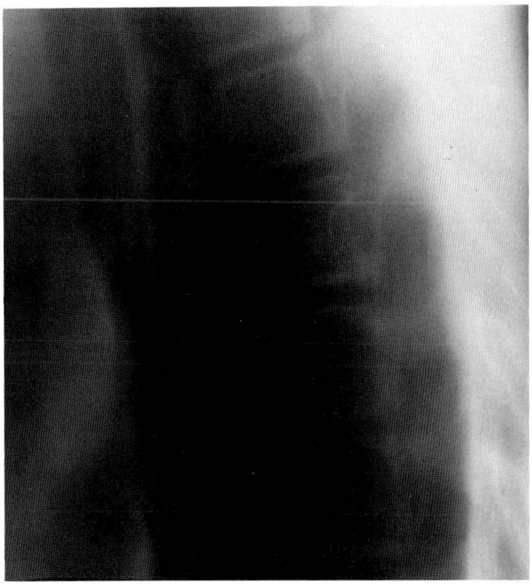

Fig. 7.6. Tomogram of spine to show erosion of vertebral body by AVM. This is one example of the occasional finding of an abnormality caused by AVM on the plain x-ray.

authors and the possible causes of which are well detailed by Aminoff.[1] The incidence of these features in the clinical course of AVM of the spinal cord are summarized in Fig. 7.5.

It is obvious from the above that there is no unique constellation of signs and symptoms pathognomonic of spinal cord AVM. In our series the shortest history was one of sudden severe back pain and paraplegia, with the final diagnosis established in less than 1 week. The longest delay between symptom onset and diagnosis was for 16 years in a patient misdiagnosed as having motor neuron disease. Differential diagnosis includes all the disease categories listed in Fig. 7.1, with multiple sclerosis and motor neuron disease being the most common mistakes. We have previously drawn attention to the value of cutaneous angiomatous lesions in suspecting and localizing spinal cord AVM (in 19% of cases), particularly when a Valsalva maneuver causes enhancement of the color intensity of such skin lesions.[7] This maneuver can also exacerbate other signs and symptoms of the AVM. Trauma, pregnancy, increase of body temperature, overeating, postural changes, and muscular effort are additional factors that may precipitate or aggravate AVM symptoms.[1] One of our patients, a successful

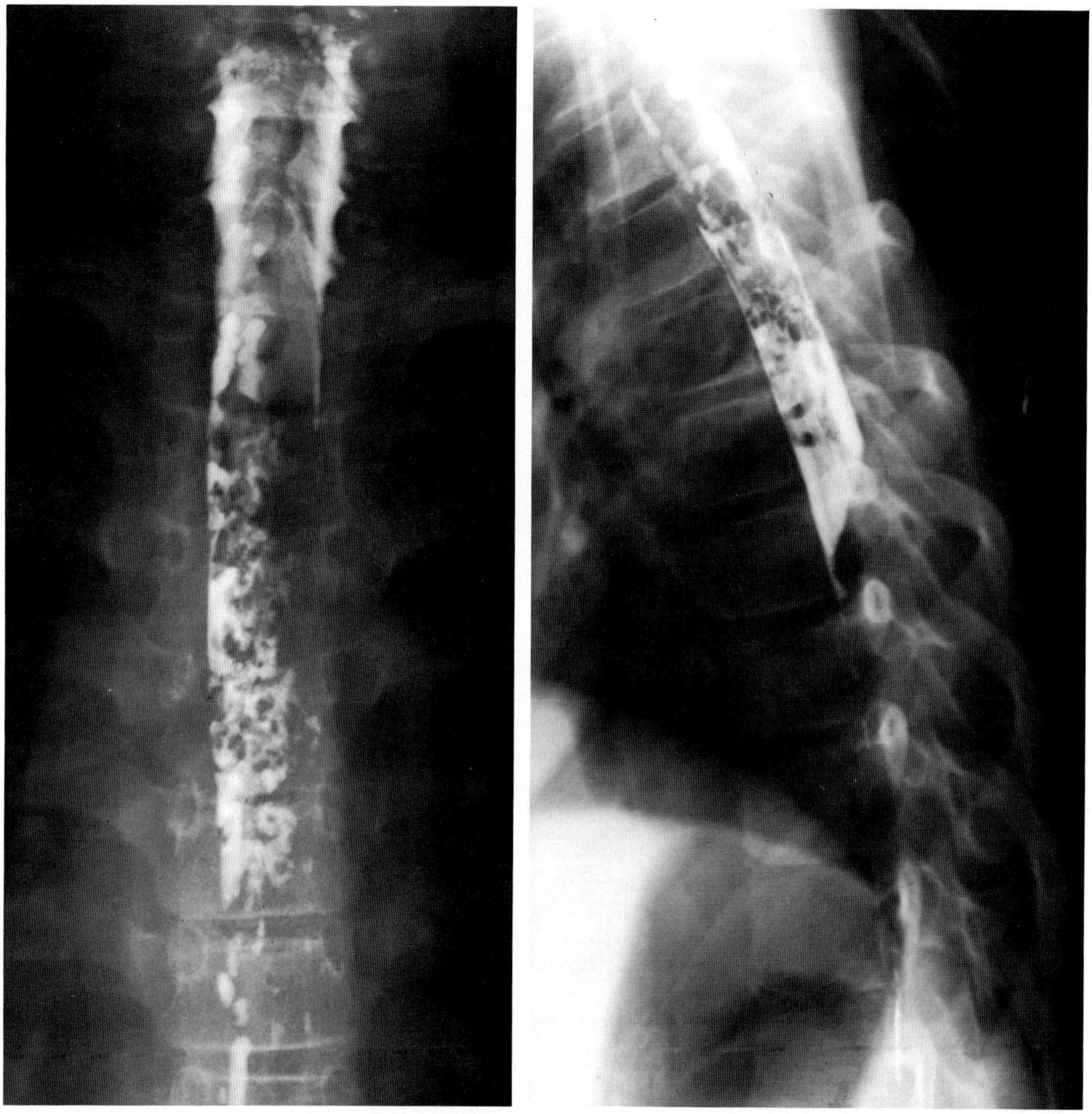

Fig. 7.7. Myelographic appearance of large spinal cord angiomas (high-flow).

fund raiser for a well-known university, had three episodes of postprandial transient paraplegia that spontaneously reversed four to six hours after the meal. Only two patients in our series had audible buits over the AVM; both had extensive extradural and extraspinal components.

Radiologic Diagnosis

Since the early work reported in 1969-1970 from Paris and Bethesda, numerous contributions on this subject have elaborated in considerable detail on the techniques and efficiency of selective spinal angiography, and the reader is referred for such details to these sources.[1,4,5,14] Although angiography is essential for precise understanding of the surgical anatomy and subsequent surgical therapy planning as well as for postoperative evaluation, it should be remembered that myelography remains the major screening method of AVM. Plain x-rays were only occasionally useful in our series (6% positive versus 94% negative findings). The findings of bony erosions in vertebral elements and of interpediculate space widening in patients with motor or sensory deficits in the lower extremeties are certainly useful diagnostic clues (Fig. 7.6). Myelography, on the other hand, was positive in 97% of our cases and diagnostic for AVM in 86%, showing the characteristic serpiginous filling deficits (Fig. 7.7). The necessity for *complete* myelographic examination of the cord, including its dorsal aspect, has been repeatedly emphasized, not only for exact diagnosis but also to provide the necessary localization of the AVM, which precedes angiographic delineation of its vascular details. It should be obvious that without myelographic guidance, spinal angiography of *all* the cord blood supply would be required —a most tedious task fraught with risk. Moreover, in our series we have not had a single case in which an entirely normal myelogram was found in an AVM case. It is, therefore, recommended that selective spinal angiography not be done in patients with suspected AVM whose myelograms show no abnormality whatsoever. On the other hand, cases with abnormal myelograms *not* clearly diagnostic of AVM but with *clinical* evidence of a progressive clinical course, e.g., a case with "localized arachnoiditis," should be examined angiographically. The relative contributions of the three major modes of radiologic investigation of AVM are shown in Fig. 7.8.

Interpretation of spinal angiograms must include a clear understanding of the normal intraspinal structure just as it does in the intrepretation of myelograms. Selective angiography was successful in demonstrating the lesion in 89% of our cases. Failure to show by angiogram an AVM that has been suspected both clinically and myelographically suggests a bad prognosis.

	Positive	Negative
Plain Spine Films*	6%	94%
Myelography**	97%	3%
Arteriography***	89%	11%

* Widening of Interpedicular Space and Bone Erosions

** Six did not Show Typical Serpiginous Defects. Four Had Complete Blocks. Two of the Negative Myelograms Suggested Arachnoiditis Only With Subsequent Positive Angiography.

*** Six Studies were Incomplete.

Fig. 7.8. Contribution of plain spine films, myelography, and angiography to the radiologic diagnosis of spinal cord AVM.

Results of surgical removal of such "nonfilling" AVM in our series were not attended by any significant benefit to the patient. Examples of myelographic and angiographic findings that are relevant for the radiologic diagnosis of AVM are shown in Figs. 7.9–7.11. Spinal angiography is a time-consuming procedure, and a careful examination of blood supply and vascular anatomy of a large AVM may require two or even three angiographic sessions.

Surgical Treatment and Results

In the course of two decades of neurosurgical experiences the author has tested and used all the various modes of surgical therapy for AVM. These include arterial ligation for certain low-flow lesions,[13] microsurgical total excision for both low-flow and certain high-flow lesions,[11] as well as the use of embolization in collaboration with Doppman,[6] both as a preoperative maneuver and as a sole or supplementary mode of therapy. As discussed below, each of these methods alone or in combination has to be known by the neurosurgeon who wishes to provide optimal management to all his patients with spinal cord AVM. The evolution of microsurgical technique in neurosurgery led by the pioneering efforts of R. Peardon Donaghy and G. Yasargil has resulted in a general consensus that spinal cord AVM should be resected "in toto" whenever possible. Hans Werner Pia in a comprehensive survey of the operative treatment of AVM of the spinal cord including his own extensive experience has emphasized that the operative technique for resection is not new and was first carried out in 1927 by G. Berthes, based on the first myelographic demonstration of the AVM with significant clinical improvement after surgery.[14,15] In our own series, dorsally placed lesions with primarily posterior blood supply were amenable to total resection even where significant intramedullary extensions were present. Anteriorly located or "global" lesions (invariably of the high-flow type) were not usually amenable to total resection, and partial resections and arterial ligation with and without embolization were the alternative procedures undertaken. Intramedullary lesions fed totally by the anterior spinal artery are usually not totally resectable, but partial resections are

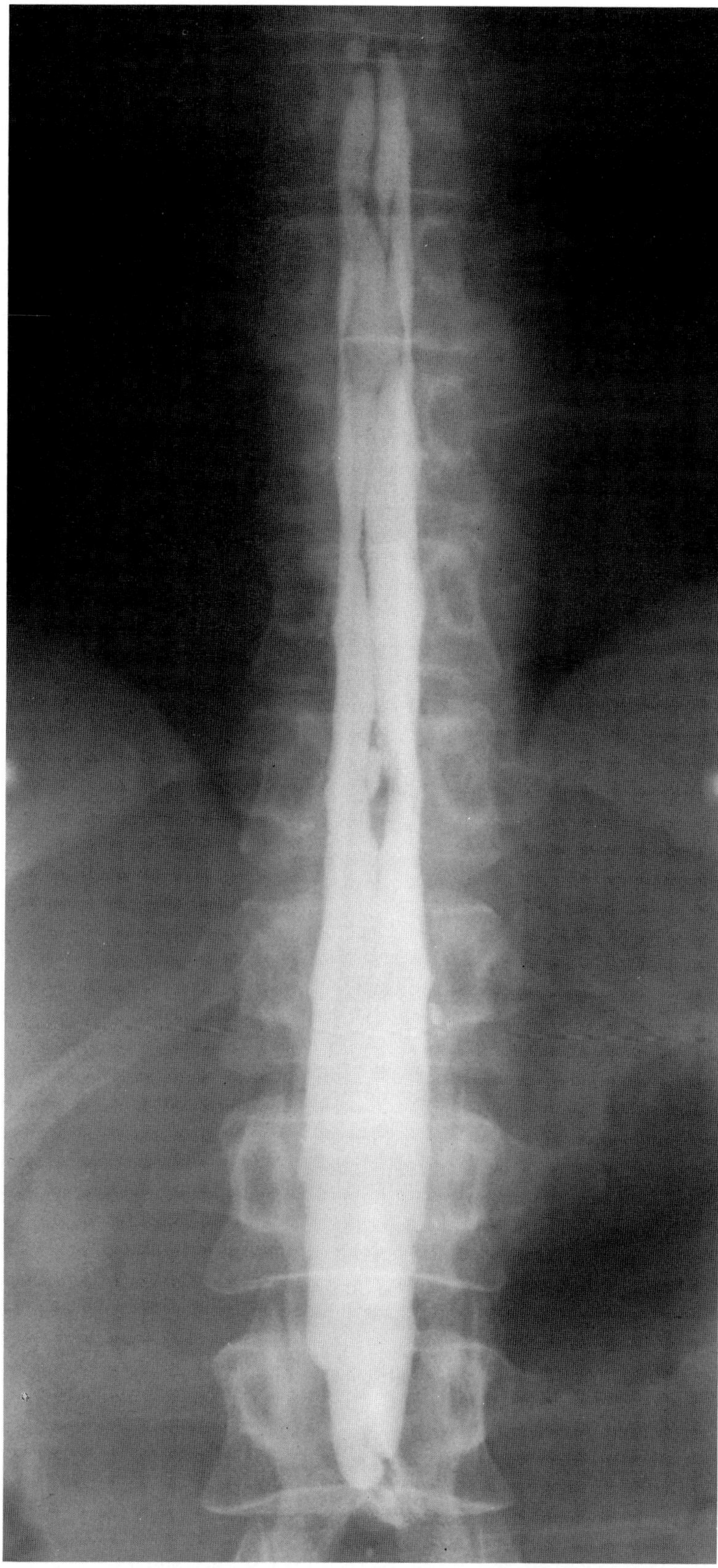

Fig. 7.9. Myelogram showing appearance of septum posticum. This normal structure may be mistaken for a vascular abnormality in some myelograms.

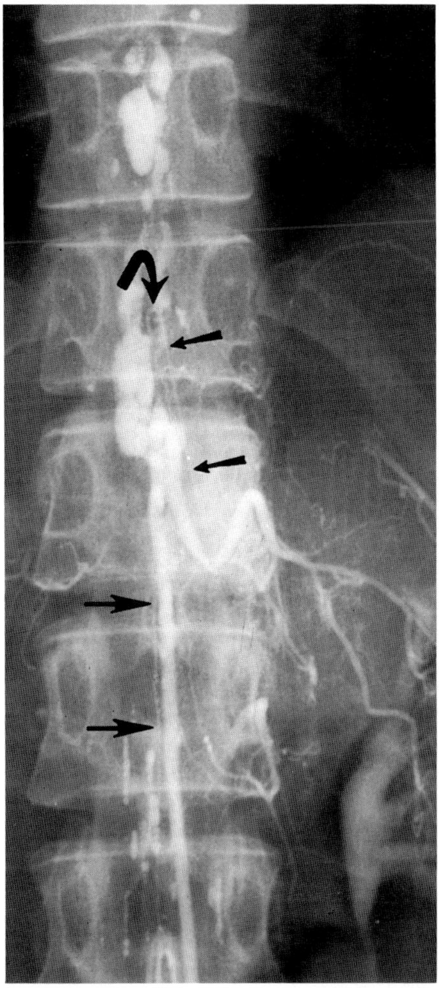

Fig. 7.10. Selective spinal angiogram to show artery of Adamkiewicz identified seperately from blood supply to AVM.

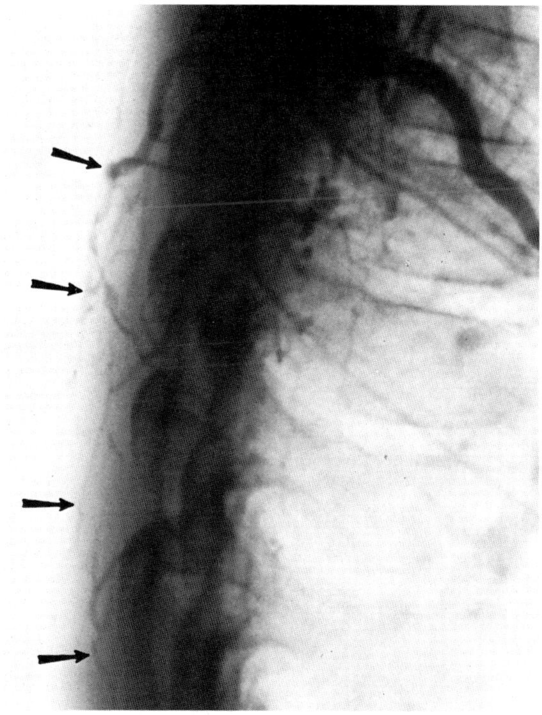

Fig. 7.11. Selective angiography of intercostal vessels feeding a spinal cord AVM (shown in the myelogram of Fig. 7.7) that also fed a cutaneous angioma overlying the AVM as seen in this illustration of a lateral view of the cutaneous zone.

often quite useful in causing neurologic improvement in patients with a short history. The results of treatment in the author's personal series of 104 cases are summarized in Table 7.1. The patients were divided into three groups according to the type of therapy used as the primary method of management. Results shown were based on clinical evaluation at a minimum of 1 year after the primary procedure. The category of results titled "unchanged" means that the previously progressive myelopathy was arrested but not reversed. This effect on the myelopathy was clear-cut in group I patients but often was temporary in groups II and III patients, who were followed up over 3 to 4 years. Delayed resumption of progressive myelopathy was especially noted in patients over the age of 60 in whom all results were qualitatively less satisfactory.

Our best results were obtained in low-flow lesions situated over the dorsum of the spinal cord where total resection and intradural ligation produced almost equally good results. In high-flow lesions total resection achieved within the first year of lesion presentation (by history) also produced good results, provided cord myelopathy was noted to be minimal and present for less than 6 months. Our worst results occurred in patients in whom angiography (often repeated) failed to reveal the myelographically diagnosed AVM in patients with progressive myelopathy of more than 12 months' duration and in patients with high-flow lesions in whom total resection was not achieved (Table 7.2).

The critical role of symptom duration on the result of treatment is shown in Fig. 7.12, where the results in 41 of our 64 group I patients with at least 5 years follow-up are shown.

Table 7.1. Results.

Types of surgical therapy	Total number of patients	Improved	Unchanged	Worse
I. Microneurosurgical Total Resection	64	50	12	2
II. Arterial Ligation ± Partial Resection	28	16	8	4
III. Embolization	12	2	9	1
TOTALS	104	68	29	7

Overall Results: Improved = 65.4%, unchanged = 34.6% or worse

The course of recovery after surgical treatment was often quite variable as illustrated by the following four case histories.

Case No. 68 in our series underwent a total excision of a low-flow dorsally placed AVM fed by the iliolumbar arteries bilaterally. Only slight improvement was noted at 1 year postoperatively but this continued so that at the fifth anniversary he was completely normal and has remained thus in the subsequent 5 years.

Case No. 80 also had a low-flow thoracic AVM completely resected at aged 55 with immediate worsening of his neurologic deficits postoperatively. However, after 3 years he had improved significantly and at 6 years postoperatively showed marked restoration of neurologic function. This type of delayed improvement after an initial worsening was never seen in patients who underwent intradural arterial ligation with or without subtotal resection.

Case No. 72 in our series (aged 44) underwent ligation of all angiographically demonstrated feeders of a low-flow thoracolumbar AVM. His immediate postoperative improvement was steadily maintained and when seen 4 years after surgery was working full time as a dentist. However 7 years later his symptoms recurred and a dural component had to be resected for recovery to return.[12]

Case No. 76, at age 64 also had a low-flow thoracolumbar AVM and received similar surgical treatment. Despite significant improvement maintained beyond the first anniversary, the patient showed progressive deterioration starting at 3 years and ending in complete paraplegia at 11 years postoperatively. Repeat myelography and angiography showed no recurrence of AVM. Significant cord shrinkage and arachnoiditis suggested a Foix-Alajuanine syndrome secondary to delayed thrombotic and ischemic changes in an intermedullary component of the AVM.

Table 7.2

Best results	Worst results
1. Total resections in Patients with Less Than 6 Months of Myelopathic History and Associated Aneurysms (5 Cases).	1. Resection of AVM in patients with Myelopathic History >1 Year and Inability to Show AVM Anatomy Angiographically.
2. Slow-Flow AVM with 6 Months History of Myelopathy. (Equivalent Results of Resection and Ligation).	2. Any AVM with >1 Year History of Myelopathy.
3. High Flow AMV with 6 Months History of Myelopathy, Totally Resected.	3. High-Flow Lesions with Incomplete Resections.

Microsurgical Technique for Total Excision (12)

Despite the best radiographic data, it is important to note that true operability of a difficult spinal cord AVM can be determined only when the lesion is inspected at surgery. It is crucial, therefore, that the exposure should be carried

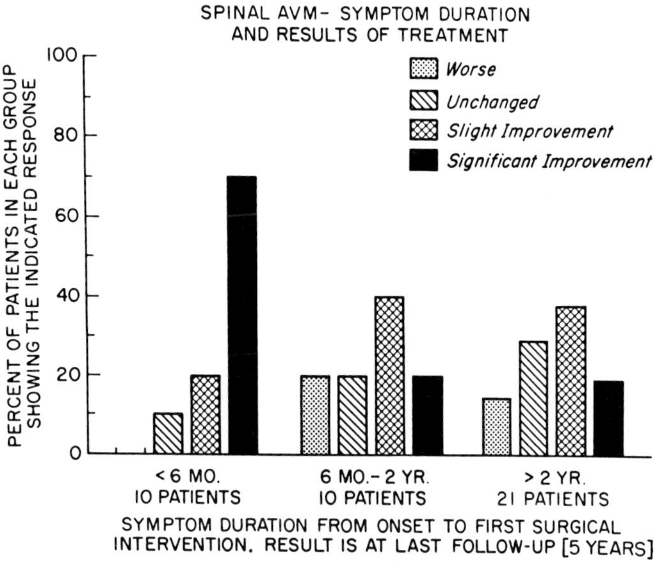

Fig. 7.12. Tabulation of results of total microsurgical excision of AVM in 41 cases followed up for at least 5 years versus duration of symptoms before diagnosis of the AVM. Note that significant improvement occurred most often in patients with a history shorter than 6 months.

out with meticulous attention to hemostasis. It is the practice of the author to use an air-powered rongeur for completion of the bone work, exposing the dura as widely as possible without removal of the facet joints. It is not necessary to expose more than what is necessary of the dura, i.e., over the main mass of the AVM or so-called "nidus" of the lesion. It is true that in certain cases the draining veins are so inextricably entwined that large exposures are necessary. At this stage the microscope is introduced and the dura is opened in the midline while preserving the arachnoid membrane and preventing escape of CSF at this stage. After the dura is tacked up to the muscles with retaining sutures, the arachnoid is opened in the midline and in turn is tacked up to the dural edges using small metal clips. In the "easy" case, a dorsally placed lesion lies primarily in the subarachnoid space and sharp discetion is used to cut arachnoidal bands holding the lesion to the cord. Arterial feeders are sought for, guided by the angiographic data, and divided between clips with bipolar coagulation of the cut ends. Arterial feeders can usually be identified as they enter the dural sheath in the lateral gutter. The cut end of the artery attached to the AVM is then used as a "handle" to aid in the further subarachnoidal dissection and removal of the AVM mass "in toto." If the lesion has subpial and intramedullary extensions, these can be pursued using a combination of bipolar coagulation to shrink bulging vascular components and both sharp and blunt dissection with microprobes and dissectors. Intramedullary AVMs fed mainly from the anterior spinal artery or by anteriorly placed vessels such as the vertebral artery branches to the anterior spinal artery as seen in one of our cases may have to be approached via a careful median myelotomy and extraction from within the cord with careful attention to preservation of the anterior spinal artery as described by Yasargil.[18] Although this is often possible in the cervical region where high-flow lesions tend to be more compact, more caudally placed thoracolumbar lesions may be only subtotally resectable because of extensive anterior intramedullary portions.[12]

Our increasing experience with these lesions over the past decade and a half has not eased the difficulties one faces with these highly variable lesions. Resection of a dorsally placed low-flow extramedullary lesion with exact correspondance of angiographic and surgical anatomy is usually an "easy" case and an undoubtedly joyful microneurosurgical experience. The high-flow AVM with major intramedullary and anteriorly placed components and dense cicatricial attachments to normal structures remains a major challenge to the neurosurgeon, and although increasing experience frequently converts the "impossible" to the merely "difficult" case, the hazards to the patient are correspondingly much greater. Our only mortality in this series occurred in such a case (No. 82 in our series) in which after a subtotal resection of a large lesion under total circulatory arrest and hypothermia, death occurred owing to cardiac tamponade by hemoparicardium. A similar case with an AVM at the cervicomedullary junction causing quadriplegia and respiratory failure was, however, successfully treated under deep hypothermia (16°C) and total circulatory arrest for 45 minutes. At his third anniversary the patient is ambulatory and able to work on his farm, although with minimal residual weakness on the right side of the body. Two extramedullary and extraspinal recurrences have been successfully excised.

We believe that emoblization is an effective preoperative technique to facilitate surgical resection of difficult lesions probably by converting high-flow to low-flow lesions. It may be quite useful as the only recourse in patients with previous incomplete surgery, with severe arachnoiditis making further surgery hazardous. In a few low-flow cases with solitary feeders, embolization may well succeed in effectively occluding and preventing revascularization of the lesion and in experienced hands may be considered as part of the angiographic session. Recent advances in catheter and embolic material technology may well expand the contribution of embolization to the improved management of such lesions. In particular, the use of controlled intraoperative obliteration of flow in complicated high-flow lesions with quick setting polymers may be a useful addition to our armamentarium.

References

1. Aminoff MJ: Spinal Angiomas (with contributions by Logue V, Kendall BE). Blackwell Scientific Publications, Oxford, London and Edinburgh, 1976
2. Aminoff MJ, Barnard RO, Logue V: The pathophysiology of spinal vascular malformation. J Neurol Sci 23:255–263, 1974
3. Djindjian Michael: Le Traitement Chirurgical des Angiomes Intra-Medullaires. Thesis, University of Paris, 1976
4. Djindjian R, Hurth M, Houdart R: L'angiographie de la Moelle Epiniere (English Text by L. Kricheff). Masson & Cie, Editeurs, Paris, 1970
5. Doppman JL, DiChiro G, Ommaya AK: Selective Arteriography of the Spinal Cord. Warren H Green Inc, St Louis, 1969
6. Doppman JL, DiChiro G, Ommaya AK: Percutaneous embolization of spinal cord arteriovenous malformations. J Neurosurg 34:48–55, 1971
7. Doppman JL, Wirth FP, DiChiro G, Ommaya AK: Value of cutaneous angiomas in the arteriographic localization of spinal cord arteriovenous malformations N Engl J Med 281:1440–1444, 1969
8. Gaupp J: Casustische Beiträge zur pathologischen Anatomie des Rückenmarks und seiner Häute. Beitr Path Anat 2:510–524, 1888
9. Hebold O: Aneurysmen der kliensten Rückenmarkgefässe. Arch Psychiat Nervenk 16:813–823. 1885
10. Kaufman H, Ommaya AK, et al: "Compression vs. Steal." The pathogenesis of symptoms in arteriovenous malformations of the spinal cord. Arch Neurol 23:173–178, 1970
11. Ommaya AK: Arteriovenous Malformations of the Spinal Cord. In Youmans J (ed.): Textbook of Neurosurgery. 1973, pp 852–862
12. Ommaya AK: Surgery for arteriovenous malformations of the spinal cord (spinal angiomas) In: Modern Techniques in Surgery. Neurosurgery. 34. Installment VI. Ed. J. Ransohoff, Futura Publishing Co. N.Y. 1984
13. Ommaya AK, DiChiro G, Doppman JL: Ligation of arterial supply in the treatment of spinal cord arteriovenous malformations. J Neurosurg 30:679–692, 1969
14. Pia HW, Djindjian R (eds.): Spinal Angiomas: Advances in Diagnosis and Therapy. Springer-Verlag. Berlin, Heidelberg, and New York, 1978
15. Pia HW, Vogelsany H: Diagnose und Therapie der Spinalen Angiome. Dtsch Z Nervenheilk 187:74. 1965
16. Turnbull IM: Blood Supply of the Spinal Cord. In Vinken PJ, Bruyn GW (eds.): Handbook of Clinical Neurology Vol 12. Amsterdam, North Holland, 1972, pp 478–491
17. Wirth FP, Post KD, DiChiro G, Doppman J, Ommaya AK: Foix-Alajonanine disease: Spontaneous thrombosis of a spinal cord arteriovenous malformation. Neurology 210:1114–1118, 1970
18. Yasargil MG, DeLong WB, Guarnuschelli JJ: Complete microsurgical excision of cervical extramedullary and intramedullary malformations. Surg Neurol 4:211–224, 1975

8

Treatment of Carotid Cavernous and Vertebral Fistulas

Gerard Debrun

Carotid Cavernous Fistulas

Introduction

The first reported case of carotid cavernous fistula was a cavernous aneurysm ruptured in the cavernous sinus.[4,5] Benjamin Travers published this case in 1811. It was thought, however, that the cause of pulsating exophthalmos was aneurysm of the cavernous carotid siphon.

Baron of France presented before the Anatomical Society of Paris in 1835 the first specimen of aneurysm of the internal carotid artery ruptured in the cavernous sinus. Delens in his 1870 thesis reported on two of Nelaton's cases of traumatic carotid cavernous fistulas. These first cases were treated by carotid ligation, but the mortality was very high and few cases were cured.

Etiology

There are two different groups of carotid cavernous fistulas, spontaneous and traumatic. The spontaneous are more prevalent in women and elderly people. Pregnancy seems to have some influence on their onset. Traumatic cases happen with an equal frequency to men and women, which was not true some decades ago when men were more exposed to trauma than women. Traumatic fistulas are, in fact, a rare complication of all significant head injuries. They are often associated with basal skull fractures and rarely with a penetrating injury through the orbit.

Anatomy is different in traumatic and spontaneous cases. In spontaneous cases some fistulas probably develop on the basis of rupture of a preexisting subclinoid aneurysm. However, although cavernous aneurysm is not unusual, a complicating fistula is exceptional.

Sugar proposed that the residual remnant of the primitive trigeminal artery might be the basis of the development of an aneurysm at this site (Fig. 8.1). This case (Fig. 8.1 A,B,C) of C.C. fistula associated to a trigeminal artery, is courtesy of Dr. Berenstein (N.Y.U.). Figure 8.10A shows another case of traumatic C.C. fistula that we treated as surgery and where an hypoglossal artery reconstituted the internal carotid artery after surgical occlusion of the internal carotid with a Selverstone clamp. Most spontaneous cases are more likely a type of dural arteriovenous malformation when one thinks of the rich anastomotic plexus that normally exists between meningeal branches of the carotid siphon and meningeal branches of the external carotid artery. In these cases, selective angiography of the internal carotid artery often demonstrates many tiny branches from the carotid siphon opacifying the cavernous sinus.

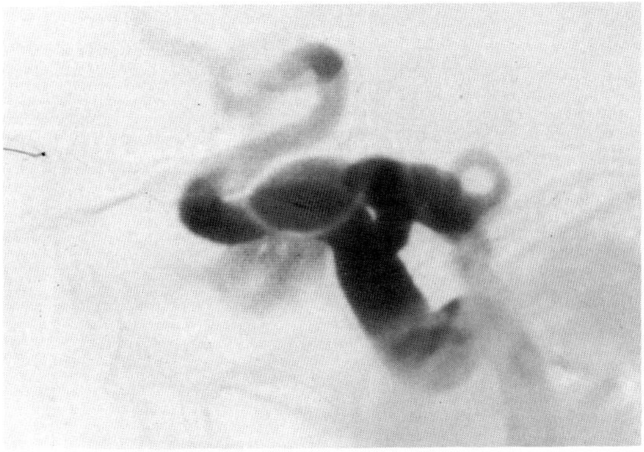

A

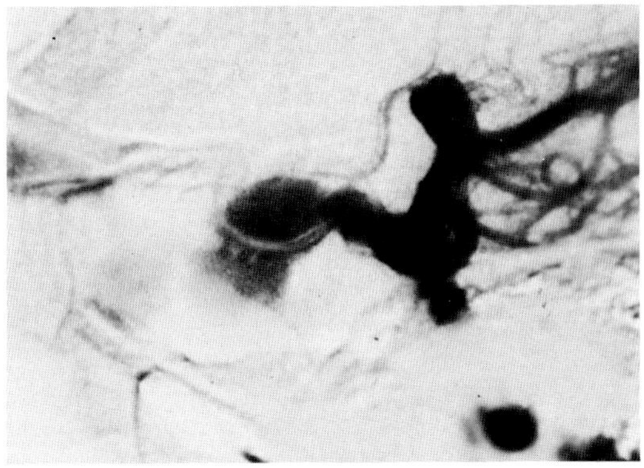

B

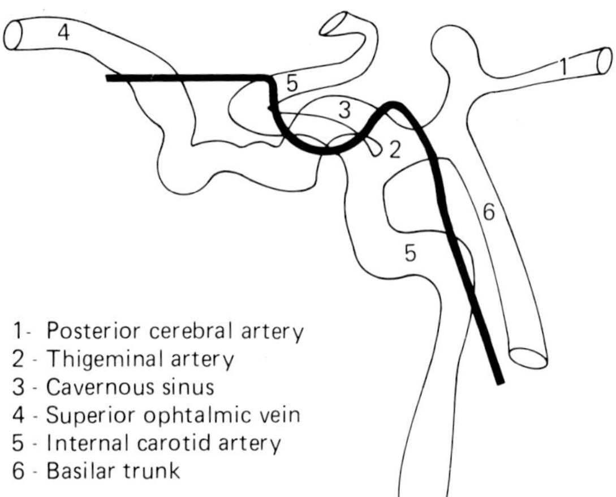

C

Fig. 8.1. Left traumatic carotid cavernous fistula associated with trigeminal artery. (Courtesy of Dr. Berenstein, New York University). **A.** Carotid angiography. The trigeminal artery opacifies both basilar trunk and cavernous sinus. **B.** Vertebral angiography. The trigeminal artery opacifies cavernous sinus and the superior ophthalmic vein. **C.** Drawing from superposition of both films.

Similarly, many meningeal branches from the internal maxillary artery and its meningeal branches, and occasionally from the ascending pharyngeal artery, can be shown on hyperselective angiography of external carotid branches.

Bilateral spontaneous carotid cavernous fistulas are not rare, with cross filling from one side to the other and without logical correlation with the side of the exophthalmos. In traumatic cases arterial rents of 2 to 4 mm have been illustrated. In Nelaton's first case as reported by Delens in his thesis, the artery was almost completely divided by the splinter of bone.

Anatomic specimens are rare and difficult to study. In 1950 Taptas reviewed 48 autopsy cases. In 22 cases he could not find the fistula and wrongly concluded that it did not exist in every case. In most cases the hole of the fistula is on the posterior ascending portion of the cavernous carotid or on the horizontal portion. The fact that the hole of the fistula can be occluded with a single balloon proves that the hole is unique (Fig. 8.2A–C). However, in my experience of 75 cases of traumatic carotid cavernous fistulas, there was one case where the principal hole was occluded with one balloon, but there were two or three tiny branches more proximal in the carotid siphon which communicated with the cavernous sinus (Figs. 8.3A–D). This type of traumatic fistula where many branches of the siphon are torn and cause the fistula is probably very uncommon. As these branches are normally anastomosed to meningeal branches of the external carotid artery, one realizes that selective external angiography may be necessary even in traumatic cases. Venous drainage depends partially on the location of the fistula. Anterior fistulas induce the most impressive exophthalmos, and the ophthalmic veins are widely distended. When the fistula is posterior, the exophthalmos can be minimal, even with a huge shunt. The superior and inferior petrosal sinuses are widely open. The contralateral cavernous sinus frequently fills (Fig. 8.4).

From the size of the cavernous sinus seen on the angiogram, it is impossible to predict the

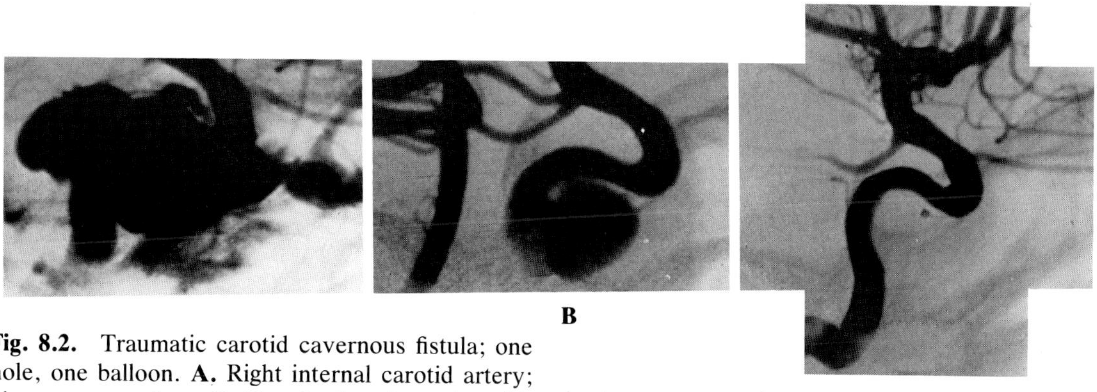

Fig. 8.2. Traumatic carotid cavernous fistula; one hole, one balloon. **A.** Right internal carotid artery; big cavernous sinus. **B.** Vertebral angiography with compression of right carotid in the neck. Retrograde opacification of the siphon, then of the fistula, and of cavernous sinus. **C.** One balloon has been detached in the cavernous sinus. Balloon is inflated with silicone and totally occludes the hole. The carotid artery is well preserved. Same stable results 6 months later.

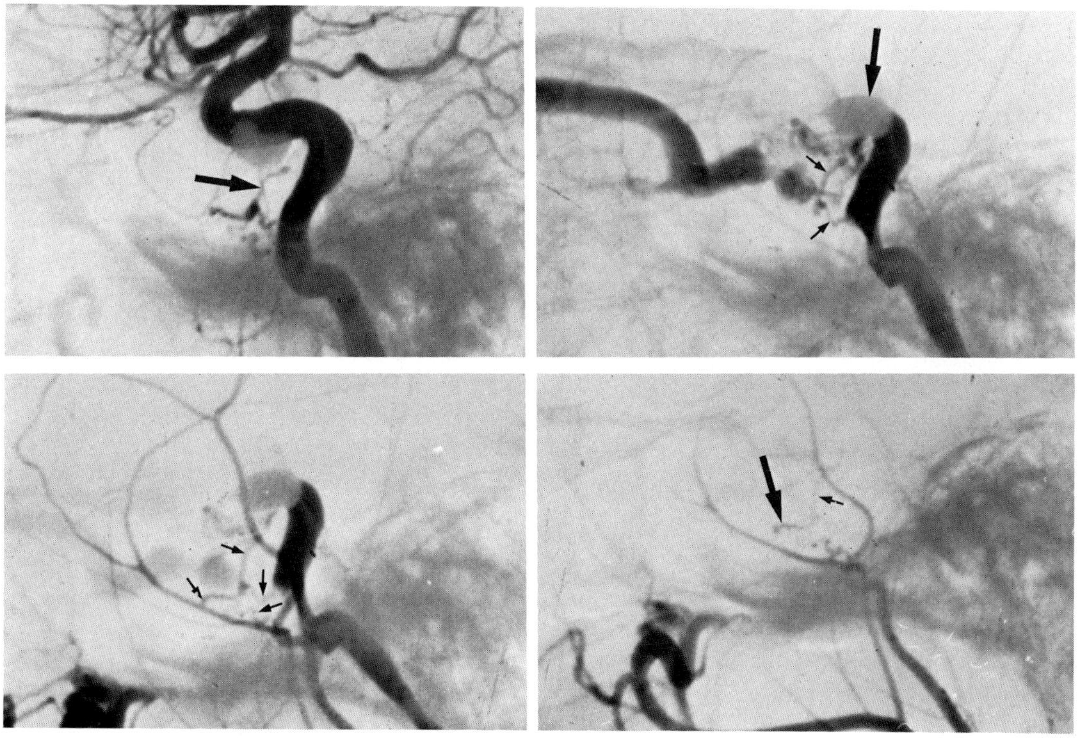

Fig. 8.3. Traumatic carotid cavernous fistula. Fistula treated with one balloon in the cavernous sinus. Excellent immediate result. Recurrence of the fistula 1 month later. **A.** Detached balloon occludes main hole of the fistula. There is, however, a tiny branch of the carotid siphon that still fills (*arrow*) without opacification of the cavernous sinus. **B.** One month later, the fistula has recurred. The balloon detached in the cavernous sinus is now totally deflated (it was filled with iodine contrast) and is not visible. This picture is obtained with another balloon catheter. To get a good selective opacification of the fistula, balloon (*arrow*) is inflated in the carotid siphon, immediately distal to new fistula. Contrast is injected into the internal carotid artery. The same abnormal vessel fills (*small arrow*). **C.** Because of transient occlusion of the siphon by the balloon, there is reflux of contrast in the external carotid artery. Anastomosis between external meningeal branch and siphon collaterals (*arrow*). **D.** Balloon is deflated and removed. Selective external carotid angiography demonstrates communication of meningeal branch (*arrow*) with collateral of the siphon (*small arrow*).

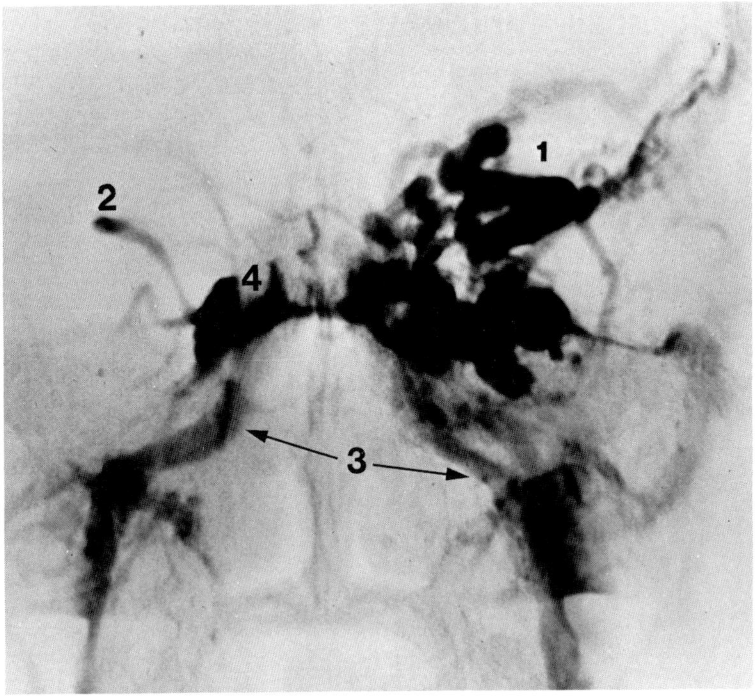

Fig. 8.4. Venous drainage of left traumatic carotid cavernous fistula. The fistula drains mainly through left side, but also through right cavernous sinus. *1*. Left superior ophthalmic vein, *2*. right superior ophthalmic vein, *3*. both inferior petrosal sinus, *4*. right cavernous sinus.

size of the fistula and the number of balloons that will be needed, because we can overlook partitions within the sinus. Casts of normal cavernous sinuses have shown a plexus of veins, but in cases of carotid cavernous fistulas, these veins are extremely dilated and the partitions of the sinus more or less ruptured, especially in long-term untreated cases. The angiogram only shows the overall size of the cavernous sinus when the shunt is fast, and it is at the time of treatment with a balloon catheter that we know the number of balloons needed to occlude the fistula. Also unknown is the necessary volume of the balloon, even if only one is needed to occlude the fistula.

Clinical Presentation

Traumatic carotid cavernous fistulas present as the following:

1. Pulsating exophthalmos and bruit appear immediately or weeks after trauma. Exophthalmos, edema of the eyelids, and chemosis are sometimes very impressive and more severe than in spontaneous cases. Pictures of the eye must be taken before treatment.
2. Diplopia is often present owing to paresis of the sixth nerve. Less often there is complete ophthalmoplegia with paresis of the fourth and third nerves. These findings must be carefully noted before starting treatment that may induce oculomotor palsy.
3. Some patients complain of pain in the orbital and sinus area by irritation of the fifth nerve. This subjective feeling must also be noted because treatment may induce retro-orbital and facial pain during the ensuing weeks. Vision remains normal during weeks or months and then gradually decreases. It is important to note the degree of vision at the time of treatment. Rarely the optic nerve will have been damaged by a spur of bone and the eye blinded.

Spontaneous carotid cavernous fistulas present as the following:

1. Pulsating exophthalmos, chemosis, and bruit are often minimal.
2. Patients are often elderly, with women more often afflicted than men.
3. Bilateral fistulas are encountered more often than in traumatic cases.
4. In this type of fistula there is often contralateral venous drainage and pulsating exophthalmos on one side; this does not prove that the fistula is on that side.

5. Both internal and external selective angiograms on both sides are absolutely necessary.
6. When treatment is decided because of intolerable pain or bruit, keep in mind that spontaneous healing occurs more frequently in spontaneous cases than in traumatic cases.

Radiologic Evaluation

As vertebral angiography is always necessary, the radiologic evaluation of a carotid cavernous fistula is better achieved by Seldinger's technique through the femoral artery. A heparin-coated 5 Fr. catheter is directed to the internal carotid artery on the side of the pulsating exophthalmos and bruit. Using an automatic syringe, 10 ml of contrast material is injected in 1 second. Lateral films can be coned on the area of interest. Anteroposterior films are coned transorbital views. The number of films per second depends on many factors. In institutions where magnification is routinely used, no more than two films per second might be taken. With most film changers, without magnification, it is risky to get more than four films per second, and six films per second are exceptional. With this cadence, the cavernous sinus fills very quickly, and the exact location of the fistula can hardly be determined. At that time it is possible to analyze the type of venous drainage—anterior with big ophthalmic veins, posterior with big inferior and superior petrosal veins, or both. It is also worthwhile to note that some fistulas, where the steal is fast and massive, fail to opacify the internal carotid artery above the level of the fistula (Fig. 8.5A). In such a case the location of the fistula is easier to predict, but the mistake would be to think that the internal carotid is not functional above the level of the fistula and that the only treatment is to occlude the siphon at the level of the fistula with a Fogarty catheter without trying to save the carotid artery. When attempting to occlude the artery at the level of the fistula, one must be sure that the fistula does not fill from above. One can realize this risk by getting a vertebral angiogram or contralateral carotid angiogram with compression of the carotid artery on the side of the fistula. In most cases the fistula gets blood from above through the posterior communicating artery or through the anterior communicating artery or through both, and the carotid siphon above the level of the fistula is retrogradely opacified until the level of the fistula, which is nicely demonstrated (Figs. 8.5B,C). This is to say that contralateral carotid angiogram and vertebral angiogram with ipsilateral compression of the carotid artery are needed in all cases to demonstrate the location and size of the fistula and to demonstrate the quality of the communicating arteries in cases where it is decided to occlude the carotid siphon. The aim of modern treatment of a fistula is to always save the carotid artery, either by detachable balloon technique or by surgery of the cavernous sinus.

When the vertebral angiography with compression of the carotid artery in the neck fails to demonstrate the location and size of the fistula (this happens in only 5% of cases), it is possible to use a double lumen 5 Fr. balloon catheter, which is maneuvered inside the introducer. The balloon is inflated above the tip of the introducer at the C2 or C3 level until it occludes the internal carotid (Fig. 8.6A). Contrast material is injected through the other lumen and slowly fills the fistula. If while attempting to enter the fistula with the balloon we do not immediately penetrate the cavernous sinus with the detachable balloon, we can inflate it at different places of the carotid siphon and each time inject some contrast material in the carotid artery. If the balloon is inflated below the fistula or occludes it, the angiogram shows occlusion of the internal carotid artery. If the balloon is above the fistula, the angiogram shows fast opacification of the cavernous sinus and no opacification of the carotid artery above the fistula. Bilateral external carotid angiograms are also necessary. In traumatic cases the external carotid angiogram is generally normal. In the rare cases where small siphon branches are torn in the cavernous sinus and sectioned, distal branches of the external carotid can be demonstrated. In spontaneous fistulas, some tiny branches of the carotid siphon communicate with the cavernous sinus and are demonstrated by selective internal carotid angiogram. There are also often tiny meningeal vessels from the internal maxillary artery demonstrated by hyperselective external angiogram (Fig. 8.7). As injection of hypertonic contrast material into the external carotid artery is painful, isotonic contrast material is better tolerated; 2 ml/second is enough, with a

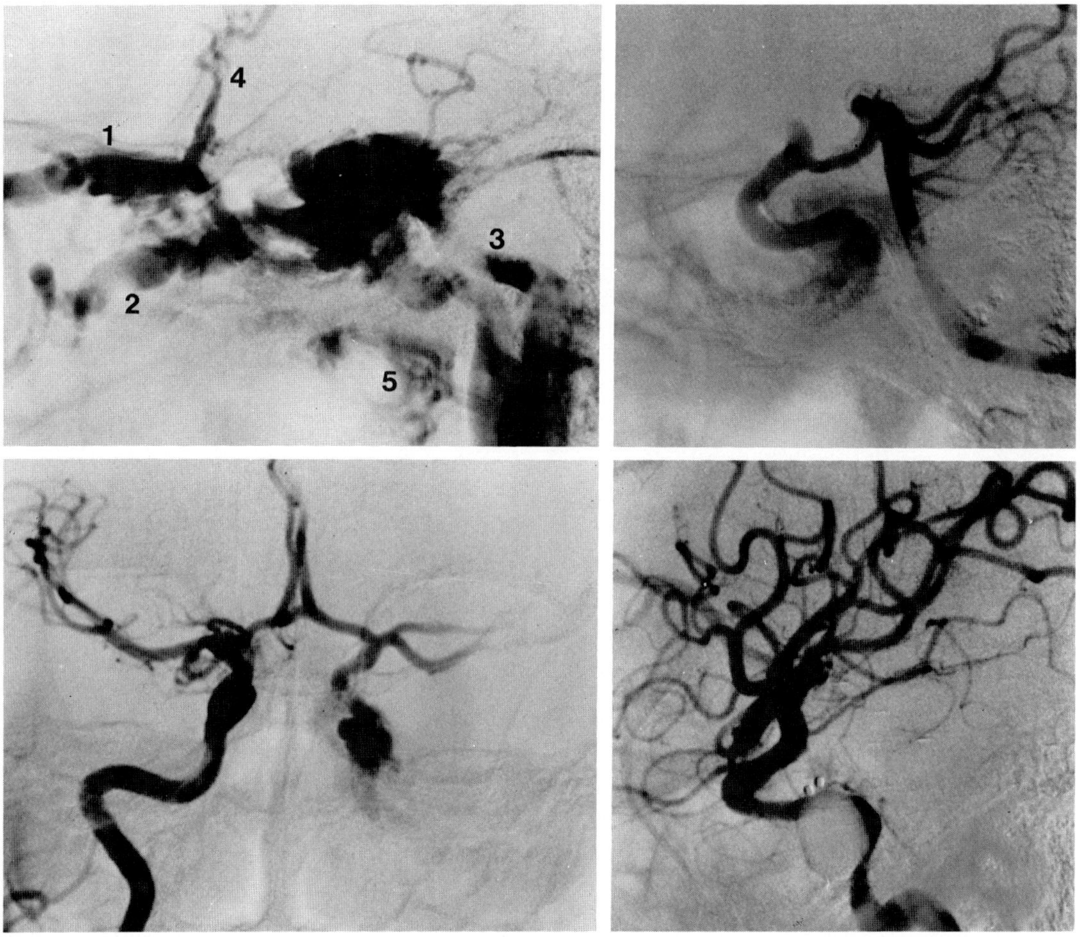

A B C D

Fig. 8.5. Left traumatic carotid cavernous fistula. Total steal. **A.** Left internal carotid angiography. Total steal without opacification of the siphon above the fistula. It does not prove that the carotid artery is occluded above the fistula. *1.* Superior ophthalmic vein, *2.* inferior ophthalmic vein, *3.* inferior petrosal sinus, *4.* middle cerebral vein, *5.* pterygoid plexus. **B.** Vertebral angiography with compression of left carotid in the neck. The distal portion of the siphon now fills and we get the level of the fistula. **C.** Right carotid angiography with compression of left carotid in the neck demonstrates both a good cross filling and retrograde opacification of the siphon until the fistula. **D.** Occlusion of the fistula with two balloons detached in the cavernous sinus. The siphon above the fistula fills now nicely.

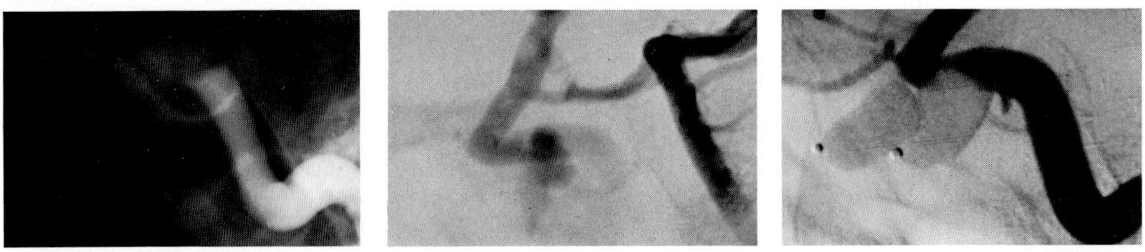

A B,C

Fig. 8.6. Demonstration of the location of the fistula by two different methods. **A.** Double-lumen balloon catheter inflated in the internal carotid artery and occluding it; through the second lumen, injection of contrast material. The fistula is located where we loose the picture of the siphon. **B.** Vertebral angiography with compression of the carotid in the neck (on the side of the fistula); retrograde filling. **C.** Occlusion of the fistula with two balloons detached in the cavernous sinus.

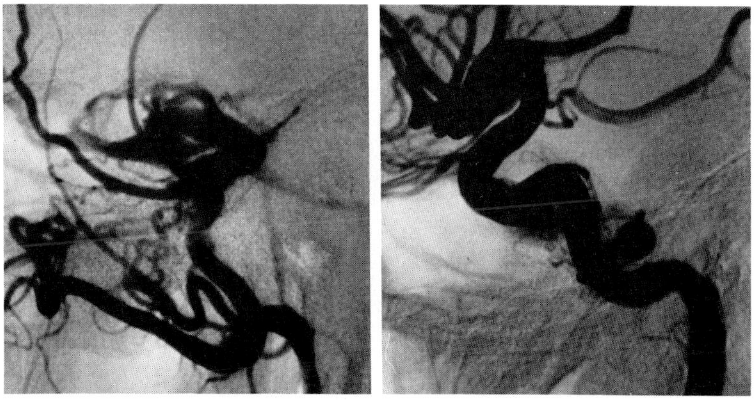

Fig. 8.7. Spontaneous carotid cavernous fistula **A.** Selective angiography of internal maxillary artery. Meningeal branches get the dura of the cavernous sinus. **B.** Selective internal carotid angiography. Network of meangiography. Network of meningeal branches of the siphon getting the cavernous sinus.

total injection of 8 ml. The balance of participating carotid siphon and external carotid branches is different from one case to the other. In some instances the only feeders of the fistula are branches of the external carotid artery, frequently including the ascending pharyngeal artery as well as the middle meningeal artery and distal branches of the internal maxillary artery.

When evaluating a carotid cavernous fistula, the status of the bifurcation of the carotid artery must be carefully noted, because stenosis or distorted origin of the internal carotid would complicate catheterization. In the same way, severe kinking or a complete loop of the internal carotid artery in the neck are of major importance because the treatment by balloon catheter becomes more difficult and risky. On rare occasions, the internal carotid in the neck has been dissected by the injury, and this lesion could be a contraindication to balloon catheterization.

Treatment of a Traumatic Carotid Cavernous Fistula

The many different types of procedures that have been proposed can be divided into two groups. The first group consists of all procedures that occlude the fistula but that sacrifice the internal carotid artery. Among these are the following:

1. Ligature of the internal carotid artery at the level of the anterior clinoid process, with or without ligature of the ophthalmic artery, associated with ligature of the internal carotid artery in the neck, without or with embolization of the fistula.
2. Occlusion of the carotid siphon with a nondetachable balloon (Fogarty's or Prolo's catheter) catheter or with a detachable balloon. The balloon is long enough to completely occlude the neck of the fistula and the cavernous carotid.

These two types of procedures are possible when the anterior communicating or posterior communicating arteries are widely open. Otherwise, if the patient does not tolerate occlusion of the carotid artery an external carotid to internal carotid bypass has to be done before occlusion of the siphon.

The second group of procedures occludes the fistula and saves the carotid artery. All these techniques have been made possible by tremendous improvement in the surgical approach to the cavernous sinus, in anesthesiology, and in the hyperselective catheterization of external and internal carotid arteries.

1. Surgical approach to the cavernous sinus: Mullan[11] nicely demonstrated that the cavernous sinus could be packed by different techniques, i.e., through the superior ophthalmic vein at its entrance to the cavernous sinus when the fistula is anterior or through the superior petrosal sinus when the fistula drains posteriorly (Fig. 8.8). The lateral wall of the cavernous sinus can be punctured with small needles and the sinus packed with phosphor-bronze wire. The neck of the fistula can be occluded with thrombogenic needles. These techniques induce thrombosis of the cavernous sinus with occlusion of the fistula. They are simpler than direct ligature of the fistula done in some cases by Parkinson[12] but with deep hypothermia and under

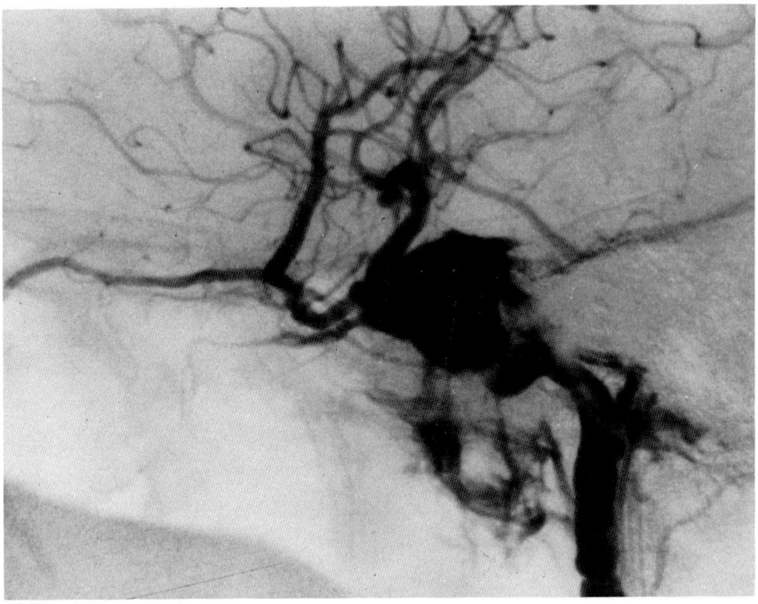

Fig. 8.8. Left traumatic carotid cavernous fistula; posterior venous drainage. The left superior ophthalmic vein is not dilated. The patient had no proptosis, nor chemosis.

cardiac arrest. One case of bilateral carotid cavernous fistula was successfully treated by Charles Drake who packed both cavernous sinuses with pieces of muscle (Fig. 8.9A–D).

Hosobuchi[5] gets electrothrombosis of the cavernous sinus. I treated three cases of traumatic carotid cavernous fistulas with the collaboration of neurosurgeons (two cases with Charles Drake and one case with Roberto Heros). Two of the three cases were treated 15 and 20 years earlier by occlusion of the internal carotid with a Selverstone clamp. In the first case balloons were detached in the cavernous sinus at surgery by direct puncture of the cavernous sinus (Fig. 8.10), and peculiarly, the internal carotid was reconstituted through a hypoglossal artery. The second case was cured with balloons inflated and detached in the cavernous sinus through two different surgical approaches: retrogradely through the C1 portion of the carotid siphon after clipping the internal carotid above the anterior clinoid process and below the posterior communicating artery. Only one balloon could be introduced into the cavernous sinus through this route. The internal carotid was exposed in the neck above the Selverstone clamp, catheterized, and the fistula treated with two detachable balloons.

2. Intravascular navigation with a balloon catheter: The cavernous sinus can be reached with a balloon catheter maneuvered through the veins or through the internal carotid artery.
   a. Through the veins: When the superior ophthalmic vein is widely dilated, it is desirable to get to the cavernous sinus by percutaneous puncture or cut down of the angular vein (Fig. 8.11). Passing all the curves of the superior ophthalmic vein with a balloon catheter can be a difficult, if not impossible, task. However, Peterson[13] treated some cases with catheterization of the superior ophthalmic vein with an insulated copper wire. When the inferior petrosal sinus is dilated in a case of posterior fistula, it is possible to catheterize the origin of the pertrosal vein with a 7 or 8 Fr. introducer bent at the tip. The jugular vein has to be catheterized either from the femoral vein with a 90-cm introducer or through the neck by direct puncture of the jugular vein and catheterization with a sheath-type Cordis No. 7 or 8 Fr. The introducer is then easily maneuvered through the sheath. When one has reached the inferior petrosal sinus, it becomes easy to retrogradely reach the cavernous sinus with the balloon catheter. Using this method, Mullan[11] successfully occluded one case of fistula while preserving the internal

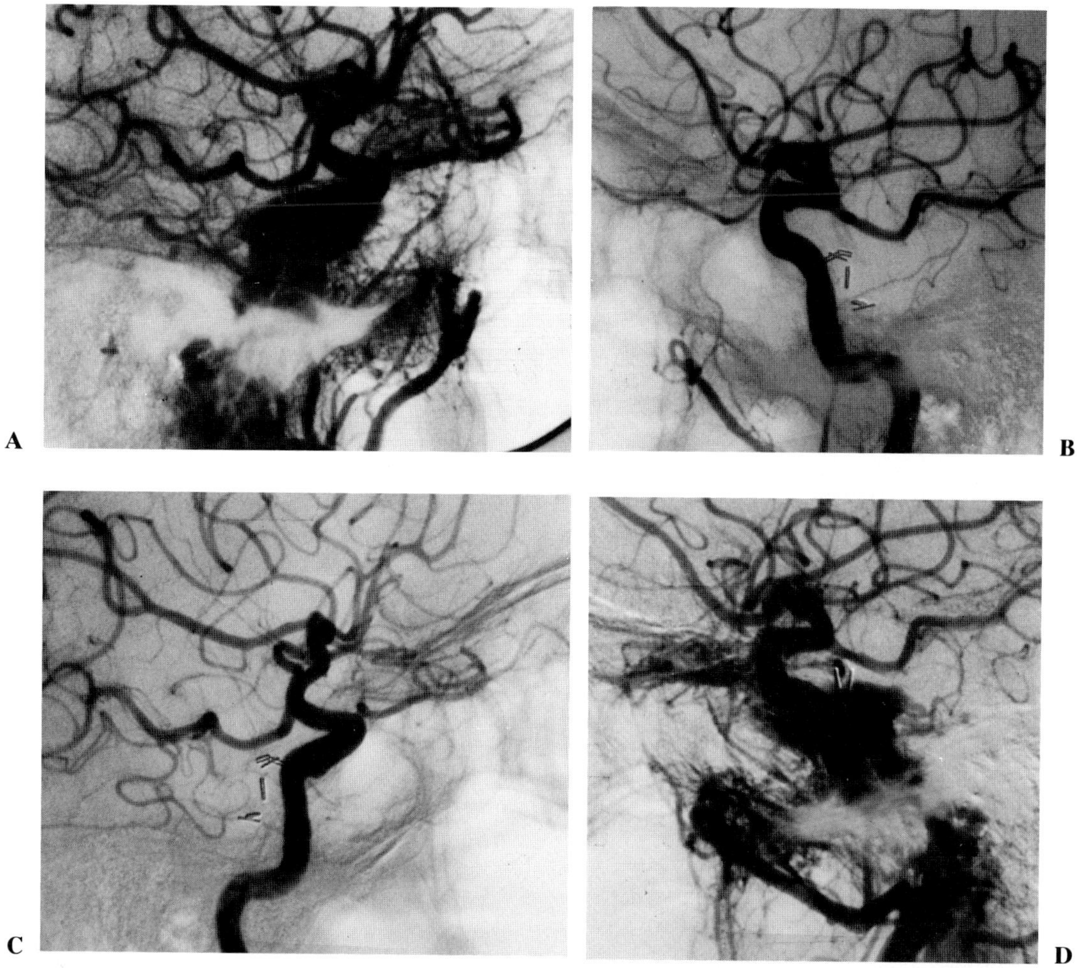

Fig. 8.9. Bilateral spontaneous carotid cavernous fistula in a 73-year-old lady. Packing of both cavernous sinus with pieces of muscle by Dr. Charles Drake. **A.** Fistula on the right side. **B.** Fistula on the left side. **C.** After packing of the right cavernous sinus. Normal internal carotid. No fistula. **D.** After packing of the left cavernous sinus. Normal internal carotid. No fistula.

carotid. In two cases I have succeeded in reaching the cavernous sinus to occlude the fistula. In several cases attempts to reach the neck of the fistula failed because of partitions of the cavernous sinus. The balloon reaches the posterior compartment relatively easily but fails to move forward. Manelfe[9] successfully treated one patient through the venous approach.

When the venous drainage of a fistula is predominantly posterior with a dilated inferior petrosal sinus of 3 mm in diameter or more, the first step should be to occlude the fistula from the venous side, which is an extremely elegant and safe procedure.

b. Balloon Catheter Maneuver Through the Internal Carotid Artery

Different types of balloon catheters corresponding to two different techniques can be used to maneuver through the internal carotid artery. One is the detachable balloon catheter first described by Serbinenko[14] and then modified and used by myself.[1,2] The second is a calibrated leak balloon catheter[8] that permits delivery of isobutyl 2-cyanoacrylate (Bucrylate), a polymerizing acrylic substance that solidifies instantaneously when it is in contact with blood. We will describe the potential risks of this technique in detail. Other balloons have been commer-

Fig. 8.10. Traumatic carotid cavernous sinus fistula treated 15 years ago by ligation of the internal carotid artery in the neck and intracranially. **A.** Vertebral angiography: reconstitution of the internal carotid artery through an hypoglossal artery (*arrow*). **B.** Later phase of the vertebral angiography shows filling of superior ophthalmic vein. **C.** Balloon inflated with iodine and detached in the cavernous sinus after surgical exposure. Bicompartmented shape of the balloon due to partition of the cavernous sinus. **D.** Vertebral angiography of the same patient one week after treatment. The hypoglossal artery no longer fills the fistula.

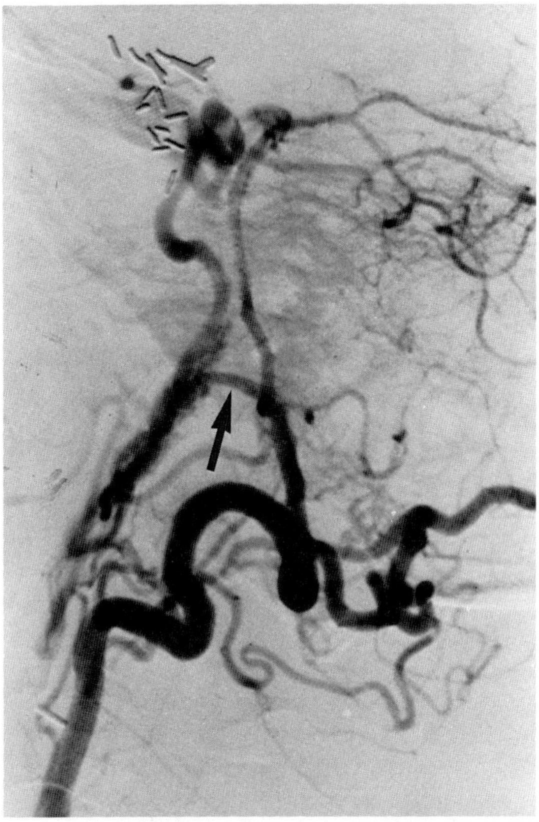

A

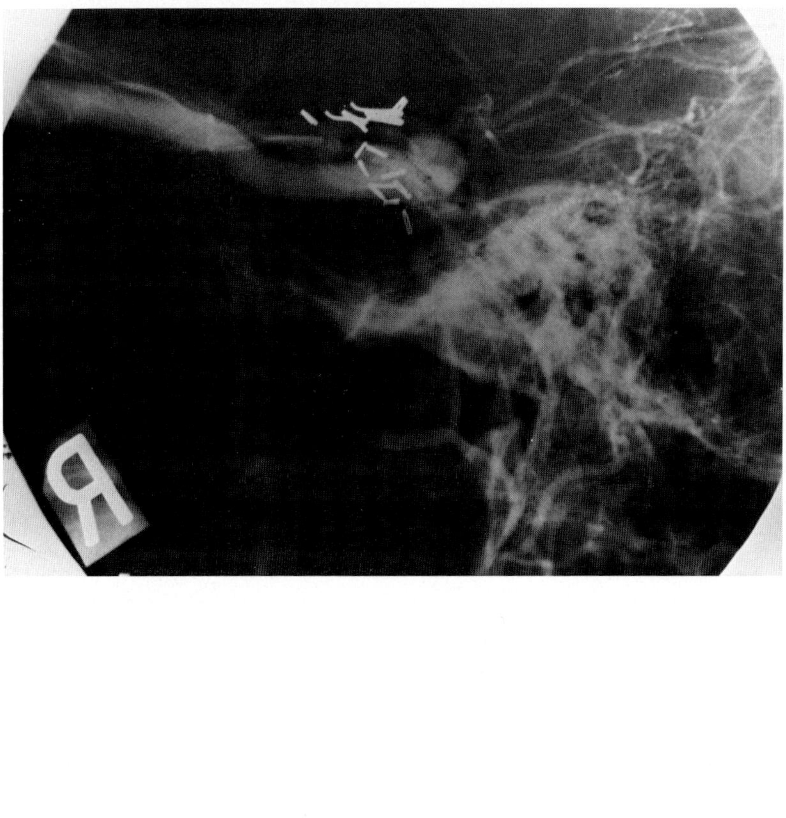

B

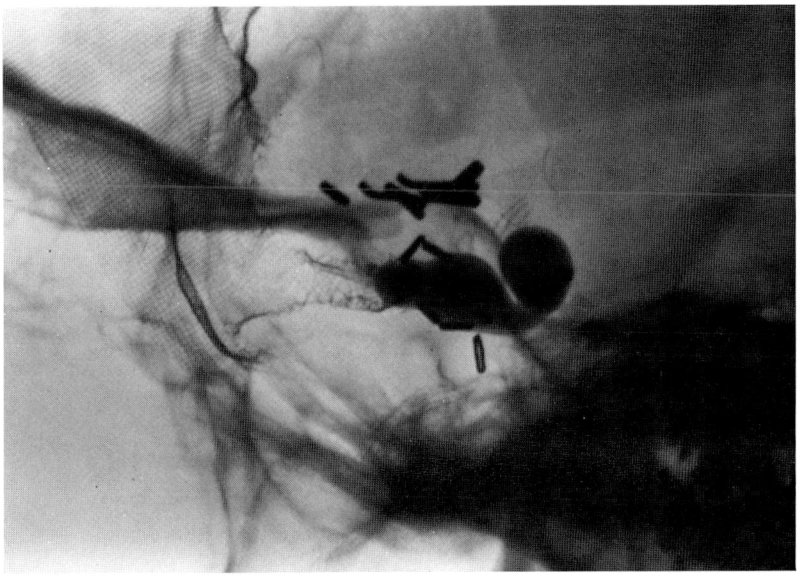

C

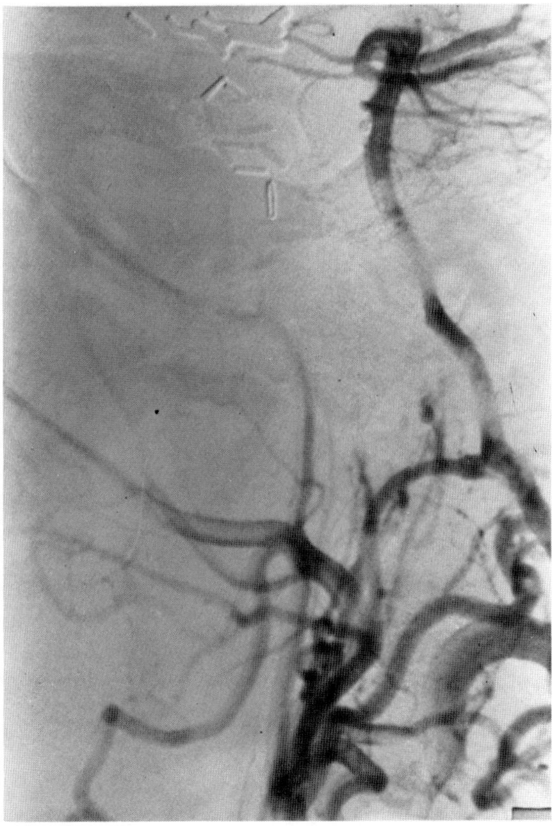

D

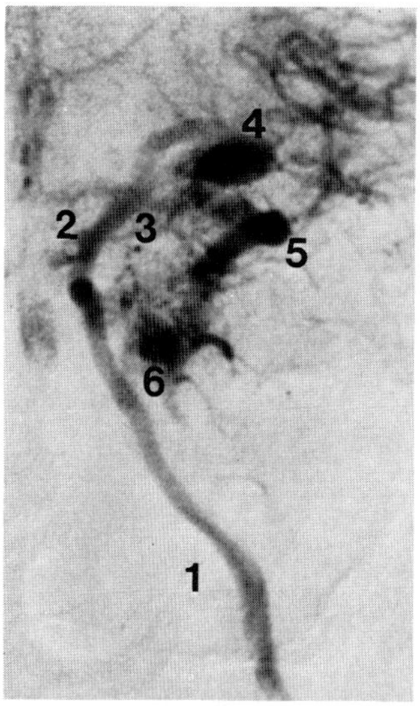

Fig. 8.11. Left carotid cavernous fistula draining anteriorly through the superior ophthalmic vein and the facial vein. It is hopeless to try to get retrogradely the cavernous sinus from the facial or angular vein. *1*. Facial vein, *2*. angular vein, *3*. origin of the superior ophthalmic vein, *4*. first loop, *5*. second loop, *6*. cavernous sinus.

cialized or are still experimental.[6,10,15,16] Our experience with these balloons is limited or nonexistent but I will describe their peculiarities and their advantages and disadvantages compared with a latex balloon.

*The Detachable Balloon Technique with Debrun's Latex Balloons**

The balloons are made from latex "fingers" of different sizes (Fig. 8.12). The diameter of the "finger" varies from 0.3 mm to 2 mm. The length of the "finger" is also variable so that one gets long or short cylindrical balloons, or even round balloons. Some "fingers" have an additional flap at the tip, where a small silver cylinder of 0.7 or 1 mm in diameter can be lodged. The balloon can be followed on the fluoroscopic screen without having to be inflated with iodine contrast.

Most of the fingers have a narrow proximal portion that grips the catheter; the balloon itself will be made of the distal expansible portion.

There are two basic types of detachable balloon. Type I (Fig. 8.13), in which the balloon is only held on the catheter by a narrow portion of the sleeve, requires no second coaxial catheter for detachment but is not self-sealing and can only be used with a polymerizing substance. Type 2, in which the balloon is tied to the catheter with latex thread, requires a second coaxial catheter for detachment but is self-sealing and can be used with iodine material or polymerizing substance as well (Fig. 8.14).

* Ingenor Laboratory, 70 Rue Orfila 75020 Paris, France.

Type 1 Balloon Catheter

The narrow portion of the sleeve simply grips the catheter through its own elasticity. One can invaginate the narrow portion into the balloon so that it grips the catheter more tightly. The advantages of this type 1 balloon are

1. The balloon is detached by simply pulling on the catheter.
2. The catheter is a double-lumen catheter made of nylon. The external diameter is 0.85 mm, and each lumen is 0.25 internal diameter.

The disadvantages of type 1 balloon are the following

1. The real danger is to detach the balloon prematurely by a maneuver such as pulling the catheter inadvertently.
2. This balloon cannot be detached when filled with iodine material because it would leak and deflate immediately. When the capacity of the balloon needed to occlude the fistula has been measured with iodine contrast, this quantity must be removed and replaced with an equal quantity of polymerizing substance. When this substance has solidified, detachment is performed by pulling the catheter. At that time there are three dangers. The first is that the balloon does not stay in the cavernous sinus and moves into the carotid artery through the neck of the fistula. The second is that damage to the neck of the fistula can result. The third is that a small bulge of solidified silicone forms at the neck of the balloon. The first danger is by far the most important.
3. This type of non-self-sealing balloon cannot be used when there is a need to detach the balloon inflated with iodine material. This occurs in three conditions explained below.

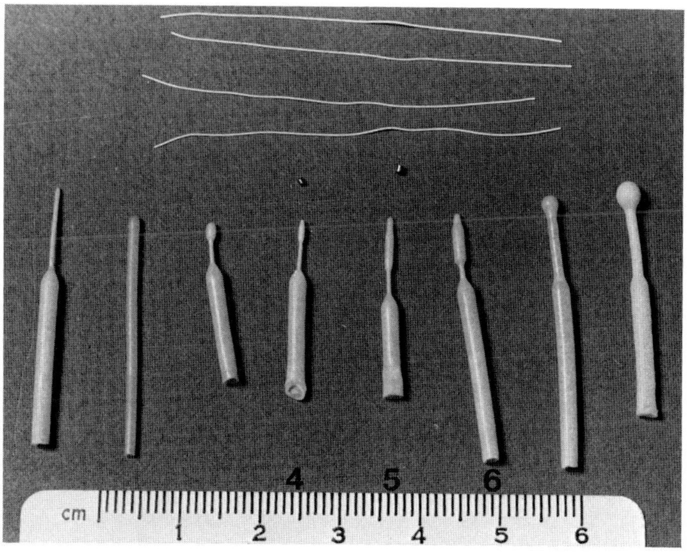

Fig. 8.12. Different types of latex fingers. Four latex threads; two silver cylinders that can be lodged in the narrow distal tip of the fingers numbers 4, 5, 6.

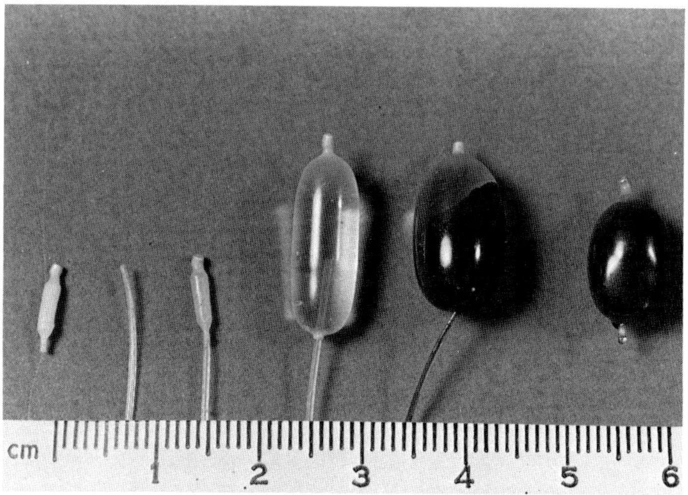

Fig. 8.13. Detachable balloon type 1. From left to right: • The sixth latex finger seen on Fig. 8.12 has been cut, keeping 2 mm of the narrow portion. The silver cylinder has been placed in the tip. • Teflon tubing 0.4 × 0.4 mm or polyethylene tubing 0.25 × 0.50 mm. • After dilatation of the narrow portion with forceps, tubing has entered the sleeve. • The balloon can be inflated with iodine contrast. • After deflating balloon and measuring its capacity, an equal quantity of silicone mixed with tantalum powder is injected. The quantity of iodine material that was inside the catheter and could not be aspirated (dead space) has been reintroduced into the balloon. • When silicone has solidified, the Teflon catheter is pulled out, the balloon is detached and generally looses its iodine contrast component.

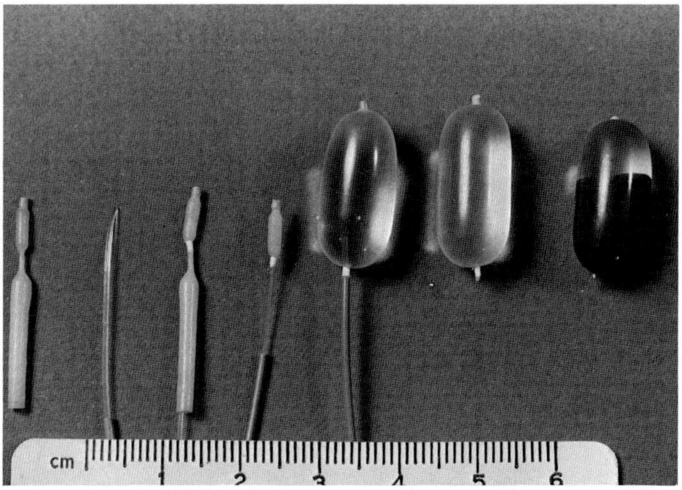

Fig. 8.14. Detachable balloon type 2. From left to right: • Latex finger with silver cylinder in its tip. • Teflon tubing 0.4 × 0.6 mm. The coaxial polyethylene tubing is seen at lower part of the Teflon tubing. • The latex finger has been ligated over the Teflon tubing with a latex thread. • Lower part of the finger below the ligature has been cut. The polyethylene coaxial catheter is visible. • Balloon is inflated with iodine contrast material. The polyethylene coaxial catheter now reaches the ligature, allowing the Teflon tubing to be pulled out without dislodging the balloon. • After detachment, the elasticity of the ligature closes the aperture of the balloon, which does not leak. • If silicone has been used, the balloon is filled with part iodine and part silicone.

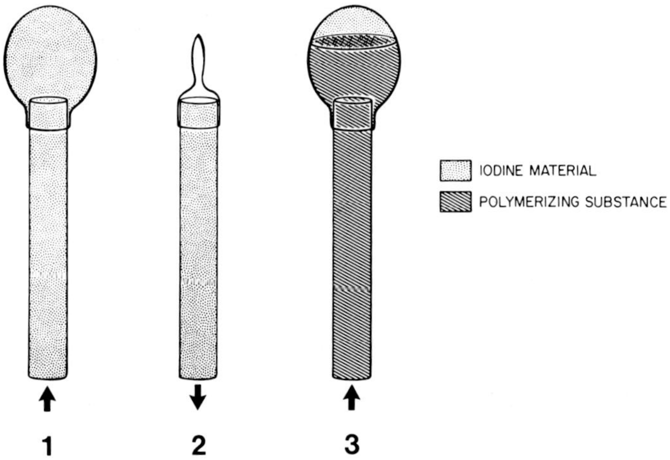

Fig. 8.15. Dead space of a single-lumen balloon Catheter. *1*. Balloon inflated with iodine material. *2*. Balloon deflated. The iodine material inside the catheter cannot be aspirated; it is the dead space of the catheter. *3*. When a polymerizing substance is injected, the iodine material in the dead space of the catheter is pushed again into the balloon. If the capacity of the balloon needed to treat the lesion is equal to the capacity of the dead space, a polymerizing substance cannot be used. The balloon has to be of type 2, inflated with iodine material, and not leaking after detachment because of the elastic thread ligature.

Type 2 Balloon Catheter

The balloon is firmly tied to the catheter with an elastic latex thread. Polyurethane tubing is not strong enough and would lengthen or rupture at the time of balloon detachment when pulling on the catheter. This is the reason to use Teflon tubing which is more resistant. Thin-wall teflon tubing is 0.4-mm internal diameter and 0.6-mm external diameter. This catheter to which the balloon is tied is called catheter A. We can get it slightly smaller and more supple by lengthening it (from 130–150 cm). To detach the balloon (which, in this type, can not be detached by simply pulling on the catheter), a second coaxial polyethylene catheter (called B) is slid up over catheter A until it is in contact with the base of the balloon, i.e., the base of the ligature. Catheter B holds the balloon in place when catheter A is withdrawn to detach it (Fig. 8.14, fifth from left to right).

The advantages of type 2 balloon are the following:

1. There is minimal risk of detaching the balloon prematurely because it is tied onto the catheter solidly.
2. The balloon is self-sealing because the elasticity of the thread is such that it closes the hole of the balloon when catheter A is withdrawn. This balloon can be filled with iodine material and detached as soon as the proper capacity of the balloon is reached. There are three situations where such a balloon is needed. First, when the capacity of the balloon needed to occlude the fistula is inferior or equal to the dead space of the single lumen catheter A (Fig. 8.15). Second, when the balloon is difficult to lodge at the proper place to occlude the fistula and is drawn away by the flow when it is deflated. It becomes risky to inject a polymerizing substance that could solidify before the balloon has been correctly located. Third, when the fistula needs many balloons to be occluded. In one case I had to detach four balloons; in a second case, three; and in two other cases, two balloons. Serbinenko showed me one case where he detached 17 balloons (personal communication, Oct. 1975). If all the balloons are filled with a polymerizing substance, the cavernous sinus will remain a huge expansive process. The oculomotor nerves will be generally compressed and oculomotor palsies will occur. If the cavernous sinus stays under pressure, terrible pain can occur. The final result is much better if all the balloons but the last one are filled with iodine material, because they will progressively return to normal size. The oculomotor palsies, if any, will improve more quickly. The major disadvantage of type 2 balloon is the need of a second coaxial catheter B to detach the balloon.

Single-Lumen Catheter A or Double-Lumen Catheter A

The problem of catheter dead space has already been mentioned (Fig. 8.15). With a single-lumen catheter, the ideal would be to start from the beginning with injection of a low-viscous radiopaque polymerizing substance that would remain liquid until some drops of catalyst were added. This idea is impractical because the proportion of polymerizing substance and catalyst must be very precise and well mixed. How can one properly mix the polymerizing substance that remains in the single-lumen catheter when the balloon is deflated?

It becomes obvious that a double-lumen catheter (Fig. 8.16) allows us to work with iodine material as long as is needed and then to inject the polymerizing substance through one lumen while the iodine material previously in this lumen is pushed into the balloon and immediately aspirated through the second lumen. Manipulation is very precise and delicate, but the final result is a balloon totally filled with the solidified polymerizing substance, whatever its size. The disadvantage of a double-lumen catheter will always be its size and its rigidity compared with a single-lumen catheter.

Because of the external diameter of the double-lumen catheter, which is close to 1 mm, it becomes difficult to use a coaxial catheter. It is a type 1 balloon catheter with all its advantages and disadvantages.

Balloons Filled With Iodine Material or With a Polymerizing Substance

The indications for use of a detachable balloon filled with iodine material rather than with silicone have been discussed. The follow-up of the

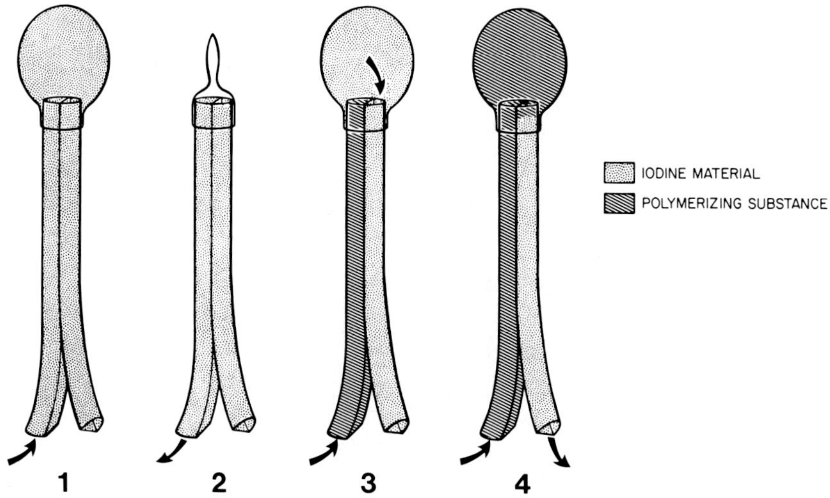

Fig. 8.16. Double-lumen catheter allows detachment of a balloon filled only with polymerizing substance. *1*. Both lumens contain iodine material as well as the balloon. *2*. The balloon is deflated through the left lumen, the capacity of which is known. *3*. Same volume of polymerizing substance is injected through the left lumen. The iodine material contained in this lumen enters the balloon again but can be aspirated through the right lumen. *4*. When the balloon is empty of iodine material, injection of polymerizing substance starts again through the left lumen until the balloon contains the appropriate volume.

two types of balloons must be explained in detail.

The latex balloon, filled with iodine material and detached, progressively deflates in a period of time very different from one balloon to the other, probably depending on how strong the ligature was. Most of the balloons are completely deflated six weeks after having been detached. Experimental work has shown that a latex balloon filled with iodine material isoosmolar with plasma does not leak if it has been tied onto the catheter with a long and solid ligature, so strong that the balloon could not be detached with the coaxial catheter (Fig. 8.17), without rupturing the Teflon catheter A. The same experiment done with balloons ligated in human conditions of use shows that the latex balloons progressively deflate after some weeks.

The fistula is always occluded because of thrombosis of the cavernous sinus around the balloon, but in 50% of cases a false venous pouch appears in place of the deflated balloon (Fig. 8.18). Three theoretical complications can occur:

1. The pouch increases in size and forms a cavernous aneurysm.
2. The pouch ruptures in the cavernous sinus and the fistula recurs.
3. The pouch induces small clots that are responsible for transient ischemic attacks.

In most cases, this pouch is small and asymptomatic.

In two cases, despite that the fistula was occluded, the patient complained of retro-orbital pain, which disappeared as soon as we occluded permanently the internal carotid artery with a second balloon. Sometimes the false venous pouch reduced in size from one year to the other (Fig. 8.19).

The advantage to using an iodine-filled balloon is that the pressure in the cavernous sinus and to the oculomotor nerves produced by the balloon will progressively decrease.

A silicone-filled balloon keeps its size indefinitely if one uses a double-lumen catheter. No false venous pouch occurs. An oculomotor nerve palsy is generally transient. A single-lumen catheter allows injection of a quantity of silicone, which depends on the capacity of the balloon needed to occlude the fistula. With a catheter A of 150 cm, the dead space is 0.25 mL. When the balloon is deflated and silicone is injected, this quantity of iodine material is in-

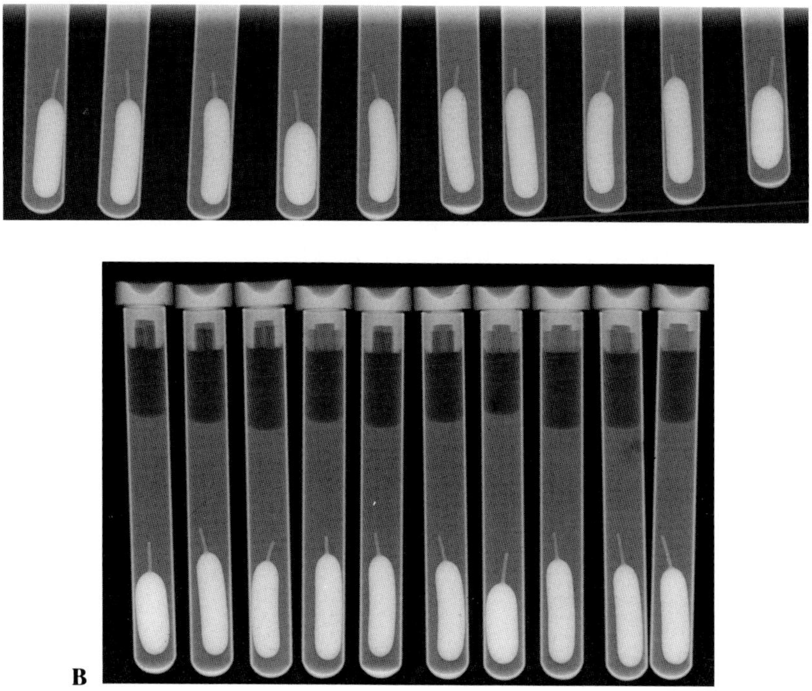

Fig. 8.17. Balloons inflated with isoosmolar iodine material and detached in plasma, **A.** Immediately after detachment of the balloon; **B,** six months later.

troduced again into the balloon. Some balloons have to be inflated with 0.3 mL. They will contain 0.25 mL of iodine and 0.05 mL of silicone. It is a negligible quantity, and there is no indications to use silicone in such a case. It becomes reasonable to use silicone when the balloon has to be inflated with 0.5 mL or more. It will then be at least half filled with silicone.

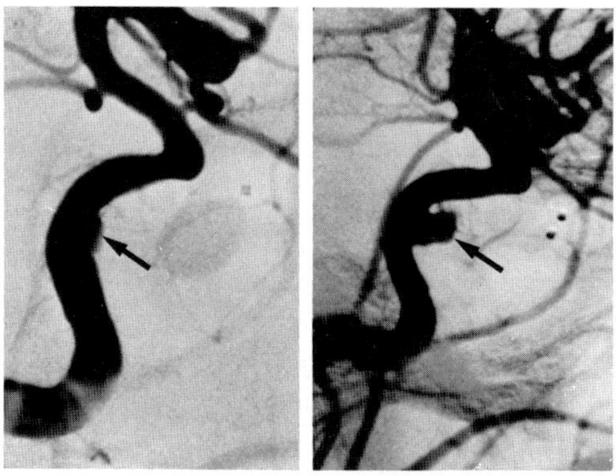

Fig. 8.18. Venous pouch after deflation of balloon. **A.** Two balloons have been detached in the cavernous sinus to occlude the fistula; minor venous pouch right after detachment (*arrow*). **B.** Three months later the venous pouch is bigger but asymptomatic (*arrow*).

Whenever the capacity of the balloon needed to treat the fistula is close to the capacity of the dead space of catheter A, it is imperative to use the double-lumen catheter if one wants to fill the balloon with silicone. If an iodine-filled balloon is preferred, a single-lumen catheter A with a tied balloon is the best.

The Introducer

Whichever balloon catheter is used (single-lumen catheter A with its coaxial catheter B, or double-lumen catheter A alone), we need a catheter that will be directed into the internal carotid artery (Fig. 8.20). The internal diameter of this catheter C has to be wide enough to allow easy maneuvers of catheter A and B as well as permanent infusion of heparinized saline and intermittent injections of iodine material. Its size depends on the size of the biggest balloon that has to be used. An inner diameter of 1.8 to 2 mm is sufficient in most cases. Thin-wall polyethylene catheter can be used with a wall of 0.2 mm. This introducer C easily passes through an 8 Fr. cordis sheath placed in the femoral artery. The introducer is 90 cm long and is straight so that its tip is exactly in the center of the lumen of the internal carotid artery. A bent

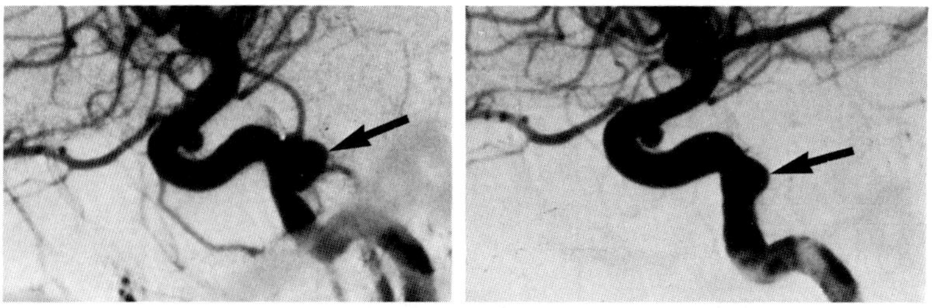

Fig. 8.19. Decrease in size of venous pouch at 1-year interval; asymptomatic patient (incidental small ophthalmic aneurysm). **A.** One month after treatment (*arrow*). **B.** 1 year after treatment (*arrow*).

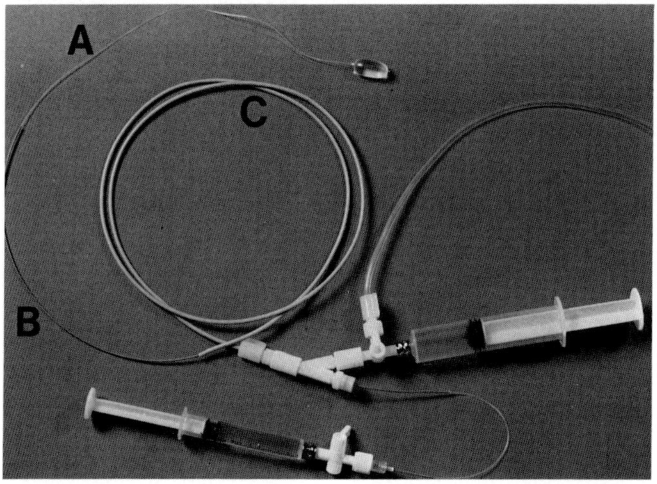

Fig. 8.20. Introducer with coaxial catheters. Teflon catheter *A* with attached balloon; coaxial polyethylen catheter *B*; introducer *C* The coaxial system (*A* and *B* catheters) enters the straight way of the side arm. The lateral way of the side arm is connected to a three-way stopcock. One way is used for permanent heparinized saline infusion. The other way is used for check angiograms.

tip would be stuck against the wall of the artery with the risk of clot formation and of difficult maneuvers of the balloon catheter. The straight introducer C will enter the common carotid artery with one of the three following techniques: (1) with a 0.52-in. C guide, (2) with a guide and a bent tip polyethylene catheter exactly fitting within the introducer, and (3) with a 250-cm guide first placed in the carotid artery and along which the introducer will slide. The introducer is connected to a side arm (Fig. 8.20). The balloon catheter enters the straight way of the side arm where a valve prevents bleeding along the catheter. A three-way stopcock is connected to the lateral entry of the side arm, giving two additional ways, one for permanent heparinized infusion, the other for iodine contrast injections.

If for some reason (atherosclerosis of the femoral or iliac arteries on both sides, tortuous and dilated aortic arch) it is impossible to catheterize the common carotid from the femoral artery, the common carotid artery is punctured in the neck with an 18G needle. An 8 Fr. sheath, 20 cm long, with guide and dilator is introduced in the common carotid artery and then directed to the internal carotid artery. This technique is difficult and dangerous, with tremendous risk of damage to the wall of the internal carotid artery with the guide, especially when there is a tortuous origin or a 380° loop of the cervical portion of the internal carotid artery. It is safer to direct the guide to the external carotid artery to avoid dissection of the internal carotid artery. The internal carotid artery, damaged by the guide, goes into spasm. The entire procedure can fail and stimulate thrombosis of the internal carotid artery.

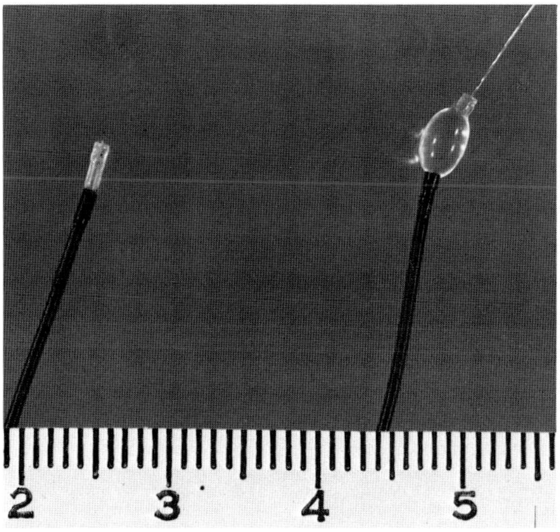

Fig. 8.21. Dr. Kerber's calibrated leak balloon. Silastic balloon stuck to the tip of the silastic tubing. Balloon has a distal calibrated leak; it cannot be detached.

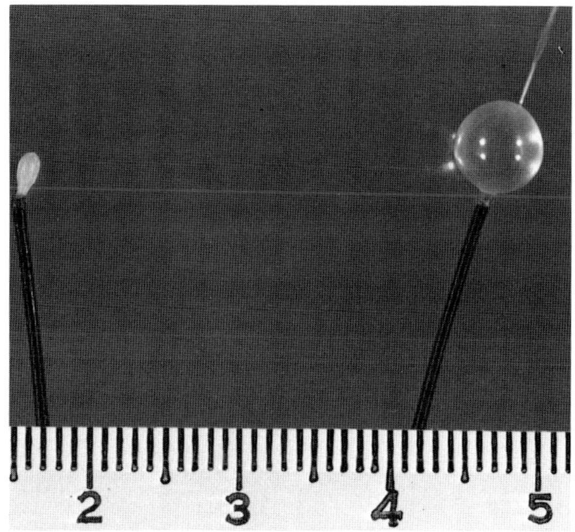

Fig. 8.22. Dr. Debrun's calibrated leak balloon. • Latex balloon gripping the tip of the silastic tubing without being attached or stuck. • Calibrated leak. • The balloon can be detached by pulling the tubing.

Embolization of the Cavernous Sinus With Isobutyl 2-Cyanoacrylate (Bucrylate) Through a Calibrated Leak Balloon

The balloon has a small leak at the tip which opens when the balloon is fully inflated. (Figs. 8.21, 8.22).

When the balloon is in the cavernous sinus, Bucrylate is injected through the balloon and solidifies in the cavernous sinus. As soon as the Bucrylate is injected, the balloon must be quickly removed to avoid having it stick in the cavernous sinus.

This technique has been used by Kerber[8] in a few cases of traumatic carotid cavernous fistulas. In my opinion it is a dangerous technique in cases of traumatic carotid cavernous fistulas for the following reasons:

1. When the flow is fast and the cavernous sinus is wide, it is hopeless to expect a complete thrombosis of the cavernous sinus. The quantity of Bucrylate that would be necessary to achieve thrombosis would be much more than we are allowed to use.
2. An unknown quantity of Bucrylate passes through the veins of drainage and embolizes the lungs. When the sinus is wide, almost all the injected Bucrylate returns solidified to the lungs.
3. There is a tremendous risk to have some Bucrylate escaping from the cavernous sinus through the neck of the fistula and embolizing the internal carotid with the risk of catastrophic strokes. The only case that I treated by injection of Bucrylate into the cavernous sinus at surgery woke up with a hemiplegia and Broca's aphasia, which regressed without sequelae.
4. When Bucrylate is injected and the balloon catheter quickly withdrawn, there is again the risk of detaching particles of Bucrylate in the internal carotid artery.
5. If ever used, this technique should be reserved to slow flow fistulas with small cavernous sinus, with almost intact partitions so that the quantity of Bucrylate needed to occlude the neck of the fistula is minimal.

These warnings, however, are not applicable to embolization of brain arteriovenous malformations where the calibrated leak balloon finds its best indications.

Other Types of Balloons

Becton-Dickinson Detachable Balloon.*[16] This is a silicone rubber balloon that has, when not inflated, a diameter of 2 mm with an advised maximum capacity of 0.6 mL. There is also a smaller balloon with a diameter of 1 mm when

* Becton-Dickinson, Rutherford, New Jersey 07070.

not inflated and should not be filled with more than 0.15 mL. The catheter holding the balloon is coiled inside a plastic chamber and injected into the artery through the introducer. The inner diameter of the catheter introducer must be at least 2.2 mm for the 2-mm balloon and 1.2 mm for the 1-mm balloon. The balloon is detached by pulling the catheter.

The advantages to this type balloon are that it and materials are sterile and ready for use. The semi-permeable property of silicone rubber theoretically allows the balloon to remain inflated after detachment for at least one month if iodine contrast isoosmolar to blood filled the balloon.

The disadvantages are that the balloon is not strongly attached and can be lost more easily than with a tied balloon. Its maximum inflated diameter is 8 mm, which is four times its diameter when not inflated. Latex has twice as much elasticity as silicone rubber. A 2-mm latex balloon can become a 16-mm diameter when inflated. A maximum diameter of 8 mm is insufficient for occlusion of large vessels or large fistulas. The valve pin mechanism inside the neck of the balloon makes this part stiff and can be a problem when negotiating hairpin loops of a vessel or when entering a narrow fistula.

Heyer-Schulte† Detachable Balloon.[6,10] This is a silicone balloon with a miter valve at its base. It is available in two sizes: 1.5-mm o.d. and 1.8-mm o.d. There is a coaxial catheter that may slide over the catheter holding the balloon and thus detaching it. The advantages to this type balloon is that it is sterile and ready for use.

The disadvantages are that the maximum inflated diameter of the balloon does not exceed 8 mm and is too small for large vessels or fistulas. The balloon is not strongly held over the catheter and is easily detached. If the catheter has followed several loops, the traction exerted on the catheter when one tries to slide over it with the coaxial catheter detaches the balloon before reaching it with the coaxial catheter. The balloon can move when detached if it is not strongly held by the vessel walls or by the fistula. No catheter is offered with the set, and the balloon catheter with its coaxial catheter has to navigate against the flow into the aorta and then directed to the vertebral or carotid artery. This disadvantage could be easily solved by positioning a 9 Fr catheter into the vertebral or carotid artery that give access to the lesion being treated.

† Heyer-Schulte, 600 Pine Avenue, Goleta, California 93117.

Dr. Taki's Detachable Balloon.[15] I have no experience with this balloon. According to Taki et al,[15] it is made of natural rubber. The junction between the balloon and catheter is a small piece of polyvinyl alcohol tube that dissolves when heated to 65°C by two microcopper wire electrodes. This balloon must be used with a polymerizing substance, which is a gel of iodine contrast and hydroxymethylmetacrylate. The idea of melting the neck of the balloon with electric current is one of my dreams that has become a reality with this Japanese balloon. I have three comments to make: I wonder if this balloon is not extremely fragile and if the release system may increase the stiffness of the balloon. Finally, the balloon cannot be detached unless it is totally filled with polymerizing substance. It is nearly impossible to realize with great accuracy the exchange of iodine versus polymerizing substance when a single catheter is used. A double-lumen catheter would be better although bigger and stiffer.

Local Anesthesia or General Anesthesia

All the procedures can be done through the groin under local anesthesia. If the patient is very anxious, neuroleptanalgesia with the permanent presence of an anesthetist will be necessary. The patient will be still, in total relaxation, but will be able to answer simple orders.

In cases treated through the neck, anesthesia with tracheal intubation is necessary, especially if systemic heparinization is used, because of the tremendous risk of sudden cervical hematoma after removal of the introducer.

Radiologic Equipment (Fig. 8.23)

Frontal fluoroscopy is necessary until the introducer is guided from the femoral artery to the common carotid artery.

Lateral fluoroscopy is then needed to guide the introducer into the internal carotid artery and then to follow the balloon from the tip of the introducer to the cavernous carotid artery. Both frontal and lateral fluoroscopy can be ob-

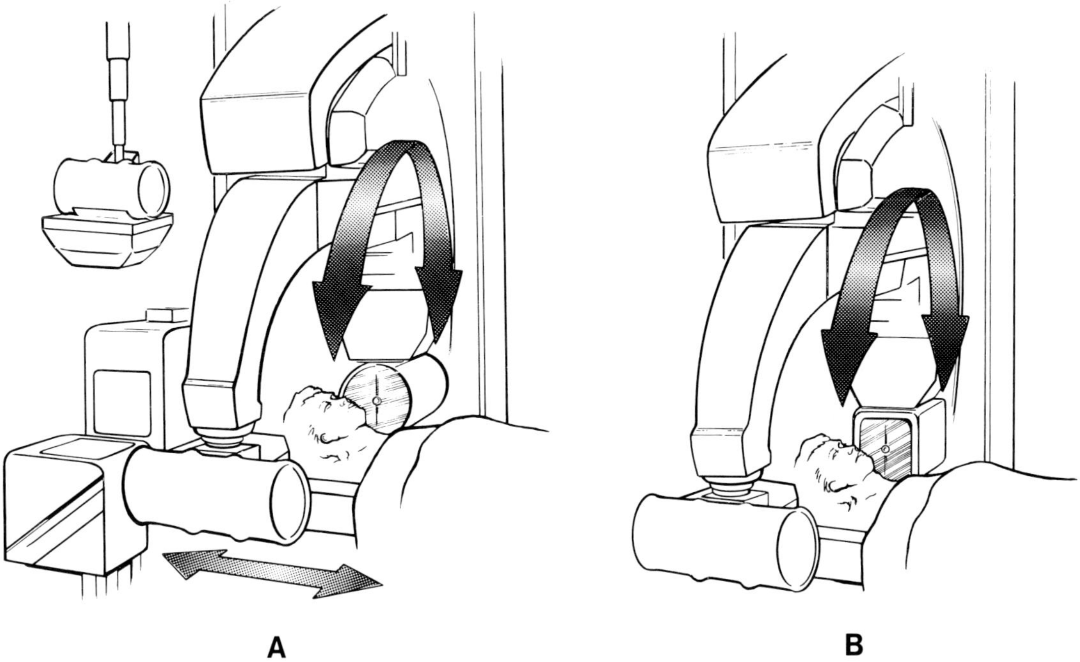

Fig. 8.23. Radiologic equipment needed for interventional neuroradiology. **A.** Conventional angiographic equipment with a C-arm getting single-plane fluoroscopy. Table and patient's head have to be moved to get angiography on the film changer. **B.** C-arm with image intensifier and film changer incorporated in the same unit. Fluoroscopy and angiography are obtained without moving the head of the patient. If the C-arm is replaced by a complete ring with two orthogonal units of image intensifier and film changer, we can get biplane simultaneous fluoroscopy and angiography without moving the head of the patient. Subtraction television with video disk is indispensible.

tained with a C arm but the ideal is simultaneous biplane fluoroscopy. High resolution of the television screen image is absolutely indispensible. Subtraction television is of great help to follow the balloon through the petrous bone.

With most C arms, only fluoroscopy can be obtained. The table and the patient's head must be moved to the film changer when angiography is needed. The ideal is to work with a C arm where fluoroscopy and serial angiography are obtained immediately without displacing the head of the patient. All phases of the treatment are followed by fluoroscopy and recorded on videotape.

The neuroradiologist in charge of this type of treatment must be particularly experienced in selective angiography. The duration of the procedure is sometimes very long, with long periods of fluoroscopy. The dose of primary radiation to the patient and of secondary radiation to the operator can be very high. Therefore, the operator has to be trained to work with a lead apron, with a lead screen between the x-ray tube and himself, and with a very small field limited to the sella turcica.

The maneuvers with the guides and with the different kinds of catheters are dangerous and must be used by a specially experienced vascular neuroradiologist to avoid catastrophic complications. One of those complications is the permanent risk of clot formation, which must be always kept in mind. This risk can be reduced by the following precautions:

1. The catheters and the guides are heparin-coated.
2. As soon as the cordis sheath is in place in the femoral artery, systemic heparinization starts with injection of 2,000 units of heparin. Partial thromboplastin time stays over 110 during the whole procedure, as long as a new injection of 1,000 units is given every hour after the first injection of heparin. At the end of the procedure, protamine sulfate

is injected through the cordis sheath to reduce hypocoagulability. Duration of compression is not changed, and there is no bleeding from the femoral artery.

3. A permanent heparinized infusion of saline with 3,000 units of heparin per 0.5L permanently flushes the introducer through one of the two lateral ways of the side arm.
4. During the entire treatment the coaxial catheter B stays inside the introducer 2 cm below its tip, so that the space between A and B catheters is also permanently flushed by infusion of heparinized saline.
5. All manipulations are meticulous but fast. The quality of the radiologic equipment, the skill of the operator, and the good training of the team of scrub assistants and technicians are essential to saving time and limiting the risk of clot formation, which is proportional to the duration of the procedure (90 minutes to 3 hours).
6. Before each injection of iodine contrast through the lateral way of the side arm, it is safe to do a double flush.
7. When the balloon is detached and A and B catheters are removed, a double flush of the introducer is indispensible before final angiography.
8. It is also possible to put an independent regular catheter in the internal carotid artery (through the contralateral femoral artery), to do all the angiograms, and to avoid injecting quickly a big bolus of liquid through the introducer.

Penetration of the Cavernous Sinus With the Balloon

Most of the balloons have a piece of silver at their tip so that they are easily followed under fluoroscopy. There is no reason to inflate the balloon with iodine material when it easily passes the curves of the internal carotid artery through the petrous bone. However, if the balloon does get stuck, even with pushing the Teflon catheter A, a slight inflation with iodine contrast and the blood flow will push the balloon downstream.

Different sizes of balloon should be prepared the day before the procedure. The first attempt is done with the biggest balloon. When the balloon has reached the level of the fistula, it is totally deflated. Sometimes it immediately enters the cavernous sinus, which is indicated by a sharp and quick change of direction of the piece of silver, which ceases to follow the curve of the siphon. When the balloon does not enter the fistula but follows the siphon above it, the catheter is withdrawn until the tip of the balloon faces the presumed entrance of the fistula. The silver clip at this time is generally moved by a quick alternating motion. Some inflation and deflation of the balloon can help the balloon to enter the fistula. When these maneuvers fail, it is dangerous to continue trying; rather, a smaller balloon should be used. If this one also fails to enter the fistula, the smallest balloon should be used and rarely will it not be able to enter the cavernous sinus.

When the piece of silver is supposed to be in the cavernous sinus, the balloon is progressively inflated with iodine material. From time to time an injection of iodine contrast in the internal carotid artery demonstrates whether the fistula is totally occluded or not. The balloon is never filled more than its maximum known capacity. If its shape becomes biloculated, a partition in the cavernous sinus is squeezing the balloon, with a risk of rupture. If the biggest balloon entering the cavernous sinus does not occlude the neck of the fistula, even at its maximum capacity of inflation, the cavernous pouch is big and needs more than one balloon. This balloon is filled with iodine and detached, and a second balloon of the same size is immediately used. If it does not occlude the fistula, it is detached and a third balloon is used and so on, until the neck of the fistula is occluded without any leak of contrast in the cavernous sinus. The last balloon is filled with silicone if possible, i.e., a double-lumen balloon catheter is used at the end of treatment or the balloon is partially filled with silicone with a single-lumen catheter. It depends on the ease with which the cavernous sinus is entered and if it is reasonable to exchange the last single-lumen balloon catheter for a double-lumen balloon catheter. When more than one balloon is necessary to occlude the fistula, the cavernous sinus is often under pressure and a third nerve palsy or a sixth nerve palsy can occur, which will reverse after some weeks or months, the sixth nerve improving quicker than the third. The iodine-filled balloons will deflate; the cavernous sinus will shrink. If the last balloon can be totally filled with silicone, no venous pseudoaneurysm will occur. If the balloon has been totally filled with iodine or partially filled with silicone, a pseudoaneurysm will occur in 50% of cases. With experience it is possible, prior to balloon detachment, to avoid doing an angiogram and to take subtracted films when the balloon occludes the neck of the fistula, thus saving time.

Detachment of the Balloon

The technique of detaching a balloon tied over the A catheter is different from that of a balloon simply gripping a double-lumen catheter.

With a tied balloon we need the coaxial catheter B to safely detach the balloon. The catheter B is pushed up so that it slides along catheter A until it reaches the base of the balloon. It can be very difficult in some cases to slide the B catheter, especially when there is a loop of 180° of the internal carotid artery in the neck. To ensure that the coaxial catheter has reached the base of the balloon, the 30-cm difference in length, which exists between the coaxial B catheter (120 cm) and the Teflon A catheter (150 cm), must be found before trying to detach the balloon. Sometimes, when the sphenoidal sinus is widely aerated, the end of the coaxial B catheter is well seen on the screen. (Subtraction television is helpful in visualizing it.) The coaxial B catheter is then held with the left hand, and the Teflon catheter A is pulled out gently until the balloon is detached. This is done under fluoroscopy. The balloon does not move and does not deflate if the ligature works nicely. The operator can feel exactly when the balloon is detached, but nothing is visible on the screen. It is the label of successful detachment.

With an untied balloon and a double-lumen catheter, successive manipulations have to be done before detachment. A 1-mL syringe is filled with catalyzed silicone (we have 10 minutes before the mixture starts to solidify). The capacity of the balloon useful to occlude the fistula is now accurately measured and the balloon is totally deflated, but there is still iodine contrast in both lumens of the catheter. The silicone-filled syringe is tightly adapted to one way of the catheter, directly, without any stopcock, which would add its own dead space and complicate measurement of the proper amount of silicone to be injected. Silicone, 0.3 mL, is injected, corresponding to the dead space of each lumen of the catheter. One sees the balloon, which is filled again with iodine material. At that time, injection of the silicone is momentarily stopped, and a 1-mL syringe adapted on to the second lumen of the catheter aspirates this 0.3 mL of iodine. The second lumen of the catheter is now hermetically closed. Injection of silicone starts again, and the exact amount is injected. An injection of contrast checks that the fistula is occluded without any leak of contrast in the cavernous sinus. The balloon is not radiopaque, and only the silver clip is visible in the cavernous sinus. If the occlusion of the fistula is total, the first lumen of the catheter is also hermetically closed, and one waits for the silicone to solidify. When solidication of catalyzed silicone has occurred in the cup, the balloon can be detached. The double-lumen catheter is simply pulled out and if detachment is successful, the piece of silver will not move. An angiogram demonstrates the quality of the occlusion of the fistula. The slightest mistake during replacement of iodine with silicone can cause the balloon to not totally fill with silicone and to slightly change its volume after detachment. The result is a small leak of contrast around the balloon on the check angiogram. A small difference of 0.01 or 0.02 mL in inflation is enough to get some leak. The leak will spontaneously disappear, or will increase, and it will be necessary to use a second balloon some days later, or the balloon, smaller, will be dislodged and will move within the cavernous sinus. Here, again, a second balloon will be necessary.

Results

We treated 75 cases of traumatic carotid cavernous sinus fistulas. All patients were cured except one, who was apparently cured after we detached one balloon, small (0.10 mL), filled with iodine. An angiogram done one month later showed recurrence of the fistula because of two tiny branches of the siphon torn in the cavernous sinus. In spite of this angiographic aspect, the patient now is asymptomatic and does not need further therapy.

Carotid blood flow may be preserved in 80% of the cases. When the internal carotid artery was occluded, it was because it was impossible to enter the cavernous sinus, or because of secondary thrombosis of the carotid siphon due to stenosis of the siphon by the balloon bulging through the neck of the fistula, or because of a traumatic cervical dissection of the internal carotid artery at the time of the injury.

The complications were essentially oculomotor nerve palsies, which occurred in 20% of the cases. It happened frequently when more than one balloon was detached in the cavernous sinus. As the iodine-filled latex-tied balloons shrink and deflate after six weeks, these oculomotor nerve palsies disappear completely in most cases.

Pain from compression of the fifth nerve is generally transient. When it is a main symptom before treatment, it often instantaneously disappears as soon as the fistula is occluded.

In one case a tremendous inflammatory and edematous reaction of the eye occurred two weeks after occlusion of the fistula. Proptosis, chemosis, and edema of the lids look like an active fistula, and the first impression was that the fistula had come back despite the absence of bruit. Angiogram demonstrated the absence of fistula and a good carotid flow. All the symptoms disappeared in some weeks, with a good final result. Probably a secondary extensive thrombosis of the cavernous sinus explains this clinical presentation.

A false venous pseudoaneurysm occurred in 50 percent of the cases. The pouch, which is the compartment of the cavernous sinus close to the hole of the fistula, was filled by the iodine-inflated balloon. Thrombosis occurs around the balloon but there is no occlusion of the tear of the carotid siphon, which fills this venous pouch when the balloon has deflated. The five first cases where this complication occurred were treated a second time to occlude as completely as possible this pouch with a second balloon. Three of these cases now have a normal angiogram. The pouch did not increase in size, did not give rise to transient ischemic attacks, and spontaneously diminished in size in some cases. Now we check every year our patients who had this postoperative complication, but none of them complain of any symptom, and we do not bother them with new angiograms after the routine one-year posttreatment angiogram. Although the use of double-lumen catheters is very recent, they will probably avoid this inconvenience in the future or allow total occlusion of the venous pouch if needed.

Conclusion

Treatment of traumatic carotid cavernous fistulas with detachable balloons is an elegant endovascular way to occlude the fistula and save the carotid blood flow. It is, however, a very meticulous technique with numerous small, technical details, all having great importance. Those who have never carefully watched all the steps of the treatment, from the radiologic evaluation with excellent subtracted films to the final angiogram after detachment of the balloon, including the preparation of the material and the treatment itself, cannot realize the complexity of the technique. The operator has to develop his skill by making a great many balloons until he trusts all his ligatures. He has to perform a great deal of experimental work in the animal laboratory, using the same material and the same technique. Surgical carotid jugular fistulas in dogs are a good material to simulate a human carotid cavernous fistula, even though it is much easier to treat.

Treatment of a Spontaneous Carotid Cavernous Sinus Fistula

There are two main anatomic differences with a traumatic case: (1) The communication between the carotid siphon and cavernous sinus is made of more than one tiny branch, and (2) there are many meningeal branches of the external carotid artery communicating with the cavernous sinus. Treatment has to be different because it is almost impossible to enter the cavernous sinus with a balloon through the artery, and branches of the external carotid artery have to be embolized. The two clinical points to remember are that these fistulas are often cured spontaneously but also often recur and that the patients are often elderly women in whom bilateral fistulas are not uncommon.

One can realize that we must be less agressive with this type of fistula than with traumatic cases which rarely cure spontaneously. It would be a great mistake to decide that the first step of treatment should be the definitive occlusion of the carotid siphon for these different reasons:

1. The fistula would continue to be fed by external carotid branches.
2. Many cases are cured by embolization of the external carotid branches only.
3. Those fistulas are often bilateral and treatment of the contralateral fistula would become more difficult and risky.
4. It is always dangerous in an elderly patient to permanently occlude a carotid siphon.
5. It is often useless as these fistulas often spontaneously cure.

In our experience the first step of the treatment has to be embolization of the meningeal branches of the external carotid artery. It has to be directed by hyperselective angiography of these branches so that embolization can be as selective as possible.

The material used for embolization can be particles of Gelfoam or Ivalon or Bucrylate. One patient has been successfully treated with the latter (Fig. 8.24). Bucrylate, 0.5 mL, was injected into the internal maxillary artery. Bucrylate reached the cavernous sinus, which thrombosed secondarily but with a huge painful inflammatory reaction and transient sixth nerve palsy. All the tiny branches between the carotid siphon and the cavernous sinus were occluded, and the varix of the cavernous sinus that communicated with the siphon thrombosed.

Even after embolization with solid particles occluding the meningeal branches of the external carotid artery, spontaneous cure of the fistula often occurs probably by spontaneous thrombosis of the cavernous sinus.

When embolization of the external carotid artery is not technically realized because of severe stenosis of the origin of the external carotid or of the bifurcation of the common carotid artery in an elderly patient, direct surgical approach of the cavernous sinus can be discussed. Thrombosis can be obtained by injection of thrombogenic material (needles or wire) or particles of Gelfoam, cotton, or muscle. Figure 8.9 shows the final result of a bilateral spontaneous carotid cavernous sinus fistula in a 73-year-old lady that Dr. Drake operated on both sides with direct approach, incision of the anteroinferior portion of the cavernous sinus and insertion of pieces of muscle. Both internal carotid arteries were saved and are perfectly normal.

Conclusion

Treatment of carotid cavernous sinus fistulas has tremendously improved during the last 20 years because of better understanding of the physiopathology of different types of fistulas, because of improvement of radiologic evaluation, and because of new techniques such as detachable balloon or direct approach of the cavernous sinus, which has been made possible and safe by improvement in anesthesiology and microsurgery.

What Hamby[5] wrote in his beautiful monograph in 1966 remains actual:

> Carotid cavernous fistula is not common and it sometimes confronts surgeons unfamiliar with its complexities, leading them to the application of therapeutic principles that should be considered outmoded, complicating future management of the case. It is to be hoped that the "occasional operator" will be convinced that it is no simple lesion and that its treatment should be confined to an especially qualified neurosurgeon.

I think that there is only to add . . . "to an especially qualified team of neuroradiologist, neurosurgeon, anesthetist, and technicians."

Treatment of Vertebral Fistulas

Vertebral fistulas are also uncommon. They can be congenital or traumatic, including the iatrogenic fistulas after direct puncture of the vertebral artery. Iatrogenic fistulas are low in the neck at C4 or C5 level (Fig. 8.25). The congenital cases are at C1-2 level (Fig. 8.26). It is difficult to say that true congenital fistulas exist because a relatively mild injury can induce the fistula as in one of our cases (the patient was hurt on the right side of the neck by the stick of a parasol when he was on the seashore). Mild injury many years before discovery of the fistula may be forgotten by the patient. Obstetric injury may probably cause such a fistula.

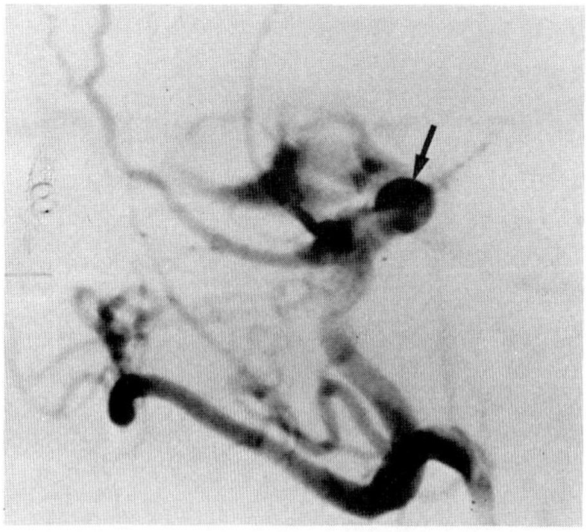

A

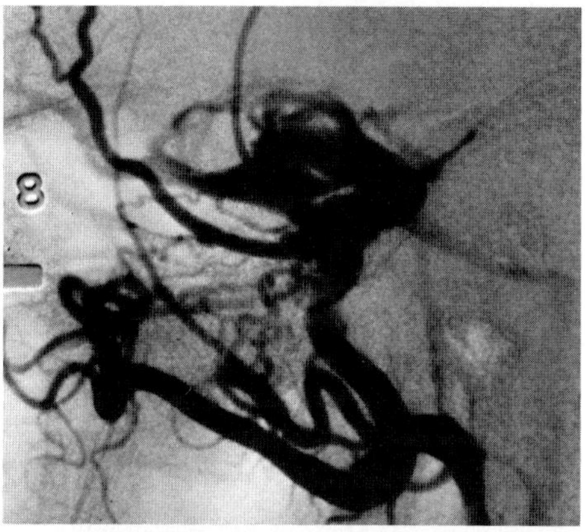

B

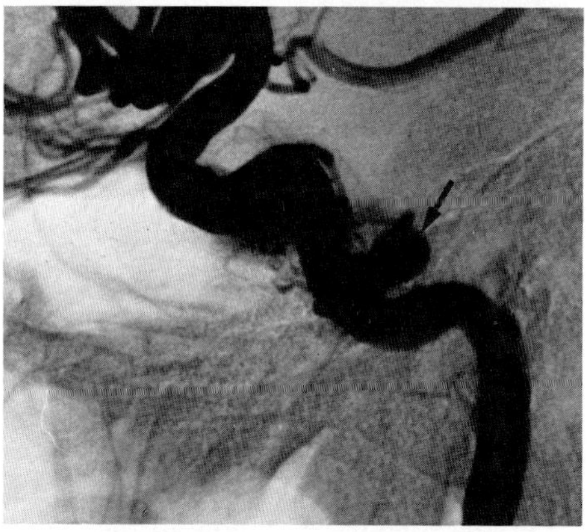

C

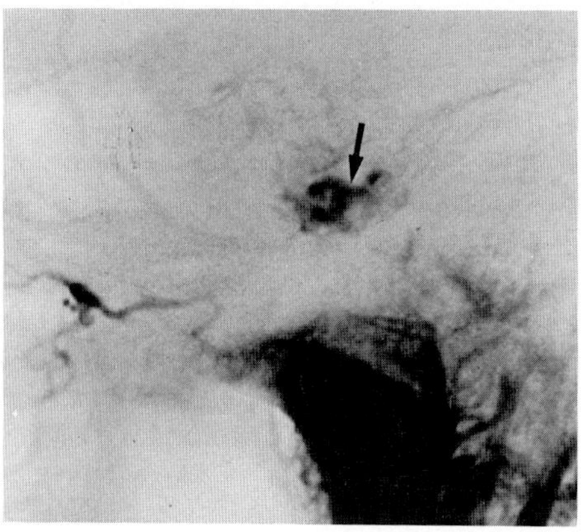

D

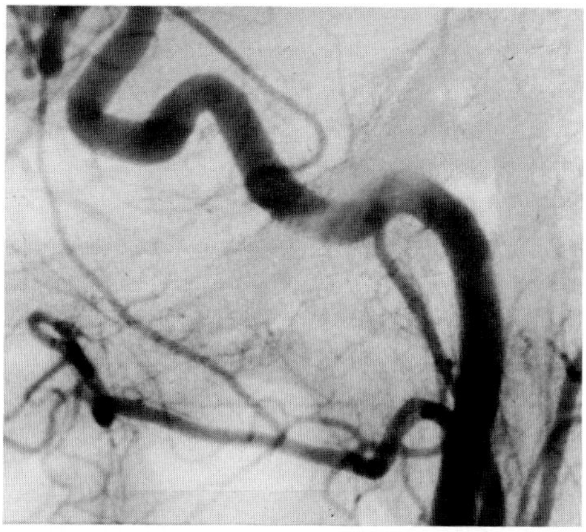

E

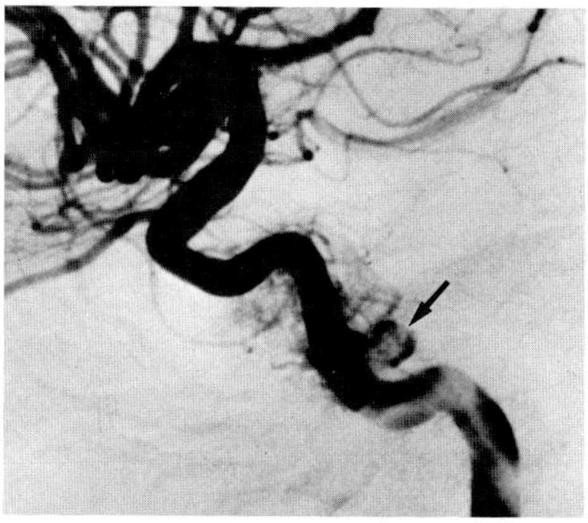

F

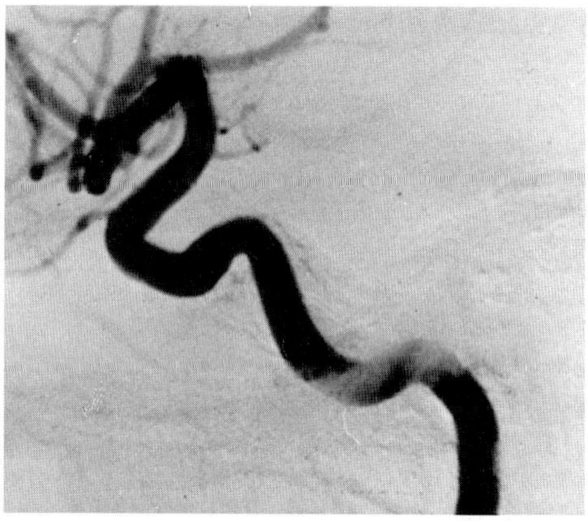

G

Fig. 8.24. Spontaneous carotid cavernous fistula in a 40-year-old woman. Retro-orbital pain and bothering bruit. **A.** Selective angiography of left internal maxillary artery. Big meningeal artery getting the cavernous sinus and filling a varix (*arrow*). Other tiny meningeal branches. **B.** Same angiography one second later. Better filling of the cavernous sinus. **C.** Selective internal carotid angiography. Tiny branches of the siphon give a blush of the cavernous sinus. Varix filled from external branches is also filled by internal (*arrow*). **D.** Left external carotid angiography immediately after embolization of left internal maxillary artery with 0.5 mL of Bucrylate. All the branches of the internal maxillary artery are

A 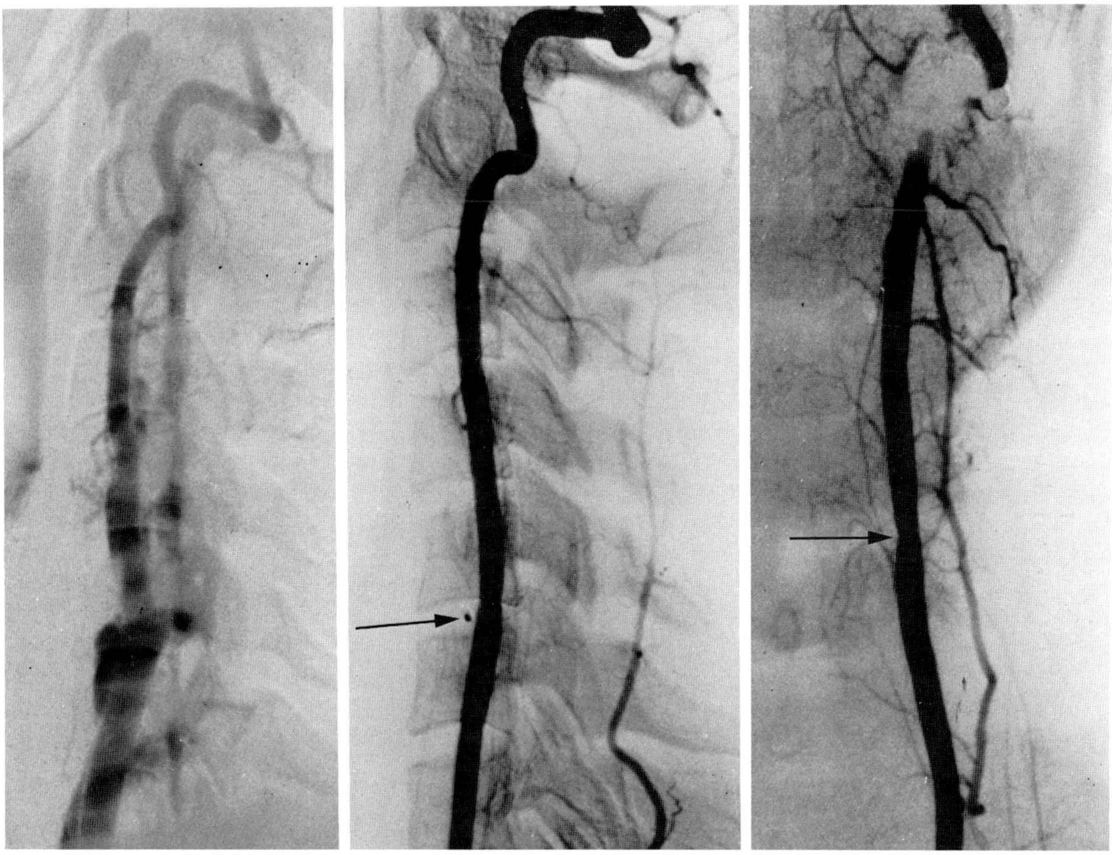 B,C

Fig. 8.25. Iatrogenic traumatic vertebral fistula at C5-6 level. **A.** Lateral left vertebral angiography. There is a difference of caliber of the vertebral artery which is wider below C5-6 than above, indicating the level of the fistula. **B.** One balloon was detached in the vertebral vein occluding the fistula and preserving the vertebral artery. This angiography is done one month later. The balloon has totally deflated and only the silver cylinder (*arrow*) is visible outside the vertebral artery. **C.** *AP* view. There is a minimal stenosis of the vertebral artery (*arrow*) where the fistula was.

The anatomic particularity of the fistulas at C1-2 is that their neck is generally very wide, necessitating a bigger introducer and bigger balloon than those used to treat a carotid cavernous fistula. There is also an almost constant participation of the ascending cervical artery and of the occipital artery, which may either converge to the neck of the fistula or join independently the venous plexus of drainage. In the first case the occlusion of the fistula with one balloon will also occlude the connection with the ascending cervical artery and the occipital

---

occluded. Huge pharyngeal blush from opacification of the ascending pharyngeal artery. Persistence of a small blush of the cavernous sinus (*arrow*). **E.** Left common carotid angiography four months after embolization. Recanalization of the internal maxillary artery. Total occlusion of the meningeal branches that fed the fistula. **F.** Selective left internal carotid angiography immediately after embolization of the internal maxillary artery. The varix (*arrow*) is partially occluded with Bucrylate. The blush of the cavernous sinus is diminished. **G.** Selective left internal carotid angiography four months after embolization of internal maxillary artery. The varix does not fill; blush of the cavernous sinus has disappeared. The patient had tremendous retro-orbital pain, inflammatory reaction of the cavernous sinus with proptosis and chemosis, transient sixth nerve palsy during two weeks after embolization. The bruit had gone. Then the patient improved and completely recovered. She is asymptomatic four months after embolization.

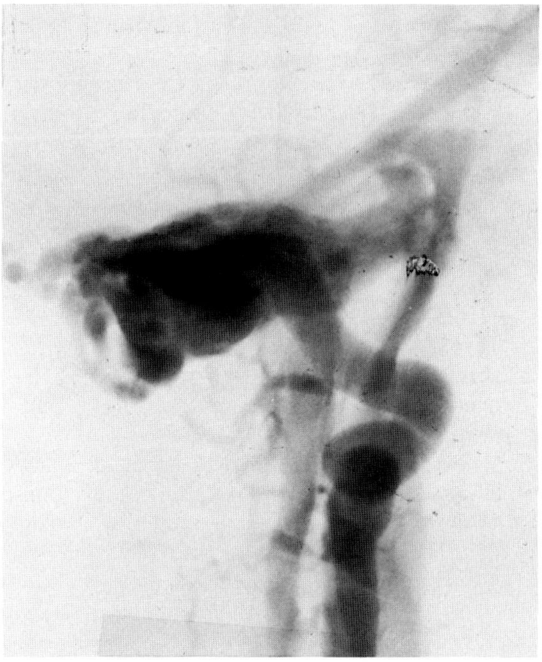

Fig. 8.26. Congenital vertebral fistula at C1 level.

artery. The balloon can even be introduced through the occipital artery. In the second case the occlusion of the neck of the fistula only closes the communication between the vertebral artery and the venous drainage plexus. The occipital artery and the ascending cervical artery have to be embolized separately. As the occipital artery may be widely communicating with the vertebral artery, as the ascending cervical artery may give an anterior spinal artery, embolization has to be very selective and prudent. Angiographic evaluation requires both vertebral angiographies and subclavian angiography so that the vertebral arteries are totally visualized from the origin to the fistula. In one case a loop of 180° below C6 prevented sliding with the coaxial catheter to the base of the balloon. Hyperselective angiography of the occipital artery and of the ascending cervical artery are also necessary.

Technical problems are slightly different. The C1-2 level fistulas have a wide neck and the balloon is a large one, 2 mm o.d., noninflated. The introducer must therefore be sufficiently large, and a number 9 Fr polyethylene catheter is used (2.4 mm i.d.). In the four cases treated, we have always used a balloon inflated with iodine material because the deflated balloon never stays in the exact position, and there is always the fear of not having enough time to position the balloon in the neck of the fistula if we use silicone. Therefore we accept the risk of a false venous pouch of the vertebral artery after deflation of the balloon. This occurred only in two cases. In the other cases, the vertebral artery looked normal. It is also possible to preserve the vertebral arteries in 80% of the cases. In my experience of 17 cases, it is almost always impossible to preserve the vertebral artery when the tear is secondary to a gunshot wound. Iatrogenic vertebral fistulas are now exceptional. I have occluded two of these fistulas at C4 and C5 level with small balloons inflated with 0.10 and 0.15 mL of iodine contrast. The vertebral artery is patent and normal in both cases without any venous pouch at the level of the fistula. Figure 8.25 shows one of these.

Conclusion

Detachable balloon occlusion of the neck of the vertebral fistula is the best way to treat those C1-2 level fistulas that are extremely difficult to treat surgically. Embolization of occipital artery and ascending cervical artery are often necessary. The clinical result has always been excellent. One patient had a cervical nerve root neuralgia for several days because the balloon compressed the root. The pain subsided completely when the balloon shrunk.

References

1. Debrun G, Lacour P, Vinuela F, Fox A, Drake CG, and Caron JP: Treatment of 54 traumatic carotid cavernous fistulae. J Neurosurg 55:678–692, 1981
2. Debrun G, Legré J, Kasbarian M, Tapias PL, and Caron JP: Endovascular occlusion of vertebral fistulae by detachable balloons with conservation of the vertebral blood flow. Radiology 130:140–147, 1979
3. Debrun G, Vinuela F, and Fox A: Aspirin and systemic heparinization in diagnostic and interventional neuroradiology. Am J Neuroradiol 3:337–340, 1982
4. Dohn DF: Carotid aneurysms and arteriovenous fistulae of the cavernous sinus. Saunders (ed.): Neurological Surgery Vol 2.

5. Hamby, WB: Carotid cavernous fistula. Monograph. Charles C. Thomas Publisher, 1966
6. Hieshima GB, Grinnell VS, and Mehringer CM: A detachable balloon for therapeutic transcatheter occlusions. Radiology 138: 227–228, 1981
7. Hosobuchi Y: Electrothrombosis of carotid cavernous fistula. J Neurosurg 42:76–85, 1975
8. Kerber C: Use of balloon catheters in the treatment of cranial arterial abnormalities. Stroke 11:210–216, 1980
9. Manelfe C, Berenstein A: Treatment of carotid cavernous fistulas by venous approach J Neuroradiol 7:13–21, 1980
10. Mehringer CM, Hieshima GB, Grinnell VS, et al: Improved localization of carotid cavernous fistula during angiography. Am J Neuroradiol 3:82–84, 1982
11. Mullan S: Treatment of carotid cavernous fistulas by cavernous sinus occlusion. J Neurosurg 50:131–144, 1979
12. Parkinson D: Carotid cavernous fistula. Handbook of Clinical Neurology Vol 12, Chapter 8, American Elsevier Publishing Co, New York
13. Peterson E, Valberg JD, Ventureyra E: Percutaneous treatment of carotid cavernous fistula with preservation of the carotid artery. Abstract, Canadian meeting of Neurological Sciences. June 19, 1975
14. Serbinenko FA: Balloon catheterization and occlusion of major cerebral vessels. J Neurosurg 41:125–145, 1974
15. Taki W, Handa H, Yamagata S, et al: The releasable balloon technique with activated high frequency electrical current. Surg Neurol 13:405–408, 1980
16. White R, Kaufman S, Barth K, et al: Embolotherapy with detachable silicone balloons. Technique and clinical results. Radiology 131:619–627, 1979

9

Surgical Treatment of Hypertensive Intracerebral Hemorrhage

Masahiro Mizukami

Introduction

The problem of whether hypertensive and/or arteriosclerotic intracerebral hemorrhage is to be treated surgically is still being debated by neurosurgeons. Since McKissock et al,[25] in 1961 published their pessimistic view on the surgical treatment of hypertensive intracerebral hemorrhage, neurosurgeons have shown a tendency to disregard this problem while favoring conservative treatment. Unfortunately, conservative treatment has proved to be of limited therapeutic value.[14,29,40,43] It therefore seems timely to reevaluate the rationale and benefit of surgical treatment. Since approximately 90,000 persons die, annually in Japan of hypertensive intracerebral hemorrhage, the Japanese experience is of particular interest.

Since 1966 we have conducted multidisciplinary studies of hypertensive intracerebral hemorrhage in an attempt to acquire knowledge of its pathophysiology. In initial stages of our research the results of surgery were unsatisfactory.[30] Later, as the pathophysiology of hypertensive intracerebral hemorrhage was clarified, the operative results improved remarkably.[30]

The purpose of this chapter is to critically evaluate the surgical treatment of hypertensive intracerebral hemorrhage. We will describe the current indications for surgery, our related studies, and a review of the pertinent literature to develop a rational basis for clinical management.

Historical Review

The operative approach to hypertensive intracerebral hemorrhage may be traced to Cushing,[9] who was the first to report the result of surgical treatment in 1903. During the ensuing three decades, up to the 1930s, there were occasional reports of patients treated surgically. Bagely,[4] in 1932, described indications for operation based on the site of hematoma. He concluded that surgical treatment was not effective for hemorrhage into the basal ganglia but was indicated for subcortical hematomas associated with increased intracranial pressure. The introduction of cerebral angiography in the 1940s provided an impetus for surgical treatment of hematomas. It allowed prospective planning and study of the problem, and several publications appeared in the French literature.[10,16] In 1947, Fazio,[12] a neurologist, first suggested a role for surgical treatment based on his extensive pathological studies. In the 1950s surgical treatment of hypertensive intracerebral hemorrhage became one of the major tasks in neurosurgery, being a main subject for discussion at the Congress of the Society of Neurosurgery of French-speaking countries in 1956 and at the Latin American Congress of Neurosurgery in 1957.

On the other hand, McKissock and colleagues[26] in 1959 reported on their own series of 244 operative cases, stating that the operative mortality was 51%. They observed the relationship between disturbance of consciousness at operation and a poorer prognosis. The mortality rate for comatose patients was 100%. Later, in 1961, McKissock et al[25] expressed a pessimistic view, reporting no noticeable difference between medical versus surgical treatment. Since then the role of surgery in the treatment of hypertensive intracerebral hemorrhage was in doubt.

In Japan, the first case of surgically treated hypertensive intracerebral hemorrhage was described by Kageyama[20] in 1944. Although the patient died 56 hours after the operation, the author was optimistic about the potential for surgical treatment. In the 1960s, Mitsuno, et al[27] advocated surgical treatment for hypertensive intracerebral hemorrhage. These authors argued that when the hemorrhage is of the lateral type, i.e., the hematoma is lateral to the internal capsule, the patient's life can frequently be salvaged.

On this basis and their own experience, many neurosurgeons in Japan actively operate on selected cases based on clinical and computed tomography (CT) data.

Location of Hypertensive Intracerebral Hemorrhage

Hypertensive intracerebral hemorrhages have been classified on the basis of autopsy and angiographic findings.[5,18,31,33] According to Fisher,[13] the approximate incidence of hemorrhages at postmortem examination has been putamen 55%, thalamus 10%, subcortical 15%, cerebellar hemisphere 10%, and pons 10%. Hemorrhage into the medulla oblongata is extremely rare (but occurs); into the midbrain it is rarer still.

The CT scan, however, has made possible the recognition of small, nonfatal hemorrhages, and this new capability calls for reassessment of the classification of hemorrhages in clinical cases (Fig. 9.1).

Table 9.1 shows the location of hemorrhages in a consecutive series of 258 cases in which CT scanning was feasible within 3 weeks after on-

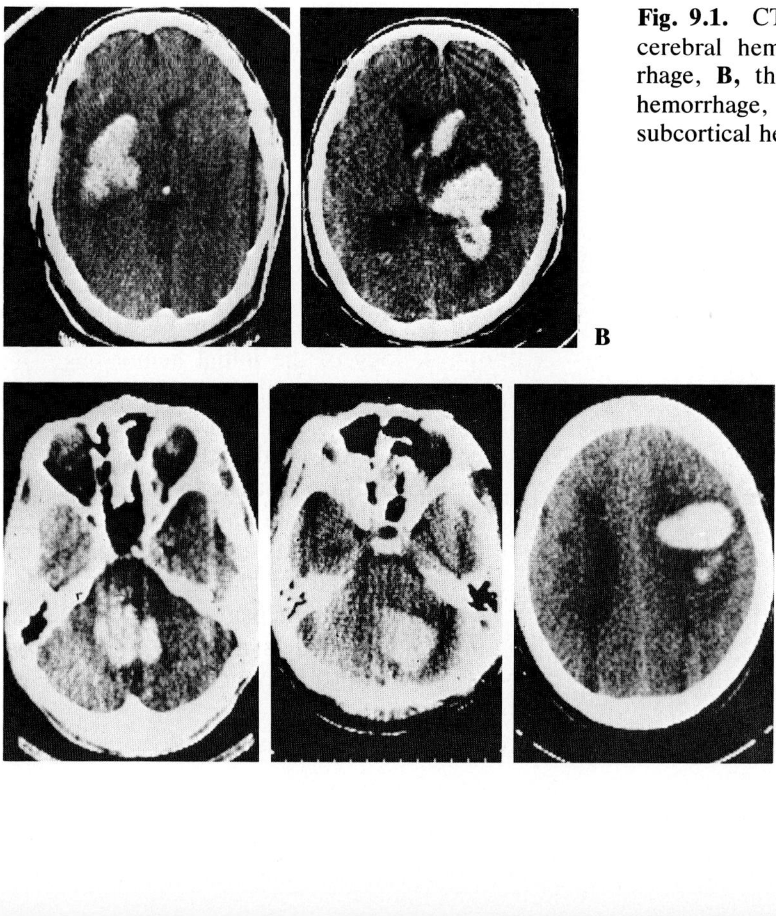

A B C D,E

Fig. 9.1. CT findings of hypertensive intracerebral hemorrhage. **A.** Putaminal hemorrhage, **B,** thalamic hemorrhage, **C,** pontine hemorrhage, **D,** cerebellar hemorrhage, **E,** subcortical hemorrhage.

Table 9.1. Hypertensive cerebral hemorrhage due to CT finding.

Classification	No of cases	%
Putamen		
external capsule	132	51
Thalamus	91	35
Subcortex	18	7
Cerebellum	8	3
Pons midbrain	9	4
Totl	258	100

[a] Evaluated within three weeks of onset.

set. On CT scanning the figure rose 35% in thalamic hemorrhage and dropped to 3% to 4% in cerebellar and pontine hemorrhage.

Pathology

Source of Bleeding

The numerous opinions on the mechanism of bleeding in hypertensive intracerebral hemorrhage may be classified into two theories, as shown in Table 9.2. One theory places special emphasis on rupture of blood vessels as primary while the other attaches importance to ischemic infarction of brain, which secondarily compromises vascular integrity.* There has long been a controversy on this subject. At the present time, however, Charcot's view[6] that the hemorrhage results from rupture of a microaneurysm has gained wide acceptance (Fig. 9.2). Matsuoka[24] was the first to advocate the theory of angionecrosis as the cause of microaneurysm. Ooneda and his co-workers[34] proposed the theory of plasmatic arterionecrosis, reporting that the morphogenesis of the arterionecrosis was the development of histolysis as well as fibrinoid degeneration caused by blood plasma insudation in the wall of the intracerebral arteries, and the plasmatic arterionecrosis formed intracerebral microaneurysms (Fig. 9.3).

According to Yoshida et al,[46] microaneurysms occur most frequently in the putamen (36%), followed by the cerebral cortex (34%), thalamus (13%), and caudate nucleus (9%); they almost never occur in the globus pallidus and internal capsule (Fig. 9.4). These authors also state that if such a microaneurysm ruptures, it usually causes minimal hemorrhagic lesions, but is extensively hemorrhagic in the putamen or thalamus. Table 9.3 shows the ruptured artery and location of hematoma based on our 60 autopsied brains with hypertensive hemorrhage.

* References 2, 6, 15, 24, 34, 41, 42, 45.

Evolution of the Hemorrhage

It is believed that rupture of an intracerebral artery of up to 100 to 200 μm in diameter results in the formation of a hematoma of 0.5 to 1.0-cm diameter at most. The question is then what is the mechanism by which a relatively large hematoma forms from the rupture of a comparatively small vessel. Matsuoka[24] and Ooneda et al[34] surmised that multiple angionecrotic arteries rupture simultaneously or in succession, and resulting hematomas become confluent to form a large hematoma. Yamamura and his associates[45] advanced a two-stage theory to explain the mechanism of a large hematoma formation. According to these investigators, the initial change is rupture of the perforating artery about 2 cm distal to its entry into the base of the brain; this rupture is followed by reactive vasospasm, which causes circulatory disturbances and a concomitant increase in vascular permeability and diapedesis of blood. The extravasated blood becomes confluent to form a large hematoma involving areas corresponding to the authors' opinion; however, hemorrhage from the initial rupture is arrested at once by the formation of a thrombus and hence does not lead to the formation of a large hematoma.

Herbstein and Schaumburg[17] studied the pathophysiology of the initial hemorrhage, its duration, and the likelihood of rebleeding by injecting erythrocytes labeled with sodium chromate Cr 51 to patients admitted shortly after the onset. They found no significant radioisotopic activities in the primary cerebral hemispheric hematomas at postmortem examination, as opposed to the terminal, mesencephalic Duret's hemorrhages. They concluded that the initial bleed is a short, monophasic process, lasting probably no more than one or two hours.

In our angiographic study of acute severe

Table 9.2. The mechanism of bleeding in hypertensive intracerebral hemorrhage.

Mechanism	→	→	Reference	Result
Theory with priority to vascular rupture:				
Rupture of microaneurysm →			(6,41)[a]	Massive hematoma
Angionecrosis →	Rupture of multiple vessels →	Fusion of small hematomas →	(24,34)	Massive hematoma
Cerebrovascular lesion (aneurysm, arteriovenous malformation, primary angionectosis, arteriosclerosis) →	Primary bleeding due to ruptured vessel, increasing venous pressure and other factors →	Secondary bleeding by extravasation or rupture of smaller vessels (↑) →	(45)	Massive hematoma
Rupture of cerebral vein →			(42)	Massive hematoma
Theory with priority to disturbance of cerebral parenchyma:				
Ischemic infarction of cerebral parenchyma due to angiospasm →	Extravasation or rupture of vessels →		(2)	Massive hematoma
Brain softening →	Rupture of ischemic vessels →		(15)	Massive hematoma
Disturbance of venous circulation →	Disturbance of cerebral parenchyma and vessels →	Extravasation or rupture of vessels	(42)	Massive hematoma

[a] Numbers in parentheses indicate the reference which reported the theory.

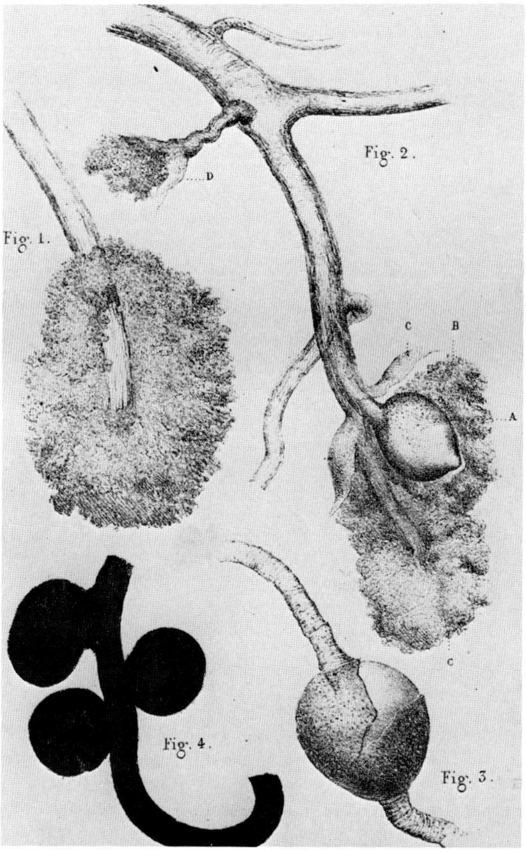

Fig. 9.2. Charcot's drawing of microaneurysm.

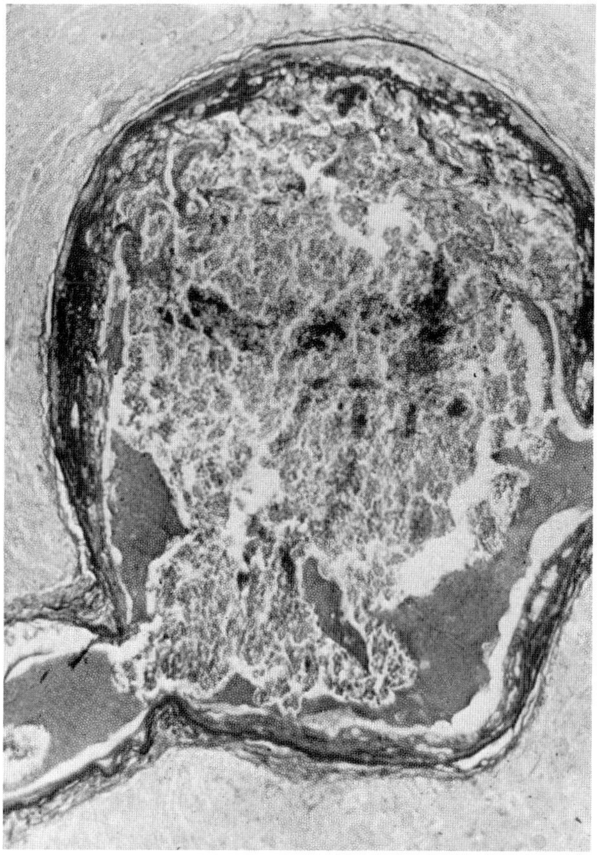

Fig. 9.3. Histologic finding of microaneurysm.

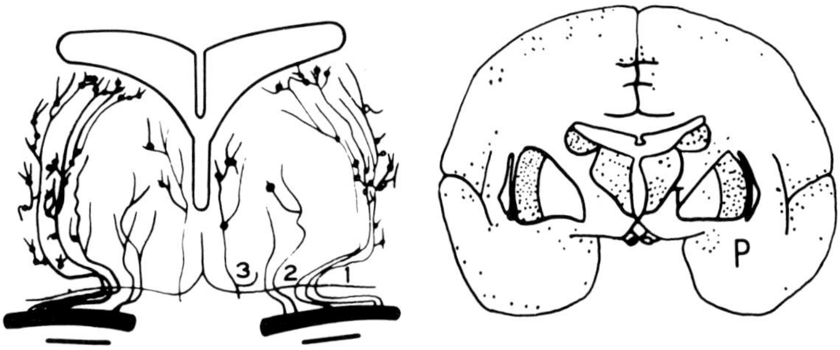

Fig. 9.4. Distribution of microaneurysm in eight cases of hypertensive intracerebral hemorrhage (Yoshida[46]). P, putamen; T, thalamus; 1, 2, lenticulostriate artery; 3, thalamoperforate artery.

Table 9.3. Ruptured artery and location of hematoma.

Ruptured artery		Location of hematoma
Lateral branch of lenticulostriate A.	→	Putaminal hemorrhage (62%)
Thalamogeniculate A. Thalamo-perforating A.	→	Thalamic hemorrhage (26%)
Perforator of superior cerebellar A. and posterior inferior cerebellar A.	→	Cerebellar hemorrhage (6%)
Paramedian branch of basilar A.	→	Pontine hemorrhage (5%)
Medullary A.	→	Subcortical hemorrhage (2%)

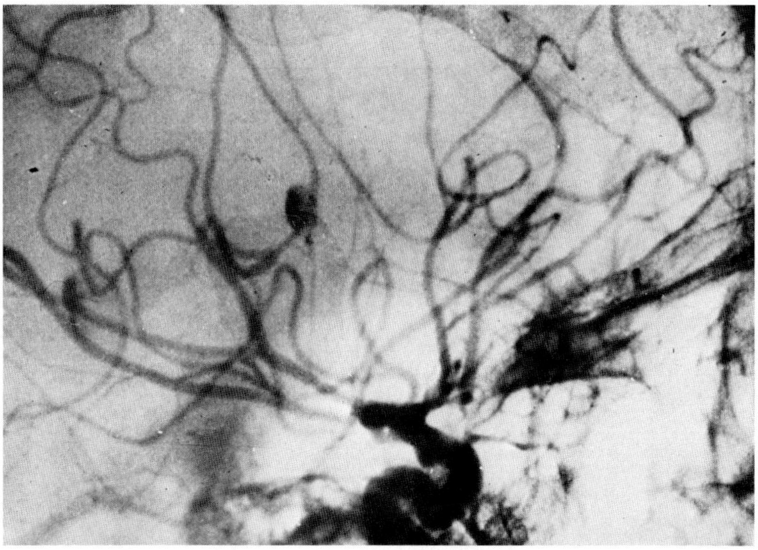

Fig. 9.5. Extravasation of contrast media from lenticulostriate artery. Carotid angiography was performed within four hours after onset.

cases,[28] however, we often observed continuous or intermittent extravasation of contrast medium from a lateral lenticulostriate artery as shown in Fig. 9.5. We also often observed the enlargement of hematoma on the CT scan when it is taken in the acute stage (within six hours after onset) (Fig. 9.6). These observations suggest that with a rapidly fatal outcome, the hemorrhage does not stop quickly but may persist continuously or intermittently for hours. In addition, an extensive hemorrhage can cause rupture of surrounding small vessels from compression and traction. It is also possible that the hematoma formation is further enhanced by necrotizing arteries secondarily compromised by acute circulatory disturbance resulting from rupture and venous stasis due to elevated venous pressure. The venous phase of serial angiograms demonstrating multiple extravasations of contrast media surrounding a large hematoma support this latter possibility. Moreover, histologic examination reveals acute angionecrosis (Fig. 9.7).

Our theory of rupture of a single blood vessel is the major rationale for surgical treatment of hypertensive intracerebral hemorrhage. In

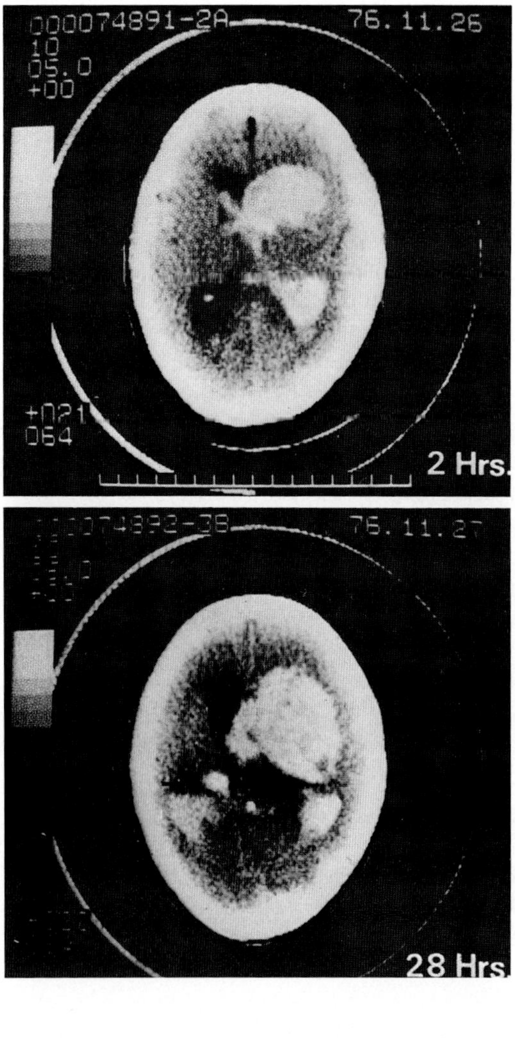

◁ **Fig. 9.6.** Growing hematoma on CT. *Upper,* CT was performed two hours after onset; *lower,* CT was performed 28 hours after onset.

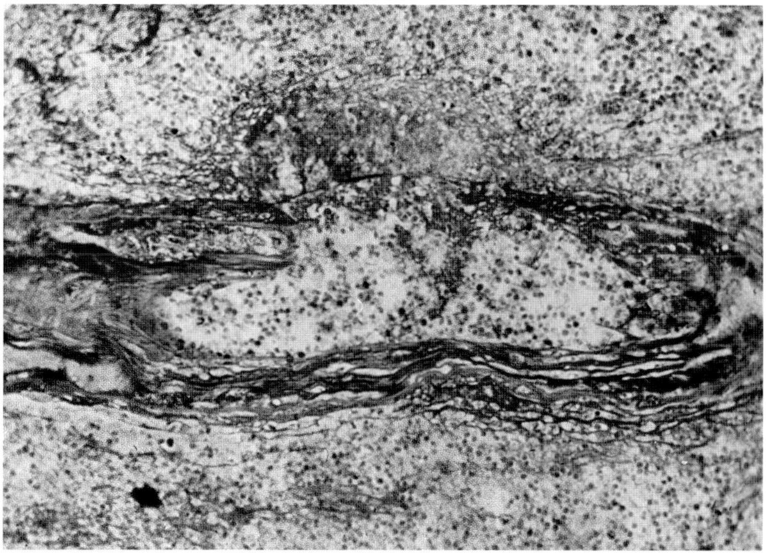

Fig. 9.7. Acute angionecrosis of the small vessel around the hematoma.

cases where the site of continued bleeding can be identified, and it is known to have only a single source, we attempt to arrest hemorrhage surgically as early as possible and to remove the hematoma.

Pattern of Hematoma Expansion

In putaminal hemorrhage arising from rupture of the lateral lenticulostriate artery, the resulting hematoma is supposed to spread along the lateral margin of the putamen in the direction of least resistance by a mechanical displacing force. This margin corresponds to the watershed area between the distribution of the lateral lenticulostriate artery and the claustrum, which is in the distribution of cortical and subcortical branches of the middle cerebral artery; blood never extravasates superficially through the cortex to reach the subarachnoid space (Fig. 9.8). Once bleeding occurs the brain tissue rendered ischemic and nonviable is softened and less resistant, making it easier for the hematoma to expand. In thalamic hemorrhage due to rupture of the thalamogeniculate artery, which supplies the lateral thalamic nucleus, the resulting hematoma readily spreads to and destroys the adjacent posterior limb of the internal capsule. Rupture of a thalamo-perforating artery, which supplies the medial thalamic nucleus, results in the formation of a hematoma that readily ruptures into the third ventricle and is apt to expand down around the subthalamic nucleus and to the cerebral peduncle (Fig. 9.9).

Subcortical hemorrhage may occur anywhere in the cerebral substance, some occurring as the result of rupture of a microaneurysm of a small penetrating artery stem in the subcortical layer (Fig. 9.10). The hemorrhage may be small (1–3 cm in extent) or may reach a size of 7 to 8 cm but does not, to any extent, penetrate the cortex to reach the subarachnoid space.

Pontine hemorrhage occurs as a result of rupture of the median pontine branch, and the hemorrhage may start in the base or tegmentum. In approximately 10% of cases the hemorrhage remains small and localized to the tegmentum and accumulates less rapidly. Rarely, a pontine hemorrhage will dissect along one or both middle cerebellar peduncles to enter the cerebellum.[13] Pathologic study has shown that as a pontine hemorrhage increases in size, numerous small arteries on its border are mechanically disrupted, each adding, in turn, its own increment of extravasation (Fig. 9.11).

Cerebellar hemorrhages originate near the dentate nucleus, where perforating branches of the superior cerebellar or posterior inferior cerebellar arteries penetrate, and the hematomas readily expand into the surrounding white matter. Further extension of the hematoma anteriorly may lead to rupture into the fourth ventricle. It is not uncommon for the hemorrhage to trek medially into the vermis and even across

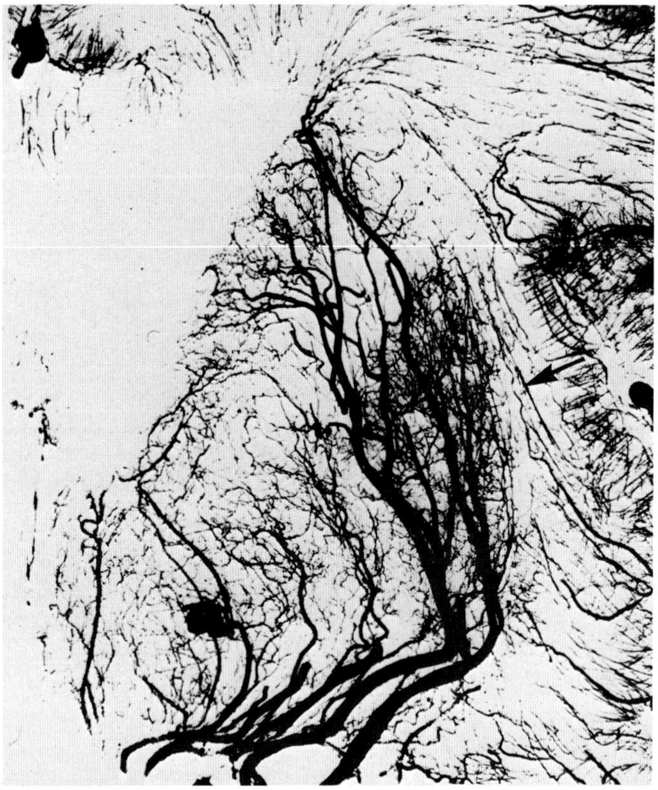

Fig. 9.8. Microangiogram of lenticulostriate artery. *Arrow* indicates watershed area between the distribution of lateral lenticulostriate artery and clastrum, which is in the distribution of cortical and subcortical branches of the middle cerebral artery.

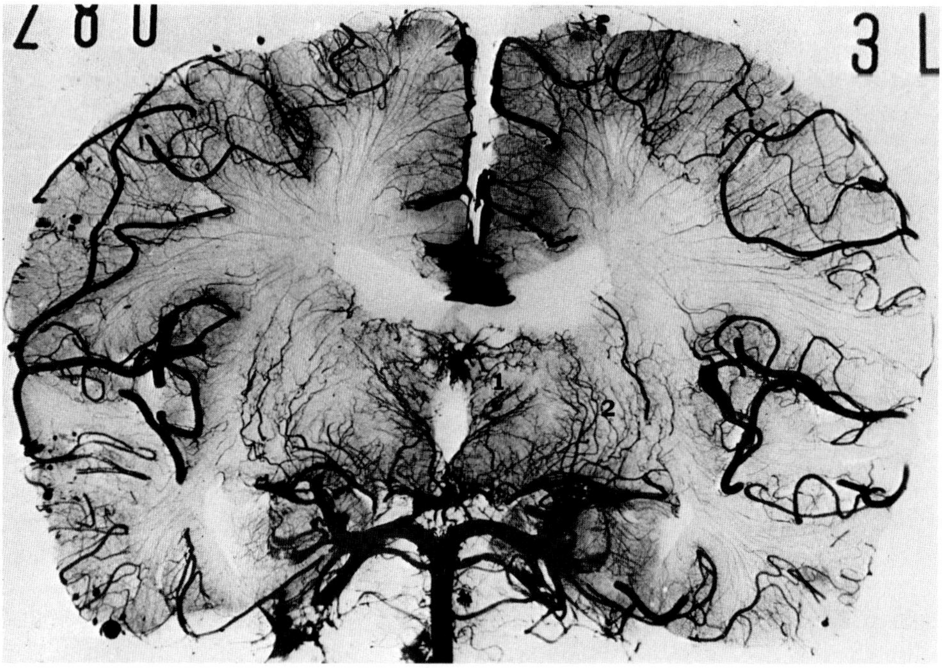

Fig. 9.9. Perforating arteries that supply the thalamus. 1, thalamo-perforate artery; 2, thalamo-geniculate artery.

into the opposite hemisphere. In a few cases the hemorrhage arises in the vermis itself and spreads bilaterally.

The progression and extension of these intracerebral hematomas were studied by frontal and sagittal sections of autopsied brains with putaminal and thalamic hemorrhages (the most frequent site of hypertensive intracerebral hemorrhages). The results are illustrated in Fig. 9.12 a,b and indicate that certain patterns of progression or evolution of the hematomas are apparent. These patterns of progression of hematoma are of great importance to the full understanding of the system of angiographic and CT classification for intracerebral hematomas and its rationale, which will be discussed later.

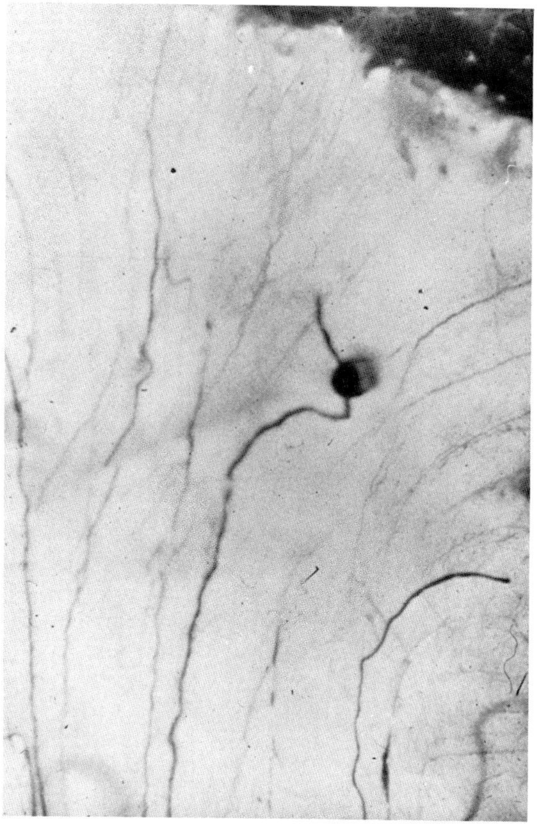

Fig. 9.10. Microaneurysm of a subcortical artery (cleared specimen).

Pathophysiology

Cause of Death

When an intracerebral hemorrhage directly destroys the midbrain and brainstem, death ensues. The presence of a large hematoma within the cerebral substance, even when it is not directly destructive to the brainstem, may frequently prove fatal through the sequence of:

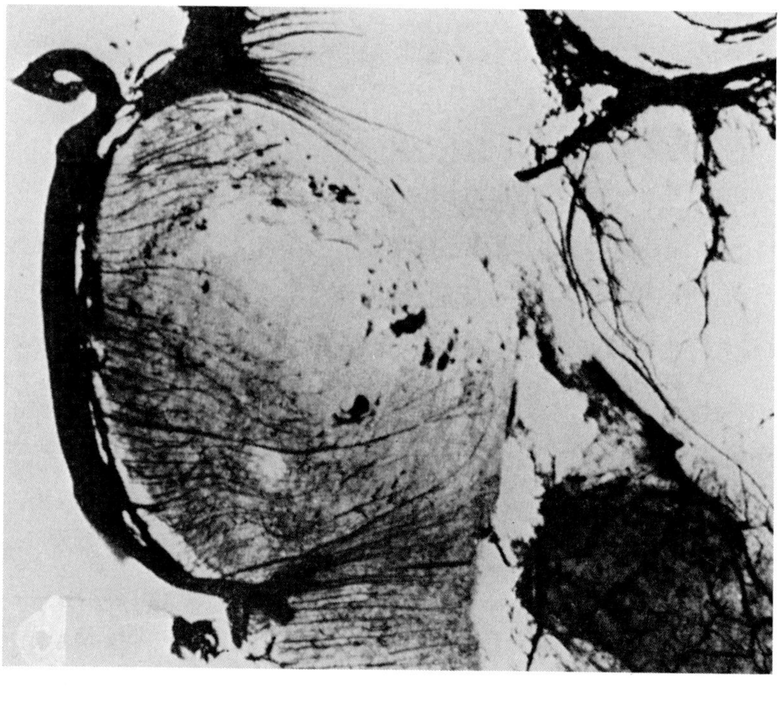

Fig. 9.11. Microangiogram of the pontine hemorrhage Courtesy of Nakajima, Research Institute of Brain and Blood Vessels, Akita, Japan.

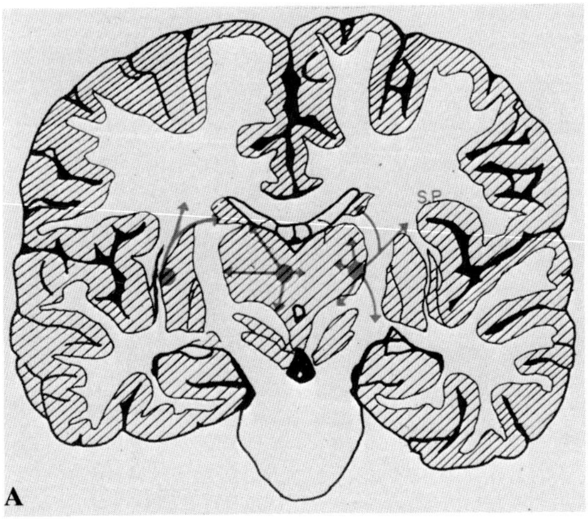

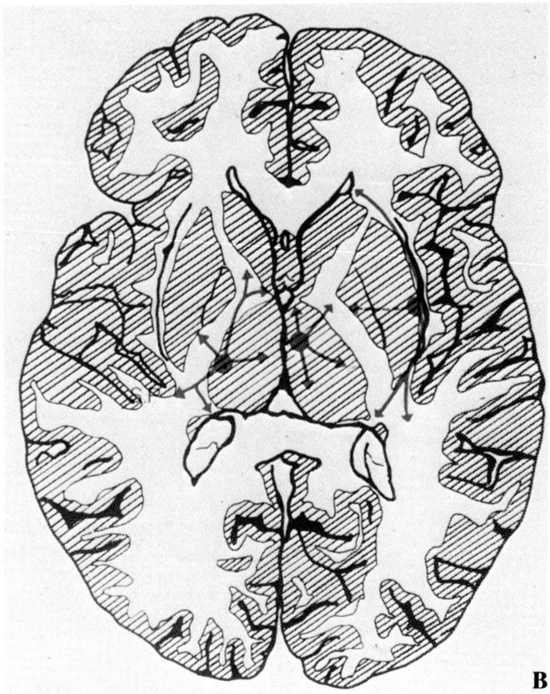

Fig. 9.12. **A.** Pattern of progression of the hematomas (coronal section), **B,** pattern of progression of the hematomas (horizontal section).

increased intracranial pressure, cerebral herniation and compression of the brain-stem. Moreover, an intracerebral hematoma compresses surrounding brain tissue and causes cerebral edema. Rupture of the hematoma into ventricles may cause acute hydrocephalus by interruption of the cerebrospinal fluid circulation. The cerebral edema and hydrocephalus in turn spur elevation of intracranial pressure. Cushing[9] drew attention to the importance of edema surrounding the hematoma. We have studied the time of onset of brain edema as determined by CT following putaminal hemorrhage. In Fig. 9.13 the size of the hematoma and the time elapsing from onset to performance of CT are plotted on the ordinate and abscissa, respectively. Open circles denote cases with no frank low density areas around the hematoma, and closed circles represent cases with clear-cut low density areas. Except in cases of so-called fulminating hematoma, which expand rapidly to fill up the ventricles like a cast, cerebral edema around the hematoma was shown to occur about six hours or later after onset. This is of great significance in determining the timing of surgery for cerebral hemorrhage, which is discussed later.

Intracranial Pressure

Intracranial pressure (ICP) is an important consideration in the treatment of hypertensive hemorrhage. Papo et al[36] also correlated the time course of ICP with clinical data and reported that the ICP remained normal or only slightly elevated in patients without noticeable disturbance of consciousness. By contrast, patients in coma with evidence of vegetative dysregulation and harboring deeply located hematomas showed very high-pressure values with a pronounced tendency to rise further. In the majority of patients exhibiting intermediate disturbances of consciousness, they noted no definite correlation between clinical condition and ICP. Therefore, the prognosis seems to depend not only on the increased pressure but also on the destruction by the hemorrhage. In fact, some comatose patients showed nearly normal ICP values. Janny et al[19] also reported that the highest pressures were recorded just after the stroke, following which the ICP decreased rapidly. Papo et al therefore concluded that from the neurosurgical standpoint, particular attention should be paid to hypertensive intracerebral hemorrhage in the very early phase

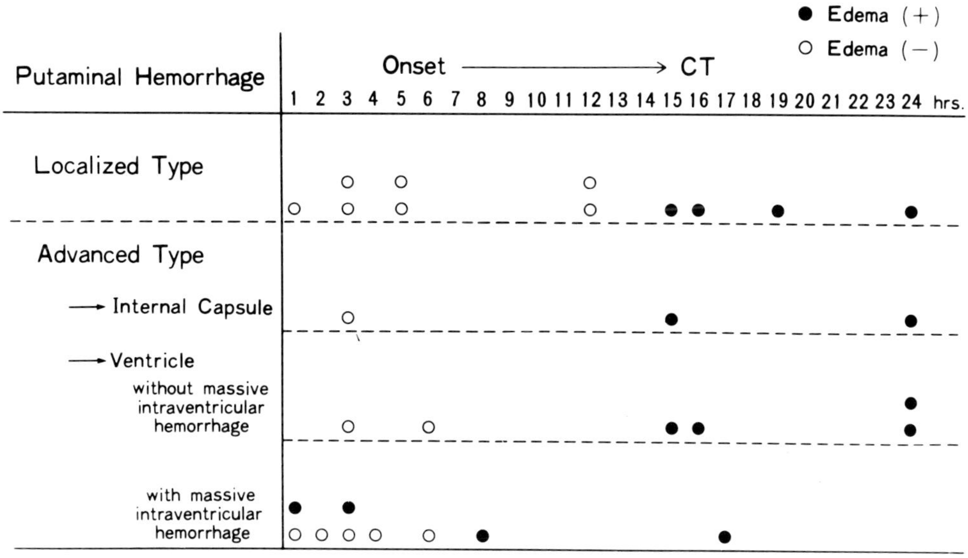

Fig. 9.13. Appearance of low-density areas around the hematoma on CT in putaminal hemorrhage.

after the stroke, for the patients rapidly become comatose. In the patients exhibiting intermediate disturbance of consciousness, neurosurgical intervention should be considered.

Mechanism for the Development of Hemiplegia

Hemiplegia arising from intracerebral hemorrhage is also a problem of serious clinical importance. In massive cerebral hemorrhage it is brought on by direct destruction of the internal capsule by the hematoma.

It seems relevant to clarify the process of destruction of the pyramidal tract by an expanding hematoma following putaminal hemorrhage that may be amenable to surgery.

In putaminal hemorrhage the hematoma is apt to develop in the direction of the distribution of the lenticulostriate artery, the direction indicated by the arrow in Fig. 9.14. In the process of this evolution the pyramidal tract that runs through the triangle is destroyed first. Hence this area may well be called the "vulnerable triangle" in putaminal hemorrhage. Figure 9.15 gives a diagrammatic representation of the extent of hematoma on CT relative to this triangle. The top of the figure shows the condition in cases with good prognosis for hemiplegia. The hematoma has not reached the triangle, and the

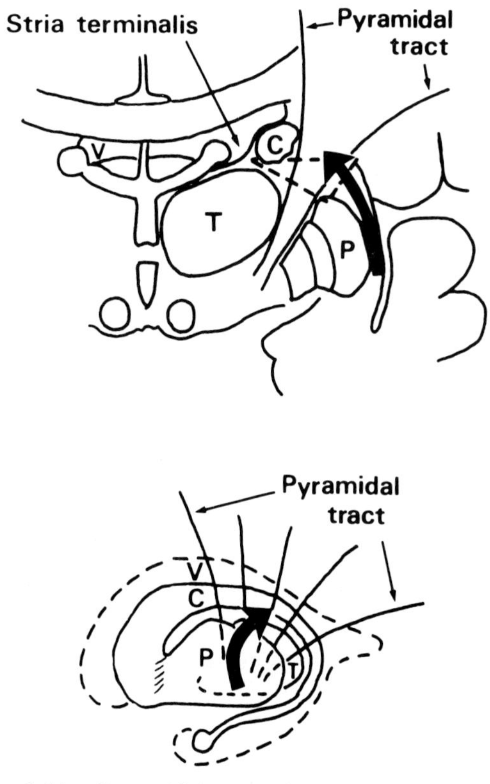

Fig. 9.14. Pyramidal tract, the ventricle and basal ganglia. Triangle indicated by dotted lines is vulnerable to hematoma. We have named it "vulnerable triangle." Hematoma tends to advance in direction of *black arrow*. C, caudate nucleus; T, thalamus; P, putamen; V, body of the lateral ventricle.

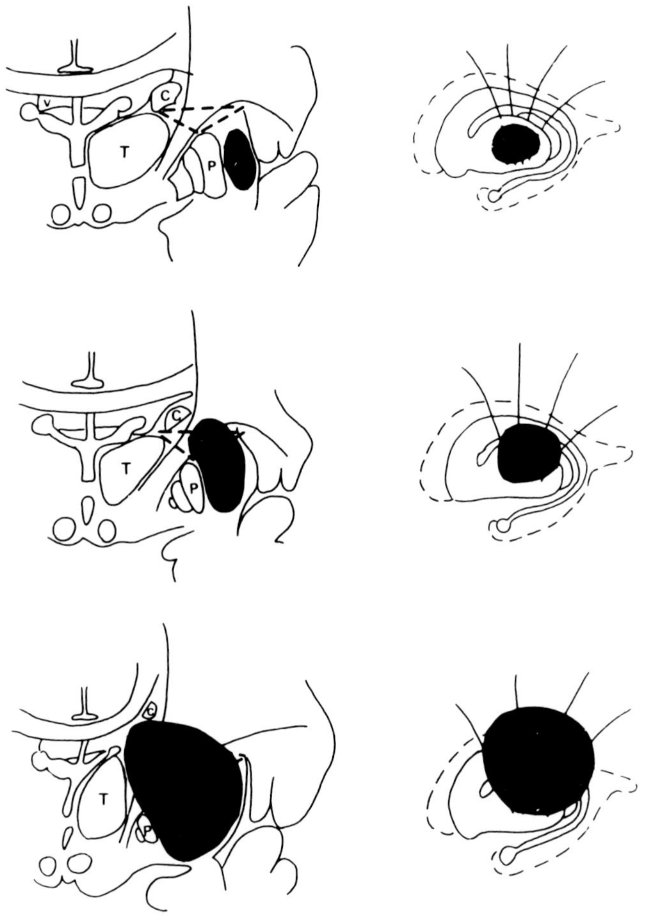

Fig. 9.15. Correlation of "vulnerable triangle" with the advancement of hematoma. *Upper part,* hematoma is localized lateral to the putamen; "vulnerable triangle" is not affected. *Center part,* hematoma progresses into "vulnerable triangle" and destroys it partially. *Lower part,* "vulnerable triangle" is destroyed completely and hematoma progresses into the body of the lateral ventricle, destroying the internal capsule.

pyramidal tract, therefore, is not destroyed. In such instances on CT no hematoma is demonstrable at the level of the body of the lateral ventricle.

In the middle of the figure are those cases in which the vulnerable triangle has been partially destroyed by a hematoma advancing upward from below. The hematoma extends beyond the upper margin of the triangle and is clearly visualized by CT at the level of the body of the lateral ventricle. Clinically, there was some delay in improvement of hemiplegia in such cases.

At the bottom of the figure are illustrated those cases in which the hematoma has perforated into the body of the lateral ventricle after causing complete destruction of the vulnerable triangle, with subsequent destruction of the posterior limb of the internal capsule.

In view of the process of destruction of the pyramidal tract by a hematoma resulting from putaminal hemorrhage, it would seem that in evaluating the prognosis of hemiplegia, the presence or absence of hematoma at the level of the body of the lateral ventricle is more valuable than the relationship of the hematoma to the posterior limb of the internal capsule. This is because the posterior limb is always displaced medially by the hematoma.

CT Classification of Hypertensive Intracerebral Hemorrhage

The system of angiographic classification was reported by us in 1976.[31] However, the CT scan has become important in the diagnosis of hypertensive intracerebral hemorrhage, as CT directly visualizes hematoma in the brain and readily distinguishes between the more medially placed thalamic hemorrhages and the more laterally situated (and more surgically accessible) putaminal hemorrhages. From the scan it is further possible to determine destruction of pyramidal tract, as mentioned before, and the presence of intraventricular hematoma. This information permits a more useful classification of hypertensive intracerebral hemorrhages than that of angiographic classification.

Table 9.4 shows a new classification of supratentorial hypertensive intracerebral hemorrhage based on CT scan. This classification of hematomas are classified into 3 types (putaminal and external capsular, thalamic and subcortical) according to the artery ruptured, and each of these types is further divided into 3 subtypes according to the direction of expansion and progression of hematoma. This classification is distinguished from the conventional classifications (which are based solely on the location and extent of hematomas on autopsy and so may be labeled as static), as it takes the dynamic process of expansion of hematomas into full account.

The classification proposed here is of great importance in the management of intracerebral hemorrhage. The rationale for this classification is explained below with the presentation of illustrative CT scans.

Table 9.4. CT classification of hypertensive intracerebral hemorrhage (supratentorial).

Putaminal hemorrhage
Localized type
Advanced type
Putamen → Pyramidal tract
Putamen → Pyramidal tract → Ventricle
Thalamic hemorrhage
Localized type
Hemorrhage in the lateral nucleus
Hemorrhage in the medial nucleus
Advanced type
Partial destruction of thalamus
Total destruction of thalamus

Putaminal Hemorrhage

Localized Type (Fig. 9.16)

Included in this type are those hemorrhages in which hematomas are within the confines of the putamen and external capsule. As mentioned earlier, the extent of hematoma in the vertical direction rather than in the anteroposterior direction is important in the evaluation of prognosis for hemiplegia.

In this type of hemorrhage the prognosis of hemiplegia is good, as no unequivocal hematoma is seen on the CT scan of brain slices through the body of the lateral ventricle, and, accordingly, the pyramidal tract is not destroyed by the hematoma.[32]

Advanced Type

Putamen → Pyramidal Tract (Fig. 9.17). In this type of putaminal hemorrhage the hematoma progresses to the point of destroying a part of the pyramidal tract. On CT scan a part of the hematoma is demonstrable at the level of the body of the lateral ventricle. Owing to edema of cerebral tissues surrounding the hematoma, damage to the pyramidal tract becomes increasingly extensive with time.

Putamen → Pyramidal Tract → Ventricle (Fig. 9.18). As referred to previously in the sec-

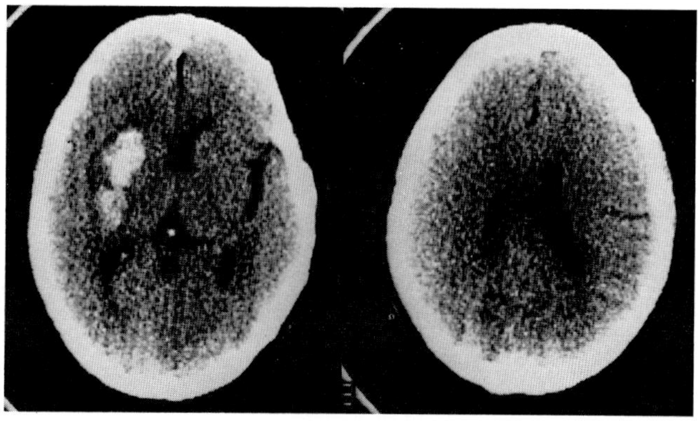

Fig. 9.16. Putaminal hemorrhage, localized type. CT scan at the level of the bodies of the lateral ventricles shows no high-density area (*right*).

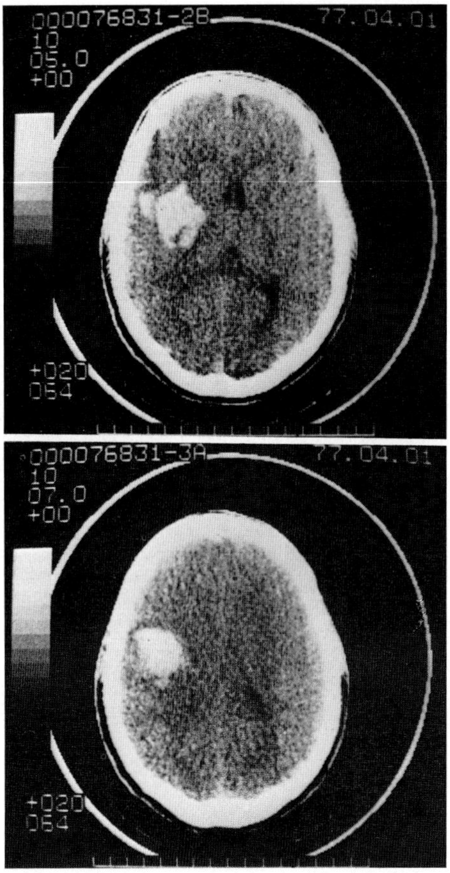

Fig. 9.17. Putaminal hemorrhage, advanced type. Putamen → pyramidal tract. On CT the hematoma is demonstrable at the level of the body of the lateral ventricle.

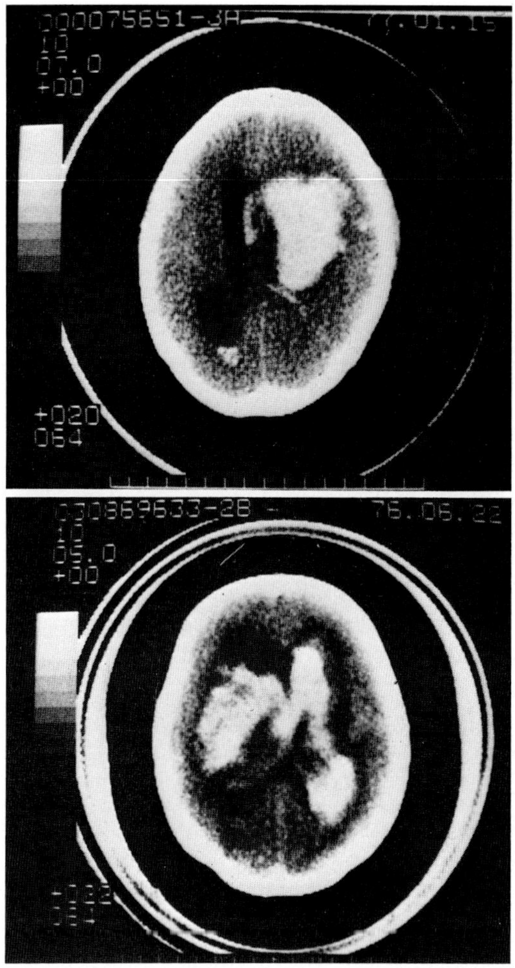

Fig. 9.18. Putaminal hemorrhage, advanced type. Putamen → pyramidal tract → ventricle. The hematoma perforates into the ventricle.

tion on advancement of hematoma, the hematoma most often ruptures into the anterior horn or trigone of the lateral ventricle.

In cases where there is a hematoma of tremendous size filling the ventricle like a cast, the patients are usually comatose within hours after onset; the prognosis is ominous, and even surgical treatment fails to salvage the patient's life. On the other hand, where only part of the hematoma ruptures into the ventricle, more than half of the cases will have a fatal outcome with medical treatment. Hence, surgical treatment is a vital necessity.

In hemorrhage massive enough to rupture into the ventricle, prognosis for hemiplegia, as a matter of course, is poor since the pyramidal tract, inclusive of the posterior limb of the internal capsule, is very likely to be destroyed by the hematoma.

Thalamic Hemorrhage

Localized Type

Hemorrhage into the Lateral Nucleus (Fig. 9.19a). In this type, the hemorrhages center around the lateral nucleus of the thalamus. Because the internal capsule is located immediately lateral to the lateral nucleus, the outward expansion of the hematoma readily results in destruction of the internal capsule, with a consequent poor prognosis for hemiplegia. However, as the hematoma is usually small, prognosis for life is good.

Hemorrhage into the Medial Nucleus (Fig. 9.19b). This type of intracerebral hemorrhage

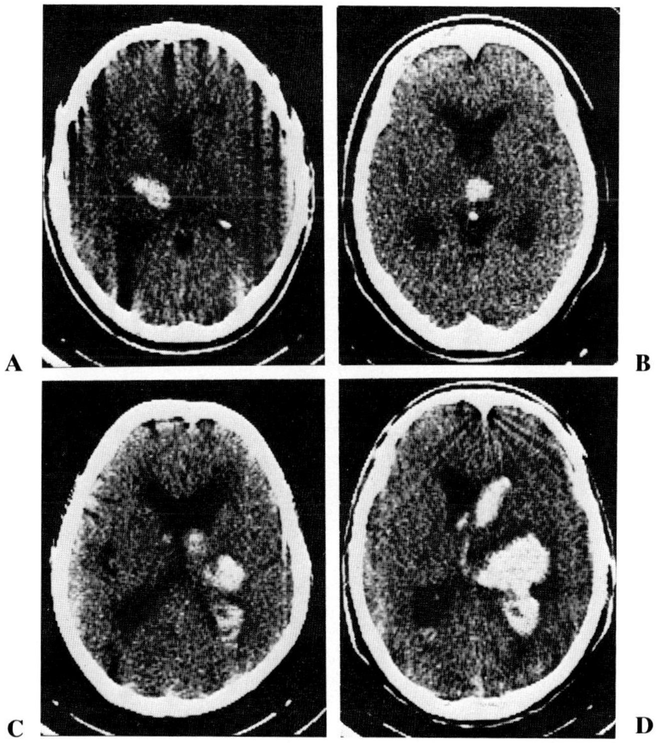

Fig. 9.19. Thalamic hemorrhage. **A.** Localized type (lateral nucleus); **B,** localized type (medial nucleus); **C,** advanced type, partial destruction of thalamus; **D,** advanced type, total destruction of thalamus.

occurs mainly in the medial nucleus of the thalamus and is often not attended by hemiplegia. Hematomas resulting from hemorrhage into the medial nucleus readily rupture into the third ventricle. When the ventricular system is completely obstructed, hydrocephalus may ensue. In this type of bleeding it is necessary to check for ventricular enlargement by serial CT scans.

Advanced Type

Partial Destruction of Thalamus (Fig. 9.19c). This type of thalamic hemorrhage perforates into the lateral ventricle and partially destroys the thalamus. Since noncommunicating hydrocephalus may occur when the foramen of Monro is blocked bilaterally, it is necessary to remove surgically the intraventricular hematoma and provide ventricular drainage with the intention of improving consciousness. As the pyramidal tract usually is partially damaged, the prognosis for hemiplegia is favorable in most instances.

Total Destruction of Thalamus (Fig. 9.19d). This type of hemorrhage causes almost complete destruction of the thalamus. In most cases the hematoma ruptures into the third and lateral ventricles. Prognosis for life, and also hemiplegia, is very poor even with surgery.

Surgical Treatment

Preoperative Clinical Classification of Patients

Hitherto, there have been scattered reports of the classification of patients according to survival probability as indicated by the neurologic status and hematoma location.* Most reports were, however, retrospective studies with undisclosed factors in the selection of cases. Luessenhop et al[23] performed early direct surgical evacuation of the hematoma for a consecutive, unselected series of cases in which angiography demonstrated the hematoma. They operated on 37 out of 64 patients with hypertensive intracerebral hemorrhage. Their operative mortality was 32% in 37 patients, with only a 4% mortality in those patients with hematomas located in the subcortical white matter, as com-

* References 7, 8, 22, 23, 35, 37–39, 44.

pared with an 89% mortality for hematomas located deep in the capsular region of the hemisphere. They included the external capsular hematomas, with forward and backward extension as lobar. The state of consciousness of patients operated on ranged from drowsy to deep stupor, without evidence of diencephalic or mesencephalic involvement by extension or compression. They operated on 13 patients with clear-cut upper or lower brainstem signs consistent with extension of hemorrhage to these areas or compression from beginning uncal herniation and saved three patients. Among the 10 operative deaths, three were apneic at the time of induction of anesthesia, and at autopsy the brain showed reaccumulation of the clot with extension into the third ventricle and hypothalamus. This indicates that regardless of how rapidly the patient is brought to surgical treatment, it is very difficult to salvage the patient with large medially arising hemorrhages that promptly dissect into the thalamus and ventricles. This is consistent with recommendations first advanced by Fazio.[11] Two patients died postoperatively with medical complications. The remaining four patients showed some clinical improvement following surgery, but within a few days gradually deteriorated and expired with upper brainstem improvement. In all of these there were marked reaccumulation of the clot and extension to the ventricular system. They have stressed that the most important surgical complication was reaccumulation of the clot. This complication indicates that one of the reasons for McKissock's high surgical mortality was due to the reaccumulation of the clot, accounting for their failure to achieve operative benefits in predominantly lobar clots.

The prognosis of intracerebral hemorrhage depends primarily on the site of hemorrhage, the direction of its progression, and the size as well as speed of hematoma formation. Clinical symptoms that are brought on by the hematoma, notably the degree of sensorial impairment, are indicators of prognosis for life. Therefore, any attempt to classify the severity of intracerebral hemorrhage must take into account the location and extent of the hematoma as well as the degree and time course of the disturbances of consciousness. We have developed a system classifying the severity of putaminal hemorrhages that are accessible to surgical treatment, as shown in Table 9.5. This grading is based on the degree of disturbed consciousness reached within six hours after onset. The rationale for this assumption is as follows: (1) the formation of a hematoma following hypertensive intracerebral hemorrhage is completed in less than six hours. As already pointed out, cerebral angiograms taken early in the course of the disease often demonstrate extravasation of contrast medium. This phenomenon is observed almost exclusively during six hours after onset. This implies that the formation of hematoma is complete within six hours after bleeding. (2) Disturbance of consciousness attains its highest level within six hours after onset. In about 90% of putaminal hemorrhages treated by us, disturbance of consciousness reached its height by six hours after onset. This fact suggests that the degree of disturbance of consciousness is determined by the severity of primary injury to the brain (hematoma formation) and a consequent increase in intracranial pressure during the initial six hours after onset. For ensuing periods the secondary damage such as brain edema and hydrocephalus become a major determinant factor.

It is possible, therefore, to classify hypertensive intracerebral hemorrhage into five grades, grade I through grade V, according to the degree of disturbance of consciousness and also on the extent of hematoma. Experience has shown that 80% of grade III cases in the over-60 age group are poor surgical risks. Especially in those cases with impairment of the dominant hemisphere, surgery, even if it is life-saving,

Table 9.5. Classification of patients with putaminal hemorrhage according to surgical risk. (M. Mizukami, 1976)

Grade I: Alert or mild disturbance of consciousness with localized type
Grade II: Mild or moderate disturbance of consciousness with pyramidal type
Grade III: Moderate or severe disturbance of consciousness with ventricular type
Grade IV: Grade III + over 60 years old + dominant hemisphere
Grade V: Very severe disturbance of consciousness with ventricular type

[a] Level of consciousness which reaches the lowest level within 6 hours after onset. Source: Mizukami M.[31]

usually does not ensure recovery to the point of being started on a rehabilitation program, and the patients remain bedridden all their life. Such cases are categorized as grade IV.

This system of classification according to severity was found to apply to 94% of 187 operated cases of putaminal hemorrhage in our present series. The remaining 6% of cases did not clearly fit the grading so they were graded solely on the basis of the degree of disturbance of consciousness.

The Results of Surgical versus Conservative Treatments and Operative Indications

Since 1966 the author has operated on more than 250 patients with putaminal hemorrhage. Since introduction of the CT scan, from 1974 to 1975 almost all patients who had disturbance of consciousness were treated surgically except for deeply comatose patients. From 1976 to 1979 conservative treatment was a first choice in almost all cases. The results of two groups consisting of 187 surgical and 165 medical patients are shown in Table 9.6.

In an attempt to evaluate the results of operation in hypertensive intracerebral hemorrhage, not only the mortality but the degree of recovery of function (classified by the system proposed by Millikan et al[1]) was determined 1 year after onset in all cases in our series. Since it is difficult to compare the medical and surgical treatment in each individual grade, the survival rate and the degree of functional recovery were compared in the combined group of patients in grades I, II, and III, which reflect patients who can manage their daily-living activities.

As indicated in Fig. 9.20, there was no difference in mortality and morbidity between surgical and medical treatments in grade I cases. In grade II cases surgical treatment was better than medical treatment, but the difference was not statistically significant.

Surgical treatment was found to be definitely superior in both mortality and morbidity to medical treatment in grade III, the difference being significant notably in grade III cases ($p < 0.05$). In grade IV and grade V cases no significant difference was observed between the treatments, but it should be mentioned that recovery to grade III was attained in three cases undergoing operation within six hours after onset.

Timing of Operation

Bagely[4] advised waiting a few days before operating, when the clots start to disintegrate, are less adherent to the wall of the cavity, and are

Table 9.6. Comparison of medical and surgical management.

Consciousness	Classication of Hematoma	Management	Fully independent in ADL		Semidependent in ADL (Requiring some assistance)		Semidependent in ADL (Requiring lifting assistance)		Fully dependent in ADL		Death		Total	
			M	S	M	S	M	S	M	S	M	S	M	S
GRADE I	Alert ~ Drowsiness	localized	36	11	6	3	1	—	—	—	—	—	43	14
GRADE II	Drowsiness ~ Stupor	advanced (Pyramidal tract)	1	1	22	23	20	28	16	11	5	8	64	71
GRADE III	Stupor ~ Semicoma	advanced (Ventricle)	—	—	1	12	5	30	6	17	17	14	29	73
GRADE IV	Stupor ~ Semicoma	GRADE III + over 60 y.o. + dominant hemisphere	—	—	—	—	—	3	4	8	6	3	10	14
GRADE V	Coma	advanced (Ventricle)	—	—	—	—	—	3	—	—	16	12	16	15

* Evaluated 1 year after the onset

162 187

total 349 cases

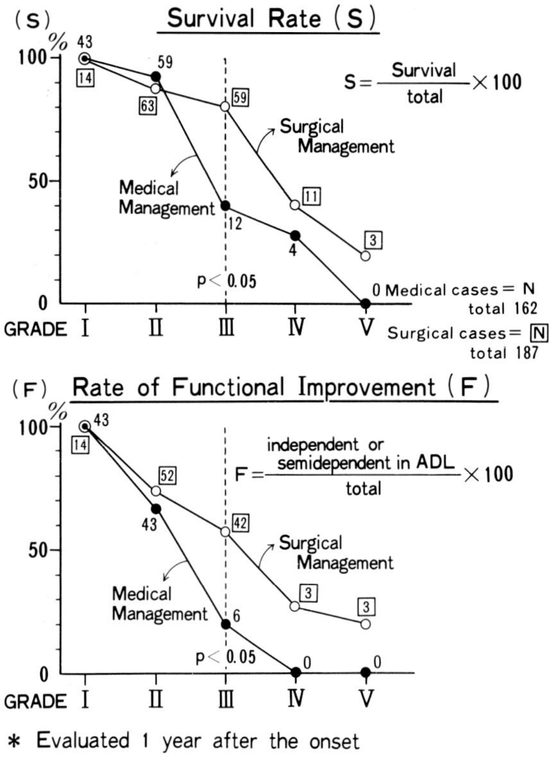

Fig. 9.20. Comparison of medical and surgical management.

easier to extirpate, and, further, because there is less risk of the hemorrhage starting again. Lazorthes[22] distinguished the date of operation as follows: (1) Routine surgical treatment carried out, if possible, on the third or fourth day, after the dangerous period of the first 48 hours has passed with the help of medical treatment; (2) emergency surgical treatment, sometimes useful by the end of the first day or in the course of the first 48 hours. This means ranking the surgical treatment of cerebral hemorrhage as urgent as that of serious visceral hemorrhages.

We have recommended early operation to free the brain from compression by the hematoma and secondary edema.[30] Recently, Kaneko et al[21] advocated early operation on hypertensive intracerebral hemorrhage using microsurgical technique within seven hours after the stroke. Papo et al[36] also concluded that the results of early operation were better than that of delayed operation, based on their monitoring of intracranial pressure.

To clarify the optimal timing of operation, survival and the quality of recovery were analyzed in our total series of 187 surgical patients. There was no distinct correlation between the timing and outcome of operation. In our series there were a few cases that were operated on within six hours after onset. To minimize the secondary brain damage, e.g., brain edema, early operation with six hours after onset is recommended, as it will improve the operative results with an increase in the number of viable cases. In fact, recovery to grade III was achieved in three of five grade IV or V cases undergoing surgical removal of hematoma within six hours after onset.

Operative Procedures

Preoperative Management

Since intracerebral hemorrhages, in most instances, occur in elderly persons with a history of hypertension, the preoperative examination of the heart, lung, and kidney is mandatory. At least ECG, chest x-ray, and phenolsulfonphthalein (PSP) test should be performed. In cases with pronounced disturbance of consciousness, nasal intubation rather than tracheotomy is preferred to avoid a rise in blood pressure and intracranial pressure. Rapid intravenous drip infusion of 300 mL 15% glycerol should be started 30 minutes before operation to minimize expansion of the brain at the time of incision of the dura mater.

Patient's Position

In cases of putaminal hemorrhage the supine position is allowable. Since, however, turning the head to one side may cause obstruction of the contralateral internal carotid artery, especially in patients of advanced age, it is recommended that a pillow be placed under the shoulders. As is always the case with operations on the brain, the head should be held at a slightly higher level than the heart.

In cerebeller hemorrhage cases the operation is performed with the patient in a sitting position as a rule, but the recumbent position in emergency cases is acceptable.

Approaches to Hematoma

The routes of surgical procedure on subcortical and cerebellar hemorrhage are the same as those for brain tumors and, hence, are omitted here. Mention will be made only of the approach to putaminal hemorrhage.

There are three time-honored approaches to this type of intracerebral hemorrhage: (1) transfrontal lobe approach, (2) transtemporal lobe approach, and (3) approach through the Sylvian fissure. Regardless of the type of approach, attack on the hematoma is invariably by a craniotomy performed under direct vision.

The *frontal approach* is almost obsolete, having the disadvantages that the operative field is not close and does not permit direct visualization of the bleeding artery. The *temporal approach* is currently the most commonly employed. It is the approach of choice in cases of hemorrhage in acute stage where brain swelling is marked. The *Sylvian fissure approach* affords the advantage of permitting access to the hematoma without causing damage to the intact brain substance, unless there is a high degree of brain swelling. In cases with marked brain swelling, the temporal approach is preferred since otherwise additional compression of brain tissue would be produced.

Recently Backlund and Holst[3] developed a new instrument for stereotactic evacuation of intracerebral hematoma and reported a successful case using this technique. The aim of this operation is not to totally remove the hematoma, but rather to evacuate only that volume considered threatening to the vitality of the brain. According to our experience, however, the mere release of the intracranial pressure reinitiated bleeding from the hematoma wall in some cases. We believe that the hematoma should be removed completely, and any bleeding from the hematoma wall should be coagulated, especially in acute cases.

Skin Incision

Whether the transtemporal lobe approach or approach through the Sylvian sulcus is employed, it is necessary to perform a small osteoplastic craniotomy through question mark incision to obtain an operative field adequate for manipulation. By using this procedure the operator can readily cope with any possible variations of the location of the sylvian sulcus. According to the author's experience, a large osteoplastic craniotomy is unnecessary for a patient even if he had a large hematoma and severe impairment of consciousness. The detached skin is turned inside out and lifted with a hook. Then a longitudinal incision of the temporal fascia and muscle is made with an electric knife along the zygomatic arch anteriorly and up nearly to the skin incision posteriorly. The attachment of the temporal muscle is incised with an electric knife, preferably leaving part of the attachment intact for later suturing.

Craniotomy

In a small craniotomy, two to three burr holes are usually placed, and the bone is excised at the base of the cranium by means of a rongeur. Cutting bone in other places is done by a neuroairtome. The bone strips so prepared are turned inside out together with the muscles attached to them.

Incision of the Dura Mater

When the dura mater is exceedingly tense, caution must be exercised in cutting it open, as this may cause expansion of the brain with resultant injury to it. It is recommended, therefore, to make a small incision, about 5 mm long, of the dura mater (over the temporal lobe) through which to perform electrocoagulation of brain surface and then to make an attempt at aspirating the hematoma. Usually a 3.5 to 4-cm puncture of the brain substance will suffice to reach the hematoma. If the first attempt fails, repeat the puncture in another direction. The best way to reach the hematoma is to puncture in a direction diverging a little to the operator's side. The dura mater is incised crosswise in parallel with the Sylvian sulcus.

Access to Hematoma (Fig. 9.21)

Transtemporal Lobe Approach

A cortical incision, about 2 cm long, is made in either the middle temporal gyrus or the superior temporal gyrus, depending on whether the Sylvian sulcus is displaced upward or downward. Prior to this incision an attempt is made to puncture the hematoma. Since in either case an additional incision of the insular cortex is to be made later, it is necessary to effect hemostasis thoroughly in this area so that postoperative rebleeding may be forestalled.

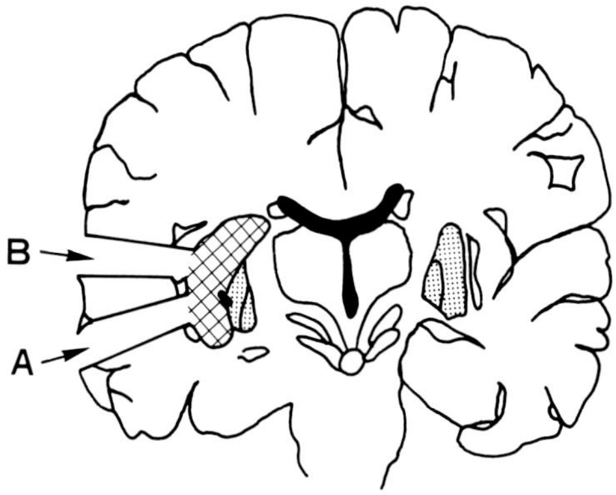

A = transtemporal

B = transsylvian

Fig. 9.21. Access to hematoma.

Approach Through the Sylvian Sulcus

As the Sylvian sulcus is more extensible in its anterior portion, the rim of the sphenoid bone is removed sufficiently from below. The arachnoid over the Sylvian sulcus is cut sharply while being tensed and stretched about 2 cm backward. The Sylvian sulcus is held open by pushing a piece of cotton through it with the aid of a brain spatula and aspirator. Small veins and venules are coagulated as soon as they come in sight. On reaching the insula, the cortical branch of the middle cerebral artery is found. Puncture of the insula with a needle (for use in ventricular puncture) to a depth of about 0.5 to 1 cm (while taking care not to cause damage to the artery) gives access to the hematoma. Incision of the insular cortex is made by coagulotomy.

Procedure for Removal of Hematoma

There is an invariable principle concerning the removal of hematoma, that is, the hemorrhagic globe attached to the bleeding artery (striate artery in the case of putaminal hemorrhage) must not be detached carelessly. This is because resultant bleeding may seriously interfere with operative manipulation. It is mandatory, therefore, to first aspirate the hematoma with the suction tube held in a direction opposite to the hemorrhagic globule.

Blood clots that cannot be aspirated are removed by the use of a pituitary clamp. Small vessels on the walls of the hematoma are coagulated. Since the hematoma is located in the posterior limb of the internal capsule, utmost caution should be exercised not to cause damage to the brain tissue surrounding the hematoma. Even if the ventricle is perforated it should not be opened through the perforation. Then, the anterior portion of the hematoma is treated in the same manner as described above. The hematoma extending toward the anterior horn of the lateral ventricle, which is out of the operator's sight, must be aspirated cautiously with the suction tube bent. If this fails to effect satisfactory drainage, it is advisable to use the small mirror used in operating for pituitary tumor. This instrument will prove of value in evacuating a blind portion of the hematoma.

Lastly, the floor of the hematoma is managed. This area corresponds to the putamen, hence injudicious aspiration may cause bleeding. The hemorrhagic globe is the last to be aspirated. On removing it, an underlying artery comes into sight. It is the ruptured vessel. This artery only is clipped. At times the main trunk of the lenticulostriate artery underneath it may be seen. Care must be taken not to injure this artery. On complete removal of the hematoma, its lumen is washed with physiologic saline. Hemorrhage of arterial origin, if any, should be arrested by coagulation, never by compression, for example, with the use of Gelfoam.

Suction tubes of varying size should be at hand. Suction should be adjusted to the consistency of the hematoma by closing, half closing, or unclosing the hole of the aspirator with the thumb. Application of vigorous suction to the walls of the hematoma must be strictly avoided.

In our experience, the reaccumulation of hematoma postoperatively is best prevented by elevating blood pressure to its preoperative level with the use of pressor drugs upon confirmation of effected hemostasis. Since the blood pressure is lowered during operation in most instances, its rapid rise following recovery from anesthesia may result in re-bleeding. The above-mentioned manipulations are greatly facilitated with the use of a microscope.

Closure of Operative Wound

The dura mater is tightly sutured. Use of an intralesional drain is unnecessary. The muscle,

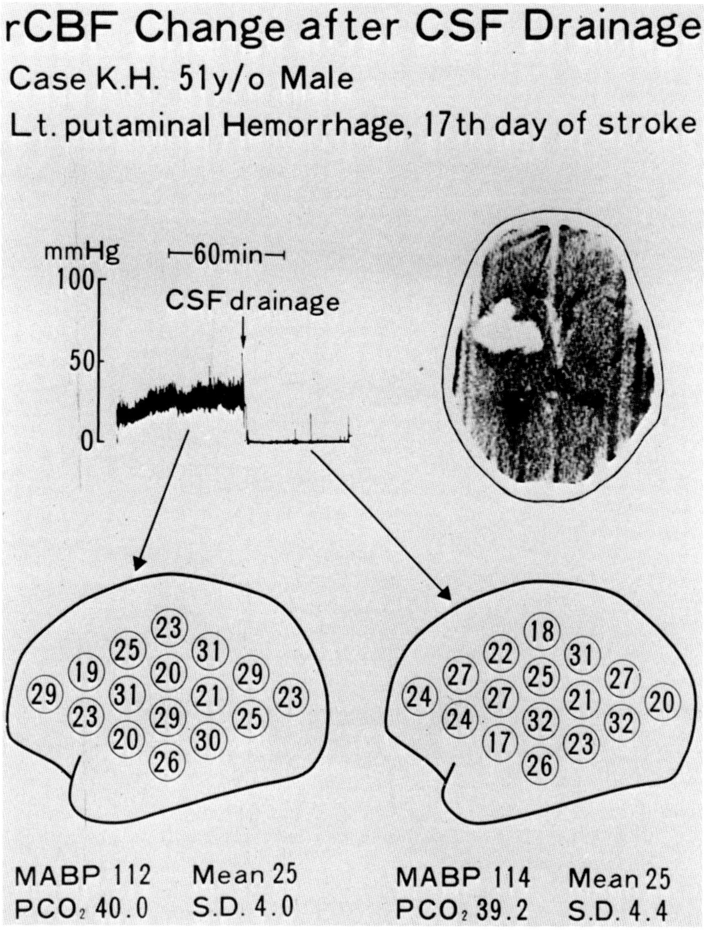

Fig. 9.22. Regional cerebral blood flow study shows no changes of flow value after CSF drainage in a case of putaminal hemorrhage on the 17th day of stroke.

fascia, and skin are sutured in that order with a drain held in place in the subcutaneous tissue, then brain swelling following the operation especially in cases with profound impairment of consciousness.

Rationale of Surgical Treatment (Intracerebral Squeeze Concept)

It was believed that ICP is high in cases of hypertensive intracerebral hemorrhage. As pointed out by Pappo et al,[36] however, ICP is not always correlated with the patient's clinical condition. Some comatose patients often show normal ICP. To clarify this discrepancy, a study of ICP changes in patients was undertaken. Figure 9.22 shows the change of the regional cerebral blood flow (rCBF) after cerebrospinal fluid (CSF) drainage. Before CSF drainage, mean rCBF was 36 mL/100 g/min; after drainage no changes of rCBF was noted. This means that rCBF did not increase even if ICP decreased. Figure 9.23 shows rCBF change after glycerol infusion. After glycerol infusion, rCBF surrounding area of hematoma remarkably increased, meaning that tissue perfusion pressure increased after glycerol infusion.

Based on these data, we would like to propose the "intracerebral squeeze concept" in hypertensive intracerebral hemorrhage, as shown in Fig. 9.24. This concept indicates that tissue pressure surrounding hematoma is more important that ICP in the management of hypertensive intracerebral hemorrhage.

Theoretical treatment for hypertensive intracerebral hemorrhage is, we believe, to reduce the tissue pressure surrounding the hematoma by giving hypertonic solution like glycerol, or by removing the hematoma surgically, as early as possible.

The value of surgical treatment for hyperten-

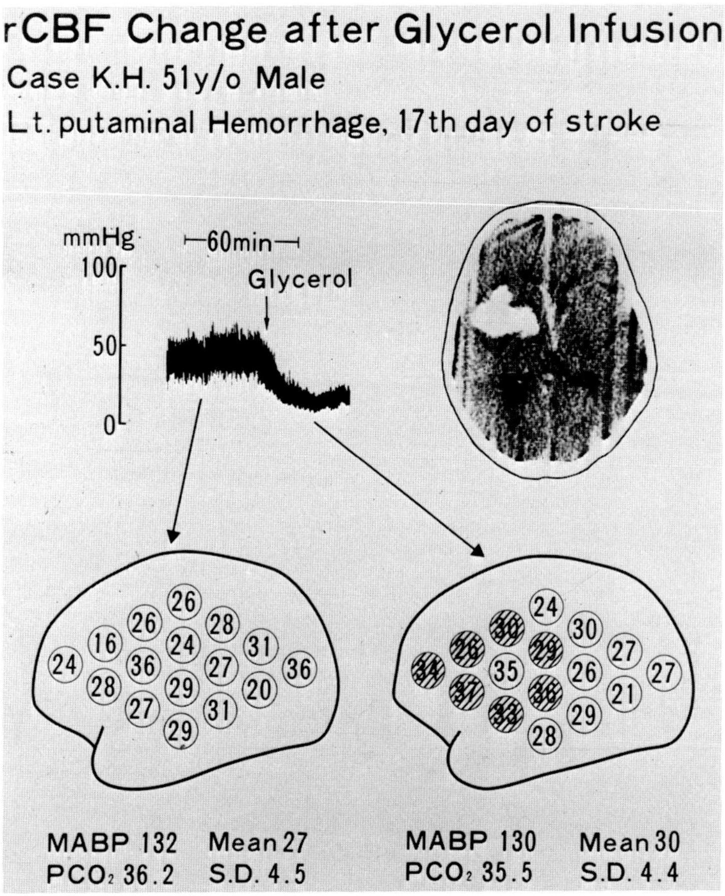

Fig. 9.23. Regional cerebral blood flow study shows the increase of flow value in the areas surrounding hematoma after 15% glycerol infusion in the same case.

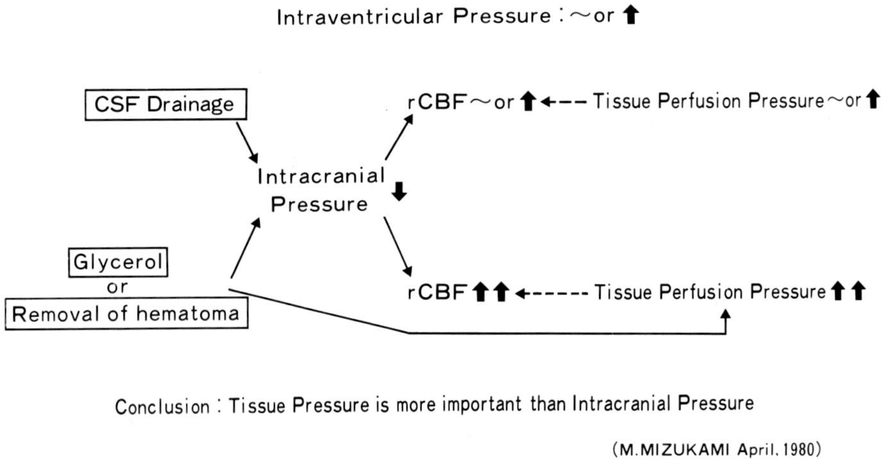

Fig. 9.24. Intracerebral squeeze concept in hypertensive intracerebral hemorrhage.

sive intracerebral hemorrhage will be evaluated by a randomized study which is currently in its planning stage.

References

1. Ad hoc committee on cerebrovascular disease: A classification and outline of cerebrovascular diseases. II. Stroke 6:564, 1975
2. Aring CC: Vascular disease of nervous system. Brain 68:28–55, 1945
3. Backlund E, Holst H: Controlled subtotal evacuation of intracerebral haematomas by stereotactic technique. Surg. Neurol 9:99–101, 1978
4. Bagley C Jr: Spontaneous cerebral hemorrhage. Discussion of four types, with surgical consical considerations. Arch Neurol Psychiat 27:1133–1174, 1932
5. Benes V, Koukobk F, Obrovsha D: Two types of spontaneous intracerebral hemorrhage due to hypertension. J Neurosurg 37:509–513, 1972
6. Charcot JM, Bouchard CH: Nouvelles recherches sur la pathogénie de l'hémorrhagie cérébrale. Arch de Physiol norm et Pathol 1:110–127, 643–665, 725–734, 1868
7. Cooke A W, Plaut M, Browder J: Spontaneous intracerebral hemorrhage: Factors related to surgical results. Arch Neurol 13:25–29, 1965
8. Cuatico W, Adib S, Baston P: Spontaneous intracerebral hematomas. A surgical appraisal. J Neurosurg 22:569–575, 1965
9. Cushing H: The blood-pressure reaction of acute cerebral compression, illustrated by cases of intracrenial hemorrhage. Am J Med Sci 125:1017–1044, 1903
10. David M: Nouvelle contribution à l'étude clinique et thérapeutique des hématomes intracérébraux spontanés. Presse Médicale, 27:371–372. 1945
11. Fazio C: A neurologist's study of problems concerning surgical treatment of spontaneous cerebral hemorrhage. Sc Med Ital 1:101–110, 1950
12. Fazio C, Carolei A: Le emorragie cerebrali. Estr Minerva Angiol 1:109–118, 1976 (in Italian)
13. Fisher CM: Pathology and pathogenesis of intracerebral hemorrhage. In Fields WS (ed): Pathogenesis and Treatment of Cerebrovascular Disease. Springfield, Illinois, Charles C Thomas, pp 295–310, 1961
14. Fisher CM: Diagnosis and management of cerebrovascular disease. Postgrad Med 38:130–140, 1965
15. Globus JH, Straus I: Massive cerebral hemorrhage, its relation to preexisting cerebral softening. Arch Neurol Psychiat 18:215–239, 1927
16. Guillaume J, Ribadeau-Dumas, Ch, Rogé R, Mazars G: Hémorragie cérébrale aiguë guérie chirurgicalement. Rev Neurol 78:30–32, 1946
17. Herbstein DJ, Schaumburg HH: Hypertensive intracerebral hematoma. An investigation of the initial hemorrhage and rebleeding using chromium Cr 51-laveled erythrocytes. Arch Neurol 30:412–414, 1974
18. Huckman MS, Weinberg PE, Kim KS, et al: Angiographic and clinicopathologic correlate in basal ganglionic hemorrhage. Radiology 95:79–92, 1970
19. Janny P, Colnet G, Georget AM, Chazal J: Intracranial pressure with intracerebral hemorrhages. Surg Neurol 10:371–375, 1978
20. Kageyama I, Komoda S, Tanaka T, Kai H: A case of surgically treated hypertensive intracerebral hemorrhage. Seishinkeishi 49(2):7–10, 1946 (in Japanese)
21. Kaneko M, Koba T, Yokoyama T: Early surgical treatment for hypertensive intracerebral hemorrhage. J Neurosurg 45:579–583, 1977
22. Lazorthes G: Surgery of cerebral hemorrhage. Report on the results of 52 surgically treated cases. J Neurosurg 16:355–364, 1959
23. Luessenhop, A.J., and Kachmann, R.: Surgical treatment of primary spontaneous intracerebral hemorrhage. Georgetown Univ Med Cent Bull 18:117–119, 1964
24. Matsuoka S: Morphological pathology of apoplexia cerebri based on vascular changes. Tr Soc Path Jpn 39 Ed gen: 1–10, 1950 (in Japanese)
25. McKissock W, Richardson A, Taylor J: Primary intracerebral hemorrhage, a controlled trial of surgical and conservative treatment in 180 unselected cases. Lancet 2:221–226, 1961
26. McKissock W, Richardson A, Walsh L: Primary intracerebral haemorrhage: results of surgical treatment in 244 consecutive. Lancet 2:683–686, 1959
27. Mitsuno T, Kanaya H, Shirakata S, et al: Surgical treatment of hypertensive intracerebral hemorrhage. J Neurosurg 24:70–76, 1966
28. Mizukami M, Araki G, Mihara H, et al: Arteriographically visualized extravasation in hypertensive intracerebral hemorrhage. Report of seven cases. Stroke 3:527–537, 1972
29. Mizukami M, Araki G, Mihara H, Tomita T: Study of surgical treatment of hypertensive intracerebral hemorrhage. Part 4: The prognosis for survival and hemiplegia based upon cerebral angiography. Brain Nerve 24:579–583, 1972
30. Mizukami M, Araki G, Mihara H, Tomita T: Study of surgical treatment of hypertensive intracerebral hemorrhage. Part 5: Operative result, method and criteria. Brain Nerve 24:695–702, 1972

31. Mizukami M, Kin H, Araki, et al: Surgical treatment of primary intracerebral hemorrhage. Part 1: New angiographical classification. Stroke 7:30–36, 1976
32. Mizukami M, Araki G, Mihara H: Angiographic sign of good prognosis for hemiplegia in hypertensive intracerebral hemorrhage. Neurology 24:120–126, 1974
33. Mutlu N, Berry RG, Alpers BJ: Massive cerebral hemorrhage. Clinical and pathological correlations. Arch Neurol (Chicago) 8:644–661, 1963
34. Ooneda G, Kishi M, Oka K, et al: The nature and morphogenesis of the so-called angionecrosis of cerebral vessels, as the direct cause of apoplectic cerebral hemorrhage. Gunma J Med Soc 8:1–31, 1959
35. Paillas J E, Alliez B: Surgical treatment of spontaneous intracerebral hemorrhage. J Neurosurg, 39:145–151, 1973
36. Papo I, Janny P, Caruselli G, et al: Intracranial pressure time course in primary intracerebral hemorrhage. Neurosurgery 4: 504–510, 1979
37. Pia HW: The surgical treatment of intracerebral and intraventricular hematomas. Acta Neurochir (Wien) 27:149–164, 1972
38. Ransohoff J, Derby B, Kricheff I: Spontaneous intracerebral hemorrhage. Clin Neurosurg 18:247–266, 1970
39. Richardson A: Surgical therapy of spontaneous intracranial hemorrhage. Prog Neurol Surg 3:396–418, 1969
40. Richardson JC, Einhorn RW: Primary intracerebral hemorrhage. Clin Neurosurg 9:114–130, 1963
41. Ross Russel RW: Observation on intracerebral aneurysms. Brain 86:425–442, 1963
42. Scheinker IM: Changes in cerebral veins in hypertensive brain disease and their relation to cerebral hemorrhage; clinical pathologic study. Arch Neurol Psychiat 54:395–408, 1945
43. Scott M, Werthan M: The fate of hypertensive patients with clinically proven spontaneous intracerebral hematomas treated without intracranial surgery: Stroke 1:286–300, 1970
44. Tedeschi G, Bernini P, Cerillo A: Indication for surgical treatment of intracerebral hemorrhage. J Neurosurg 43:590–595, 1975
45. Yamamura T: Pathogenesis of hypertensive cerebral hemorrhage with special reference to soft x-ray and histological serial section. Acta Pathol Jpn, in press
46. Yoshida Y, Ooneda G, Sekiguchi I, et al: Pathology of hypertensive intracerebral hemorrhage. Saishinigaku 25: 1221–1226,1970 (in Japanese)

10

Posterior Fossa Hematomas

George W. Sypert

Introduction

Hematomas of the posterior cranial fossa may be of spontaneous or traumatic origin. Hemorrhage into the posterior fossa may result from many etiologies, as listed in Table 10.1. Discussion of some of these diseases is given in other chapters. Spontaneous parenchymatous posterior fossa hemorrhages comprise approximately 20% of all spontaneous parenchymal brain hemorrhages.* The majority of spontaneous posterior fossa parenchymal brain hemorrhages are related to hypertension and are located in either the cerebellum or pons. Spontaneous extra-axial hematomas are rare. In contrast, space-occupying traumatic posterior fossa hematomas tend to be extra-axial (extradural or subdural) in location rather than parenchymal. Most traumatic parenchymatous hemorrhages are located in the brainstem and are secondary to brainstem contusion or transtentorial herniation from supratentorial mass effects.

The prognosis and treatment of posterior fossa hemorrhage are dependent on an early diagnosis, exacting localization, and a clear knowledge of the natural history of the individual lesion. The advent of computed tomography (CT) scanning** has recently changed the methods of evaluation and management of patients with intracranial hemorrhages. CT scanning has proved to be a reliable, rapid, noninvasive technique that demonstrates the presence, location, size, and configuration of acute hematomas. Hydrocephalus, ventricular shift and/or compression, presence of intraventricular hemorrhage, and degree of edema in adjacent cerebral tissue are demonstrated by CT scanning. Moreover, CT scanning allows precise follow-up of medical and surgical treatment of the hemorrhage. Hence, CT scanning has become the diagnostic procedure of choice immediately on admission in all patients suspected of having an intracranial hemorrhage.

* References 2, 7 12, 16, 19, 30, 37, 48, 63, 78.

** References 4, 32, 33, 42, 49, 62, 69.

Spontaneous Cerebellar Hematomas

Incidence and Mortality

Spontaneous cerebellar hemorrhage as a cause of death was first reported by Sedillot,[71] who presented three cases described by Morgagni and Lieutard. Subsequently, numerous case reports relating to cerebellar hemorrhage have appeared in the clinical literature. The earliest reports were concerned with distinguishing hemorrhages located in the cerebellum from those located in other areas of the cere-

Table 10.1. Etiology of posterior fossa hematomas.

Spontaneous
Hypertension
Saccular aneurysm
Mycotic aneurysm
AVM
Neoplasm
Hemorrhagic disorders
Miscellaneous (rare types)
inflammatory vasculitis
sickle cell disease
vasopressor medications
Traumatic

brum.[2,7,11,39,74] Unfortunately, the diagnosis has been all too frequently made at postmortem, as indicated by several large autopsy series.[16,47,48,63,78]

The true incidence of spontaneous cerebellar hemorrhages is not known. In a recent large autopsy series performed at three university-affiliated general hospitals, the rate of intracerebellar hemorrhage was 0.7%. The incidence of acute cerebellar hemorrhages in that study is similar to the incidence found by others in their clinicopathologic studies of acute cerebellar hemorrhage.[16,48,63] Thus, cerebellar hemorrhage is not a rare lesion. In fact, cerebellar hemorrhage accounts for approximately 5% to 10% of all spontaneous intraparenchymal CNS hemorrhages. This might be expected since the cerebellum makes up approximately 10% of the CNS by weight.

The importance of spontaneous cerebellar hemorrhage is further emphasized by the high mortality associated with this not infrequent problem. It is difficult to estimate the mortality exactly, since the correct clinical diagnosis was rarely made premortem prior to CT, so that the denominator (total number of cases of cerebellar hemorrhage) remains unknown. However, from the observation that only two examples of old, large cerebellar hemorrhages (compared with 39 examples of acutely fatal cerebellar hemorrhages) could be found in a large adult autopsy series,[78] it would appear that the mortality of large spontaneous cerebellar hematomas may approach 90%. Recent clinical reports[27,40,59] indicate that the incidence of smaller cerebellar hematomas (less than 3 cm) may be higher than retrospective autopsy studies predict. Therefore, mortality estimates will have to be readjusted as diagnosis can now be reliably made prior to death by using CT scanning. The clinical studies of Fisher,[23] Ott et al,[59] and Little et al,[40] suggest that the overall mortality of patients with cerebellar hemorrhages treated medically in a large general hospital may range from 60% to 80%.

Etiology and Pathology

Although spontaneous cerebellar hemorrhage may occur at any age, it occurs most frequently in the sixth and seventh decades of life.† Arterial hypertension (blood pressure higher than 140/95 mm Hg), usually of 5 years or more duration, is by far the most common predisposing factor in cerebellar hemorrhage, being present in greater than two-thirds of cases.[16,24,59] Anticoagulation therapy is also an important predisposing factor, particularly when the patient has coexisting hypertension. Additional factors involved in this type of intraparenchymal hemorrhage include arteriovenous malformations (AVMs), aneurysms, inherited or acquired hemorrhagic diathesis, hemorrhage into a tumor bed, trauma, and other undetermined factors. The causes should be considered in relation to the age of the patient in that AVMs usually occur in 15- to 40-year age group. Based on their studies of "cryptic" AVMs, McCormick and Nofziner[44] suggest that such malformations may be responsible for one-fourth of spontaneous cerebellar hemorrhages with a fatal outcome.

Most hypertensive cerebellar hemorrhages occur in or near the dentate nucleus, causing an expanding hematoma.[16] The precise assessment of the vascular source of the hemorrhage has not been possible, as the dentate nucleus may be supplied by all of the cerebellar arteries. The two main theories regarding the mechanisms responsible for hypertensive intraparenchymal hemorrhages involve leakage from microaneurysms[17] or from rupture of the vessel wall altered by segmental fibrinoid necrosis.[22] The hematoma produces considerable compression and destruction of the cerebellar gray and white

† References 6, 23, 24, 47, 48, 53, 59, 63.

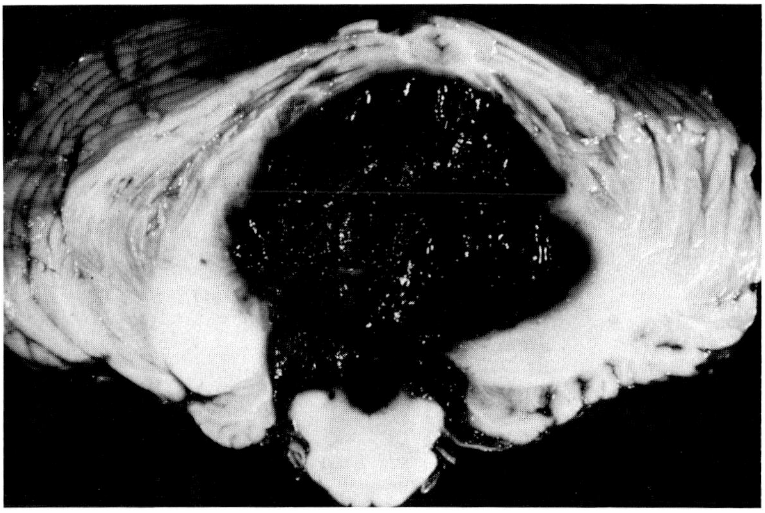

Fig. 10.1. Postmortem hypertensive hemorrhage into the cerebellum with rupture into the fourth ventricle. The patient was a hypertensive 74-year-old female who suddenly lost consciousness. She remained in coma and six hours from onset suffered a terminal arrest of cardiorespiratory function following a brief interval of flaccid quadriplegia and ataxic respirations.

matter and tends to rupture into the fourth ventricle or subarachnoid space.[16] A typical massive primary cerebellar hemorrhage is illustrated in Fig. 10.1. Hemorrhage in a site unusual for the typical hypertensive cerebellar hemorrhage should suggest an unusual cause.

At autopsy there is a notable lack of signs of anatomic disruption of the brainstem.[16] Hydrocephalus, molding and compressing of the brainstem, and tonsillar herniation are the usual findings. Death is attributed to direct medullary compression and tonsillar herniation.

Clinical Presentation

The onset of symptoms is usually sudden with acute cerebellar hemorrhage, without any premonitory symptoms or precipitating factors. In most patients, the initial symptom is a fall, with inability to stand or walk.[59,78] Nausea, vomiting, and headache of sudden onset are very common complaints. Dizziness, vertigo, dysarthria, and ataxia of the extremities are also frequent symptoms at onset.

On admission to the hospital, the majority of patients are hypertensive, with an altered state of consciousness (drowsiness or stupor). As many as one-fourth of patients are comatose when first examined. In noncomatose patients, cerebellar signs are usually prominent, including gait ataxia, truncal ataxia, ipsilateral extremity dysmetria or intention tremor, and scanning dysarthria. The pupils are usually small and reactive. Cranial nerve findings often include an ipsilateral gaze paresis, ipsilateral peripheral facial palsy, nystagmus, and depressed corneal reflex. A triad of signs—gait and/or extremity ataxia, ipsilateral gaze paresis, and ipsilateral peripheral facial palsy—should immediately alert the clinician to the possibility of an acute cerebellar vascular mass lesion. At least two of the three signs are present in three-fourths of patients in whom testing for all three signs is done.[59,78] However, it must be kept in mind that great difficulty has been experienced in the neurologic differentiation of this condition.[45,65]

Clinical Course

The clinical course of spontaneous cerebellar hemorrhage appears to occur in three basic patterns[24]:

1. Acute onset, with an immediate or rapid loss of consciousness, and rapid, progressive deterioration of brainstem function to death over a few minutes or hours. These patients, if admitted to the hospital, are in such poor condition that aggressive decompressive therapy is often considered useless.
2. Subacute onset, comprising the largest group, wherein there is progressive deterioration of brainstem function within 72 hours of onset. Evidence of brainstem deterioration is manifested by the appearance of impairment of consciousness, pupillary abnormalities, disorders of ocular motion

including gaze paresis, and motor (pyramidal-type) dysfunction that generally progresses to quadriplegia, coma, and death over a few hours or days. The deterioration of lower brainstem function may be rapid, with death occurring within a few hours of the onset of stupor or coma.

3. Chronic, wherein onset of symptoms may be gradual or episodic, with or without late deterioration. Cerebellar type signs and symptoms are frequently prominent. Spontaneous recovery with no substantial neurologic deficit may occur. However, delayed deterioration of brainstem function may occur from three days to two weeks after onset.

In all of these groups, the development of stupor and coma are essentially irreversible stages in untreated cerebellar hemorrhage and eventually lead to death.[59] Furthermore, the rate of clinical deterioration is unpredictable in individual cases. Patients in good condition and under close observation may precipitously develop coma and suddenly die.

Diagnosis

One of the principal obstacles to the development of a successful management or therapeutic program for cerebellar hemorrhage has been the failure to make the diagnosis clinically, particularly in the early stages of the illness. In retrospective studies based on postmortem material, the diagnosis of acute spontaneous cerebellar hemorrhage was considered infrequently.[16,63] Moreover, the scarcity or reported fulminant "acute" or "subacute" cases treated surgically is impressive, particularly since this contrasts markedly with the estimated incidence of these presentations of cerebellar hemorrhage[16,28] and reflects failure to make a premortem diagnosis. However, recent clinical reports[10,23,59] suggest that the clinical appearance of spontaneous cerebellar hemorrhage shows a pattern of symptoms, signs, and courses sufficiently common to be of diagnostic value.

Most of the early symptoms and signs can be explained on the basis of destruction of cerebellar tissue. Approximately three-fourths of these patients have such symptoms and signs as vomiting, dizziness or vertigo, appendicular ataxia, extremity dysmetria or tremor, dysarthria, and nystagmus. The subsequent clinical progression is characterized by a progressive deterioration of lower brainstem function, including impairment of consciousness, ipsilateral facial and gaze palsy, motor (pyramidal-type) dysfunction, and respiratory irregularity due to mechanical compression of the brainstem by the hematoma and the associated cerebellar swelling. Once these latter symptoms and signs appear, a relentless progression to coma, quadriplegia, respiratory arrest, and death over a few hours or days is the usual course of events.

The clinical diagnosis of spontaneous cerebellar hemorrhage can be reliably made if there is a high index of suspicion and an accurate clinical evaluation. Essentially, the patient has an expanding posterior fossa mass lesion. Subdural and epidural hematoma of the posterior fossa, massive cerebellar infarction, or rapidly expanding cerebellar neoplasms may also present a similar clinical picture. However, the initial differentiation of these clinical entities may not be imperative, as they all represent treatable expanding posterior fossa mass lesions.

Fisher et al[23] and Loeb and Meyer[41] have clearly described the differentiating features of the various other stroke syndromes, and in most cases these should not offer difficulties with the differential diagnosis. Certain cases of progressive brainstem infarction or hemorrhage and subarachnoid hemorrhage from a ruptured aneurysm remain difficult diagnostic problems. Furthermore, the diagnosis is especially difficult in those patients with no accurate history who are in a stuporous state, so that the clinical examination is limited.

From available data regarding spontaneous cerebellar hemorrhage, it now appears imperative that clinicians immediately and accurately distinguish this treatable posterior fossa mass lesion from brainstem infarction. A delay in diagnosis of a patient exhibiting progressive brainstem dysfunction will, in most cases, result in irreversible brainstem damage and death. A lumbar puncture may be hazardous, needlessly delaying, and frequently confusing to the clinician. EEGs and radioisotopic scans are also of little value in arriving at a rapid, correct diagnosis.

CT scanning has proved to be a rapid and ac-

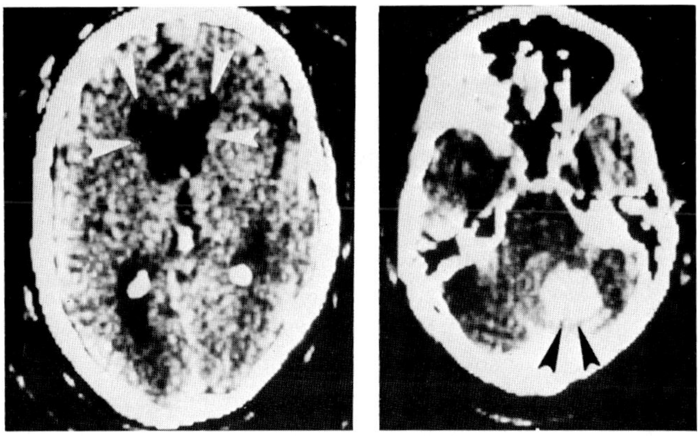

Fig. 10.2. CT scan demonstrating a right paramedian cerebellar hematoma (*right, arrows*). Hydrocephalus is shown by the dilated frontal horns of the lateral ventricles (*left, arrow*). The patient was a hypertensive 62-year-old mechanic who suddenly vomited and fell at work. Eight hours later he was found to be somnolent with a right gaze paresis, peripheral VII paresis, and moderate quadriparesis. Three years following emergency evacuation of the hematoma, he is working full-time and has a normal neurologic examination.

curate method for the diagnosis and localization of spontaneous cerebellar hemorrhages.[27,40,59,77] This study is the procedure of choice immediately on admission in all patients suspected of having a posterior fossa hemorrhage. Even in urgent situations with brainstem compression, two or three tomographic cuts can be obtained within 10 to 15 minutes. A typical CT scan of an acute hypertensive cerebellar hemorrhage is illustrated in Fig. 10.2. Ordinarily, in the case of an acute or subacute hemorrhage, the CT scan will reveal a radio-dense (+30 to +45 Hounsfield units) intracerebellar mass lesion.[40] The higher density hematoma is surrounded by a lower density rim, probably representing edematous cerebellar tissue that adds to the mass effect. If the hematoma is large (3 cm or greater in transverse diameter), then moderate to severe third and lateral ventricular enlargement may be evident. Moreover, intraventricular extension of the hemorrhage frequently results from larger hemorrhages. With smaller hemorrhages, internal hydrocephalus and intraventricular extension of the hemorrhage are often absent.

Follow-up studies in those surviving patients not undergoing surgical evacuation revealed resolution of the intraparenchymal hematoma over a four- to six-week period.[27,40] The density of the hematoma gradually attenuates with a progressive decrease in size of the hematoma.

If CT scanning is not available, then combined carotid and vertebral angiography appears to be the diagnostic procedure of choice. The use of the latter diagnostic procedure implies that angiography will be performed on some patients whose primary lesion is a brainstem infarction; however, the risk of modern contrast media and neuroradiologic techniques is sufficiently low to justify this procedure. In patients with an acute cerebellar hemorrhage, vertebral angiography should show an avascular cerebellar mass. Carotid angiography should show some degree of hydrocephalus in most cases.

Although CT scanning and, particularly, combined carotid and vertebral angiography are time-consuming, the judicious use of a single confirmatory study and good logistical planning should keep any delay in necessary surgery to a minimum and avoid an unnecessary posterior fossa exploration.

Treatment

Acute or subacute massive cerebellar hemorrhage is, for all practical purposes, uniformly fatal without neurosurgical decompression. Since possibly 20% to 40% of patients treated conservatively with close observation, bed rest, antihypertensive agents, and steroids recover without disabling neurologic deficits,[40,59] it would be ideal to develop a formula to predict which patients should recover. Unfortunately, there are no reliable data available that can yield such a formula. The clinical course cannot be predicted with certainty in individual cases.[59] The rate of deterioration may be sudden and fulminating even in the patient whose condition has remained stable for a number of days. Furthermore, the operative mortality becomes exceedingly high once the patient progresses to stupor or coma.[10,59]

When the diagnosis of spontaneous cerebellar hemorrhage with progressive brainstem dysfunction is reached, immediate posterior fossa craniotomy with evacuation of the hematoma is recommended to prevent irreversible brainstem damage and death. It appears reasonable to assume that a patient who has been rendered stuporous or comatose will not recover without surgical intervention.[10,23,45,59] Intensive and aggressive therapy is particularly indicated, since those patients treated with surgical decompression can recover with little or no disability and resume full activity despite what must have been severe brainstem compression.[10,23,59,77] For this to be accomplished, a high index of suspicion and an early diagnosis are required.

The results of aggressive surgical therapy are gratifying. Most cases and series reported prior to 1960 are concerned with the evacuation of chronic hematomas; that is, cases coming to operation one to three weeks after onset. Table 10.2 reviews my cases, as well as those cases of surgically treated spontaneous cerebellar hematomas that have been published in the English literature since 1960. The overall operative mortality of these patients is 35%. Review of these data reveals that there are several factors that appear to contribute directly to the surgical outcome. The level of consciousness at the time of suboccipital exploration had the major influence on prognosis. Where the patient was still arousable, the mortality ranged from zero to 27%. Of the 25 patients who were comatose prior to operation, only seven survived, yielding a mortality on the order of 70%—certainly better than that expected based on the natural history of these patients. The time interval between onset and definitive surgery does not appear to influence the patient's prognosis. The beneficial effect of youth may be related to the absence of hypertension and superimposed dis-

Table 10.2. Craniotomy for primary cerebellar hematoma.

	Age		Classification		Level of consciousness		
Author	< 40	> 40	Acute	Subacute or chronic	Coma	Drowsy or stuporous	Alert
McKissock, et al (1960)[45]	—	—	—	9/14	—	4/9	5/5
Odom et al (1961)[56]	3/3	—	1/1	2/2	—	2/2	1/1
Giroux and Leger (1962)[25]	2/2	—	2/2	—	—	2/2	—
Aronson, et al (1965)[5]	—	0/1	0/1	—	—	0/1	—
Fisher, et al (1965)[23]	—	2/3	2/3	—	2/3	—	—
Norris, et al (1969)[53]	—	1/2	1/2	—	0/1	1/1	—
Richardson (1972)[64]	3/3	8/15	8/12	3/6	2/5	9/13	—
Ott, et al (1974)[59]	—	—	—	—	2/10	9/13	2/2
Brennan and Bergland (1977)[10]	1/1	5/8	6/9	—	0/3	6/6	—
Little, et al (1978)[40]	—	—	4/5	—	0/1	4/4	—
Yoshida, et al (1978)[82]	—	1/1	1/1	—	1/1	—	—
Sypert (1977)	1/1	4/6	3/5	2/2	1/3	3/4	—
Percentage surviving	100	58	68	66	30	78	100

Numerator, number of patients surviving; denominator, total number of patients in category.

ease, as well as a greater capacity to regulate the blood supply to the brainstem under adverse circumstances. The higher incidence of hemorrhage from an arteriovenous anomaly in the young may also contribute, since these hemorrhages may not be as violent as a primary hypertensive hemorrhage.

The cause of death in these surgically treated patients is generally related to failure to show satisfactory recovery of brainstem function after surgery or reaccumulation of hematoma. Until recently, the differential diagnosis of these two conditions has been made only with great difficulty. However, CT scanning should presently make an accurate differentiation with a high level of confidence.

The percentage of surviving patients who are capable of making an excellent functional recovery is extremely high. Moreover, patients who are comatose at the time of operation frequently have an exceedingly worthwhile quality of survival.[23,59,64] The available data do indicate, however, that the quality of survival is inversely related to the patient's preoperative level of consciousness.

A more conservative approach may be indicated in the alert patient without symptoms or signs of brainstem compression who has a small cerebellar hemorrhage (hematoma less than 3 cm) without ventricular dilatation or intraventricular extension of the hemorrhage.[27,40] The number of such patients that has been treated conservatively is, however, small, but currently available preliminary results appear to favor such an approach. Hopefully, additional experience with CT scanning and the management of spontaneous cerebellar hemorrhage will further delineate those predictive factors that will be useful for the determination of those alert patients with cerebellar hemorrhage who may be treated conservatively.

Spontaneous Pontine Hematomas

Incidence and Mortality

The pons is not an infrequent site of spontaneous massive intraparenchymal brain hemorrhage. Dana[14] found two cases of primary pontine hemorrhage in 50 consecutive cases of massive cerebral hemorrhages. In a series of 938 cases of spontaneous cerebral hemorrhage studied in 1928, Novak recorded a pontine location in 5%.[54] Various authors have found an incidence of 3% to 13.4% in their series of intracerebral hemorrhage cases.[3,13,18,66,79,81] In a recent clinicopathologic report on a large series of cases of primary pontine hemorrhage that were derived from the neuropathologic department of a large general hospital, Silverstein[72] found that pontine hemorrhage represented 7.5% of the total number of intracranial hemorrhages. Pontine hemorrhages resulting from trauma or secondary to cerebral neoplasm, abscess, or other intracranial hematoma are also frequent terminal events.[80] Such secondary pontine hemorrhages are excluded from consideration in this chapter.

According to Dana,[14] the earliest description of pontine hemorrhage was by Cheyne in 1812. Numerous case reports subsequently appeared in the English, French, and German literature. Silverstein[73] attributes the first clear clinical definition of spontaneous pontine hemorrhage to Oppenheim.[58] In the more recent literature, Epstein[18] and Steegman[75] reported on the clinicopathologic correlations of primary pontine hemorrhage in seven and 17 cases, respectively. Subsequently, Mutlu et al[51] discussed the differential diagnosis of pontine hemorrhage as related to intracerebral hemorrhage. Dinsdale[16] reported on the differentiating features of spontaneous hemorrhage into the pons and cerebellum. Finally, Silverstein[73] presented the clinical and pathologic findings in 50 cases of spontaneous pontine hemorrhage.

The importance of primary pontine hemorrhage is further emphasized by its exceedingly poor prognosis. Previous reports[20,52,72] indicate that the prognosis for these patients is hopeless, with the mortality rate approaching 100%. The exact mortality is not known. Recently, isolated cases of prolonged survival have been reported.*

It will be possible to obtain more accurate estimates of the mortality and natural history of primary pontine hemorrhage in the future, as the premortem diagnosis can now be reliably made using CT scanning.[8,49,61,62,69]

* References 1, 8, 15, 26, 29, 31, 34, 35, 38, 43, 49, 50, 55, 60, 61, 67, 68.

Etiology and Pathology

Although spontaneous pontine hemorrhage may occur at any age, it occurs with the highest incidence in the fourth and fifth decades.[16,72] This contrasts with cerebellar hemorrhage, which tends to peak in the sixth and seventh decades. Sex and race do not appear to be causally related to primary pontine hemorrhage. Hypertension (blood pressure higher than 140/95) usually of 5 years or more duration, is by far the most common predisposing factor in spontaneous pontine hemorrhage, being present in more than 90% of cases.[16,72] Other factors such as inherited or acquired hemorrhagic diatheses and neoplastic, inflammatory, or infectious diseases appear to be involved in this condition only rarely. In the younger age groups, "cryptic" brainstem AVMs must be considered as an etiologic factor. McCormick and Nofzinger[44] documented that the pons represents one of the most frequent sites of cryptic AVMs, particularly capillary telangiectases. This high incidence of cryptic pontine AVMs may contribute to the fact that primary pontine hemorrhages occur two decades earlier than primary cerebellar hemorrhages.

At autopsy almost all hypertensive primary pontine hemorrhages appear to arise at a midpontine level.[16,18,72] The hemorrhage appears to originate near the junction of the basis pontis and tegmentum and the midline. A postmortem example of a massive primary pontine hemorrhage is illustrated in Fig. 10.3. The hematoma usually dissects the brainstem in a relatively symmetrical fashion in all directions, with a tendency to follow the planes of the fiber pathways. Rostral extension along the peduncles past the junction of the pons and midbrain is frequent, with occasional dissections of clot extending into the hypothalamus and/or thalamus. Caudal dissection into the medulla is infrequently observed. Silverstein[72,73] divided his 50 postmortem cases into three groups: unilateral pontine hemorrhage (22%), bilateral pontine hemorrhage (56%), and tegmental pontine hemorrhage (22%).

Rupture of the hematoma into the fourth ventricle is frequent, occurring in 70%[72] to 90%[16] of cases. Mild to moderate hydrocephalus may be found in about 20% of cases usually associated with rupture into the fourth ventricle.

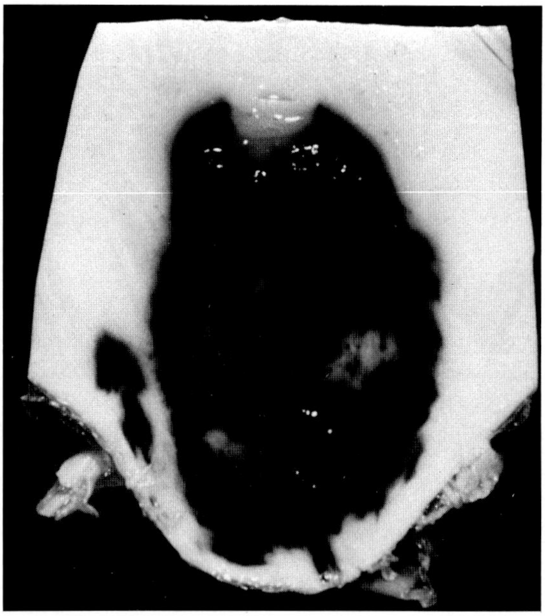

Fig. 10.3. Postmortem hypertensive massive pontine hemorrhage with rupture into the fourth ventricle. The patient was a 51-year-old male who suddenly developed a severe occipital headache and vomiting rapidly followed by coma, flaccid quadriplegia, fixed pinpoint pupils, and hyperthermia of 108°F. Death occurred nine hours after onset of symptoms.

Upward or downward herniation of posterior fossa structures is an infrequent finding.[16,72] Dinsdale[16] suggests that the hemorrhage arises, in most cases, from the distal portions of the long penetrating paramedian branches of the basilar artery. The pathogenesis of hypertensive pontine hemorrhage, however, remains controversial, as discussed in the section on cerebellar hemorrhage. Both microaneurysms and segmental fibrinoid necrosis have been found in cases of primary pontine hemorrhage.[16,72]

Clinical Presentation

In hypertensive pontine hemorrhage, the onset is abrupt and without prodromal warning in about one-half of cases, with an immediate loss of consciousness. In patients who are not instantaneously rendered comatose, severe headaches, located usually in the occipital region, are the most frequent prodromal symptom.[16,18] Vomiting is the next most frequent symptom.

Other premonitory symptoms include dizziness, dysarthria, confusion, visual disturbance, paresthesias, and generalized weakness.

On admission to the hospital, 70% to 80% of patients are in coma, with the remaining patients demonstrating some alteration in consciousness, varying from mild confusion to stupor.[16,72] Convulsive seizures occur in about 20% of patients.[18,72] The motor manifestations of the seizures are usually bilateral but can occasionally involve one side of the body.

Striking hyperthermia (temperature above 39.5°C) has been observed in about one-half of patients.[16,72] It appears that such temperature elevations in these patients are an unrelenting process usually preceding death by one or two hours.[16] This high incidence of hyperthermia is also seen in cases of pontine infarction.[72] In contrast, cases of spontaneous cerebellar hemorrhage infrequently present with substantial elevations of body temperature.[16]

Respiratory disturbance is frequently encountered in these patients on admission, occurring in approximately two-thirds of cases.[16,72] Stertorous breathing, Cheyne-Stokes respirations, and rapid, shallow breathing are observed in that descending order of frequency.[16] Ataxic respirations are frequently seen immediately prior to final respiratory failure.

Miotic and sluggish or nonreactive pupils are found in more than one-half of patients. Unilateral dilated pupils or bilateral fixed and dilated pupils have been observed in an additional 15% of patients.[16,72]

Abnormalities of eye movements have been frequently observed. The eyes midline and fixed in the position of rest have been the most often observed abnormality, described in about 20% of patients.[16] Conjugate deviations of the eyes have been described in an additional 10% of patients. "Ocular bobbing" has also been described in cases of pontine hemorrhage and infarction.[20] Although ocular bobbing has been associated with primary intrapontine lesions,[52] additional recent reports have demonstrated that this ocular motility sign may result from treatable extrapontine causes, such as acute cerebellar hemorrhage.[9,21,59,76]

More than one-half of cases of primary pontine hemorrhage present with a flaccid quadriplegia.[16,72] Spasticity and decerebrate posturing are observed infrequently. A hemiplegia, usually flaccid, has been described in 10% to 20% of patients. In some cases, an alternating hemiplegia may be observed.[72] Cerebellar signs are of little diagnostic value.

Lumbar puncture will reveal evidence consistent with an acute subarachnoid hemorrhage in about 90% of cases of primary pontine hemorrhage.[16,72]

Clinical Course

In most instances, primary pontine hemorrhage has a rapid, progressive course, terminating in death. The mortality for the first 48 hours includes greater than 80% of the patients.[16,72] The remainder of the patients generally die within the first week. Prolonged survival has been observed, however, in a few cases.**

Coma is not invariably produced by spontaneous pontine hemorrhage, and the clinical course is not always fulminating, leading relentlessly to death. In some cases the primary pontine hemorrhage is not massive, being limited to the lateral tegmentum or paramedian areas of the basis pontis such that prolonged worthwhile survivals are possible.[73] Moreover, surgical evacuation of the intrapontine hematoma and a fourth ventricular hematoma, if present, may benefit selected patients.

The presentation and clinical course of some cases of primary pontine hemorrhage may also be atypical, particularly in the younger age groups. Such patients often have a more slowly progressive or staggering evolution of pontine symptoms and signs. It is likely that some such cases represent repeated small hemorrhages from a cryptic pontine vascular malformation.

Diagnosis

The neurologic symptoms and signs of primary pontine hemorrhage depend largely on the location, size, and rate of development of the hematoma.

The usual pontine hemorrhage is abrupt in onset, with sudden collapse and coma in a patient with a history of hypertension. In such a patient, the diagnosis is almost certain if the

** References 8, 26, 31, 34, 35, 43, 50, 55, 60, 61, 67, 68, 73.

Table 10.3. Surgical evaluation of brainstem hematomas.[a]

Author	Age, sex	Symptoms, signs	Diagnostic studies	Location	Operative approach	Result	Etiology
Scoville and Poppen, 1949[10]	44,F	1.5 yr—R hypesthesia; headaches, ataxia, vomiting, stupor, bilat III, R hemiplegia; coma	Ventric	Midbrain	Supratentorial-occipital	8 yr dysarthria, mild ataxia, R hemiparesis	? Cryptic AVM
Scott and Silverstein, 1960[68]	41,M	3 wk—headache, diplopia, ataxia, L monoparesis; L gaze paresis, ataxia, papilledema, coma	Ventric	Pons	Supratentorial-4th ventricle	2 yr dysarthria, mod quadriplegia	? Traumatic
Kempe, 1964[31]	25,M	5 mo—head injury; 6 wk—fever, vomiting, vertigo; lethargy, L V, VII, VIII, IX, X, Babinski	Pneumo	Pons	Suboccipital-4th ventricle	6 mo, L dysmetria	? Traumatic
Koos et al, 1969[34]	11,F	Fall 7d—headache, vertigo, vomiting, ataxia; bilat V1, quadriparesis, L III, decerebration	Angio, ventric	Pons	Suboccipital-4th ventricle	2yr, normal	? Cryptic AVM
Obrador, et al, 1970[55]	10,M	5 d—headache, vertigo; nystagmus, anisocoria, L VII, ataxia	Ventric	Pons	Suboccipital-4th ventricle	1 yr, mild L ataxia	? Cryptic AVM
Abrams et al, 1971[1]	15,F	3 wk—headache, vertigo, diplopia, L numbness, ataxia; L VII, IX, X, R hemiparesis, hemihypesthesia, ataxia	Pneumo	Pons	Suboccipital-4th ventricle	3 yr, mild R hemiparesis	? Cryptic AVM
Kowada et al, 1972[36]	47,M	L hemiparesis; coma, quadriplegia, miotic pupils, L gaze paralysis, vomiting	Angio, pneumo	Pons	Suboccipital-4th ventricle	1.5 yr, quadriplegia, totally disabled	Hypertension
	41,M	Sudden coma, skew, miotic pupils, quadriplegia	Angio, pneumo	Pons	Suboccipital-4th ventricle	6 mo, moderately disabled	Hypertension
Murphy, 1972[50]	39,M	Headache, inability to stand, dysarthria; stupor, skew, bilat V, L VII, bilat Babinski	Angio, ventric	Pons	Suboccipital-4th ventricle	1 yr, mild ataxis, R hemihypalgesia	Hypertension

Scott, et al, 1973[67]	1.5,M	3d—clumsiness; vomiting, lethargy, L VI, VII, IX, X	Angio, pneumo	Pons	Suboccipital-4th ventricle	6 mo mild L VI	Cryptic AVM
Arseni and Standiu, 1973[6]	43,F	2 mo—headache, blurred vision, diplopia, ataxia; R hemiparesis, hemihypesthesia, L III, VI, VII, IX, X, ataxia, somnolence	Angio	Pons	Suboccipital-4th ventricle	2 mo L III, R gaze paresis, hemiparesis	Unknown
	40,F	3 wk—headache, vertigo, vomiting; drowsy, ataxia, dysarthria, L dysmetria, hemiparesis, hypesthesia	None	Pons	Suboccipital-4th ventricle	2 mo mild gait disturbance, L hypacusis	Unknown
Papo, et al, 1976[60]	35,F	3 mo—headache, ataxia; papilledema, axial ataxia, R dysmetria	Ventric	Pons	Suboccipital-4th ventricle	3 mo mild gait disturbance	? Cryptic AVM
	23,M	1 mo—diplopia; R VI, L hemiparesis	CT scan, pneumo	Pons	Suboccipital-4th ventricle	1 mo, R VI	? Cryptic AVM
Humphrey, 1978[29]	10,M	6d—headache, fever, somnolence, vomiting, inability to stand; coma, decerebration	CT scan	Midbrain	1st-suboccipital 2nd-subtemporal-supratentorial	7 mo, normal	? Cryptic AVM
La Torre et al, 1978[38]	38,F	2 yr—headache; diplopia, vomiting 1 mo; papilledema, drowsy, bilat VII, bilat Babinski, coma	Angio ventric	Midbrain	Infratentorial-supracerebellar	7 mo, normal	? Cryptic AVM
Becker and Silverberg, 1978[8]	55,F	dizziness, vomiting, stupor, dysarthria, L V, VI, VII, VIII, IX, X, R hemiparesis, R hypalgesia	CT scan	Pons	Suboccipital-4th ventricle	2.2 yr, ataxia, walk with assistance	Unknown
Sypert, 1977	64,F	4 yr—progressive R hemiparesis, hypesthesia, III	CT scan, angio	Midbrain	Supratentorial-subtemporal	6 mo, ambulatory, mild R hemiparesis, III	? Cryptic AVM

[a] Dandy[15] and Matson[43] mentioned having evacuated chronic pontine hematomas but no details were given.

examination reveals a comatose patient with hyperthermia, miotic poorly reactive pupils, and a flaccid quadriplegia. However, at least one-half of patients will not present with this "typical" history and examination. Moreover, it is imperative that pontine hemorrhage be expeditiously differentiated from conditions requiring emergency treatment, such as acute subdural and epidural hemorrhage, acute cerebellar hemorrhage, subarachnoid hemorrhage, hypertensive encephalopathy, diabetic coma, hypoglycemia, brain tumor, brain abscess, meningitis, epilepsy, and exogenous poisons, particularly alcohol and barbituates. Lumbar puncture may be hazardous in many of these latter conditions and frequently delays and confuses the clinician. EEG, echoencephalography, and radioisotopic scans are also of little value in arriving at an immediate, correct diagnosis.

CT is the most rapid and accurate method currently available for making the diagnosis of spontaneous pontine hemorrhage.[49,61,69] Figure 10.4 illustrates the typical CT scan from a patient with an acute primary pontine hemorrhage. For a further discussion of the diagnostic technique, the reader is referred to the preceding section on spontaneous cerebellar hematomas.

Treatment

Upon confirmation of an acute pontine hemorrhage, a program of medical therapy should be initiated to prevent further hemorrhage, reduce the mass effect of the hematoma, prevent complications (especially seizures and elevated intracranial pressure), and reduce elevated blood pressure. In addition, the clinician needs to maintain adequate respiratory function, prevent fluid and electrolyte abnormalities, treat other complicating medical disease, and prevent nonneurologic complications such as pneumonia, decubitus ulcers, urinary tract infections, and pulmonary embolism. Prevention of further hemorrhage may be accomplished by reducing blood pressure and correcting any abnormalities in blood coagulation if present. If the etiology is hypertension, rehemorrhage from the same site is rare. Repeated hemorrhage should

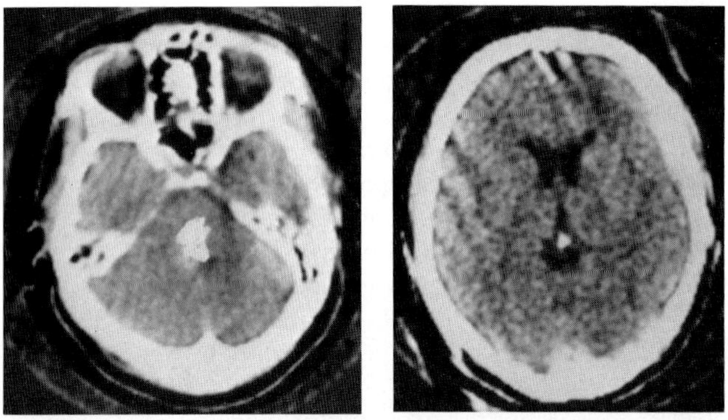

Fig. 10.4. CT scan of a primary pontine hemorrhage (*left*). Note absence of hydrocephalus on more rostral scan (*right*). The patient was a 58-year-old hypertensive male who suddenly collapsed and fell to the floor, completely unresponsive. He remained in coma with flaccid quadriplegia, stertorous respirations, and fixed pinpoint pupils until death six hours later.

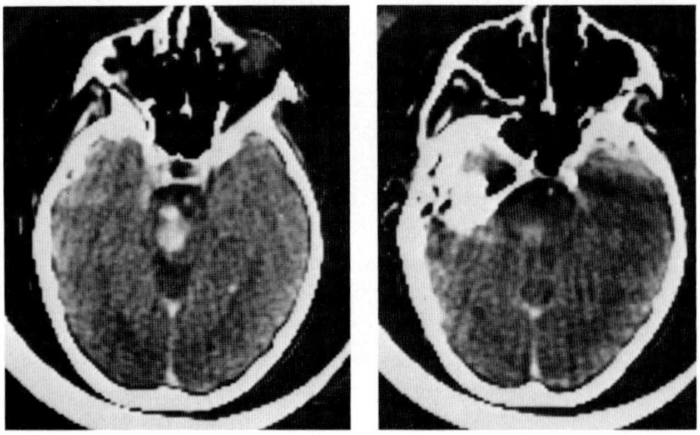

Fig. 10.5. CT scan of a chronic, calcified hematoma expanding the midbrain (*right*). Note the absence of hematoma in the pons (*left*). The patient was a normotensive 64-year-old female with a 4-year history of staggering, progressive right hemiparesis, hemihypesthesia, and left partial III palsy. Six months following partial evacuation of the hematoma via a pedunculotomy, she was ambulatory, with a mild residual right spastic hemiparesis and left partial III paresis.

suggest the presence of a vascular malformation or neoplasm. Reduction in blood pressure can generally be achieved with either methyldopa or hydralazine. Available data indicate that lowering of the systemic arterial blood pressure in patients with hypertensive intracerebral hemorrhage is beneficial.[46] Attempts to reduce the mass effect are directed principally to the use of edema-modifying agents, such as high-dose corticosteroids. The benefit of this therapy has not been documented. Seizures may be prevented by the prophylactic use of phenytoin.

Unless the patient deteriorates in neurologic function or level of consciousness, medical therapy is continued, and surgical management is not considered. In fact, the role of surgical therapy in primary pontine hemorrhage is unclear. Some neurologic surgeons feel that surgery is not indicated in patients with pontine hemorrhage.[57] It is possible, however, that temporary external ventriculostomy drainage may be of some benefit to those infrequent patients who develop acute hydrocephalus from fourth ventricular rupture. Moreover, the reported cases of surgically treated primary brainstem hematomas are listed in Table 10.3. In evaluating the success of surgical treatment in these latter cases, it must be kept in mind that these patients are highly selected, with largely atypical presentations and clinical courses (see Fig. 10.5). Furthermore, unsuccessful cases are not likely to be reported in the clinical literature.

References

1. Abrams IF, Yessayan L, Shillito J, Balow CF: Spontaneous intracerebral hemorrhage in patients suspected of multiple sclerosis. J Neurol Neurosurg Psychiatry 34:157–162, 1971
2. Abud-Ortega AF, Rajput A, Rozdilsky B: Observations in five cases of spontaneous cerebellar hemorrhage. Can Med Assoc J 106:40–44, 1972
3. Adams RD, Vander Eecken HM: Vascular diseases of the brain. Ann Rev Med 4:213–252, 1953
4. Ambrose J: Computerized x-ray scanning of the brain. J Neurosurg. 40:679–695, 1974
5. Aronson H, Shafey S, Gargano F: Intracerebellar hematoma. J Neurol Neurosurg Psychiatry 28:442–444, 1965
6. Arseni C, Stanciu M: Primary haematomas of the brain stem. Acta Neurochir 28:323–330, 1973
7. Ballance H: A case of traumatic hemorrhage into the left lateral lobe of the cerebellum treated by operation with recovery. Surg Gynecol Obstet 3:223–225, 1906
8. Becker DH, Silverberg GD: Successful evacuation of an acute pontine hematoma. Surg Neurol 10:263–265, 1978
9. Bosch EP, Kennedy SS, Aschenbrener CA: Ocular bobbing: The myth of its localizing value. Neurology 25:949–953, 1975
10. Brennen RW, Bergland RM: Acute cerebellar hemorrhage. Analysis of clinical findings and outcome in 12 cases. Neurology 27:527–532, 1977
11. Brown-Seguard CE: Diagnosis of hemorrhage in the cerebellum. Lancet 2:391–392, 1861
12. Charcot JM, Bouchard C: Nouvelles recherches sur la pathogenie de l'hemorrhagie cerebrale. Arch Phys Norm Pathol 1:110–127, 1868
13. Courville, CB: Pathology of the Central Nervous System. Pacific Press, Mountain View, California, 1950
14. Dana CL: Acute bulbar paralysis due to hemorrhage and softening of the pons. Med J Rec 64:361–374, 1903
15. Dandy W: The brain, in Lewis D (ed.): Practice of Surgery, Vol 12. WF Pryor, Hagerstown, Maryland, 1959, pp 642–643
16. Dinsdale HB: Spontaneous hemorrhage in the posterior fossa. Arch Neurol 10:200–217, 1964
17. Ellis AG: The pathogenesis of spontaneous cerebral hemorrhage. Proc Path Soc 12:197–235, 1909
18. Epstein AN: Primary massive pontine hemorrhage. Clinicopathological study. J Neuropath Exp Neurol 10:426–488, 1951
19. Fang HCH, Foley JM: Hypertensive hemorrhages of the pons and cerebellum. Arch Neurol Psychiat 72:638–639, 1954
20. Fisher CM: Clinical syndromes of cerebral hemorrhage. In Fields WS (ed.): Pathogenesis and Treatment of Cerebrovascular Disease. Thomas, Springfield, 1961, pp 318–338
21. Fisher CM: Ocular bobbing. Arch Neurol 11:543–546, 1964
22. Fisher CM: Pathological observations in hypertensive cerebral hemorrhage. J Neuropath Exp Neurol 30:536–550, 1971
23. Fisher CM, Picard EH, Polak A, Dalal P, Ojemann RG: Acute hypertensive cerebellar hemorrhage: Diagnosis and surgical treatment. J Nerv Ment Dis 140:38–57, 1965
24. Freeman RE, Onofrio BM, Okazaki H, Dinapol RP: Spontaneous intracerebellar hemorrhage. Neurology 23:84–90, 1973
25. Giroux JC, Leger JL: Hematomas of the poste-

rior cranial fossa: A report of three cases. Can Med Assoc J 87:59–61, 1962

26. Gros C, Giraud G, Latour H: Hematome spontane de la calote protuberantielle opere et queri. Presse Med 56:890, 1948
27. Heiman TD, Satya-Murti S: Benign cerebellar hemorrhage. Ann Neurol 3:366–368, 1978
28. Helpern M, Rabson R: Analysis of 2,000 cases of sudden and unexpected death. NY Med J 102:659, 1953
29. Humphrey RP: Computerized tomographic definition of mesencephalic hematoma with evacuation through penduncolotomy. J Neurosurg 49:749–752, 1978
30. Hyland HH, Levy D: Spontaneous cerebellar hemorrhage. Can Med Assoc J 71:315–323, 1954
31. Kempe LG: Surgical removal of an intramedullary hematoma simulating Wallenburg's syndrome. J Neurol Neurosurg Psychiatry 27:78–80, 1964
32. Kinkel WR, Jacobs L: Computerized axial transverse tomography in cerebrovascular disease. Neurology 26:924–930, 1976
33. Kistler JP, Hochberg FH, Brooks BR, Richardson EP Jr, New PFJ, Schnur J: Computerized axial tomography: Clinicopathological correlation. Neurology 25:201–209, 1975
34. Koos WT, Sunder-Plassman M, Salah S: Successful removal of a large intrapontine hematoma: Case report. J Neurosurg 31:690–694, 1969
35. Kowada M, Ito Z, Matsuoka S, Yamaguchi K: Primary pontine haemorrhage revealed by pneumoencephalo-roulette tomogeaphy, and a report on surgically treated cases. Acta Neurochir (Wien) 25:269–276, 1971
36. Kowada M, Yamaguchi K, Ito Z, Matsuoka S: Pneumoencephalo-roulette tomography of operated primary pontine haemorrhage with long survival: Report of two cases. J. Neurol. Neurosurg. Psychiatry 35:243–246, 1972
37. Kron I, Mintz W: Kleinhirnblutung geheilt druch operation. Dtsh Med Wochenschr 53:1054–1055, 1927
38. La Torre E, Delitala A, Sorano V: Hematoma of the quadrigeminal plate. J Neurosurg 49:610–613, 1978
39. Lichtenstein RS: Spontaneous cerebellar hematomas. Johns Hopkins Med J 122:319–328, 1968
40. Little JR, Tubman DE, Ethier R: Cerebellar hemorrhage in adults. J. Neurosurg 48:575–579, 1978
41. Loeb C, Meyer JS: Strokes Due to Vertebrobasilar Disease. Thomas, Springfield, 1965
42. Lukin RR, Chambers AA, Tomsick TA: Cerebral vascular lesions: Infarction, hemorrhage, aneurysm, and arteriovenous malformation. Sermin Roentgenol. 12:77–89, 1977
43. Matson DD: Surgery of posterior fossa tumors in childhood. Clin Neurosurg 13:263–264, 1968
44. McCormick WF, Nofzinger JD: 'Cryptic' vascular malformations of the central nervous system. J Neurosurg 24:872–894, 1966
45. McKissock W, Richardson A, Walsh L: Spontaneous cerebellar hemorrhage: A Study of 34 consecutive cases treated surgically. Brain 83:1–9, 1960
46. Meyer JS, Bauer R: Medical treatment of spontaneous intracranial hemorrhage by the use of hypotensive drugs. Neurology 12:36–47, 1962
47. Michael JC: Cerebellar apoplexy. Am J Med Sci 183:687–695, 1932
48. Mitchell N, Angrist A: Spontaneous cerebellar hemorrhage: Report of 15 cases. Am J Pathol 18:235–253, 1942
49. Muller HR, Wuthrich R, Wiggli U, et al: The contribution of computerized axial tomography to the diagnosis of cerebellar and pontine hematomas. Stroke 6:467–475, 1975
50. Murphy MG: Successful evacuation of acute pontine hematoma: Case report. J Neurosurg 37:224–225, 1972
51. Mutlu N, Berry RG, Alpers BJ. Massive cerebral hemorrhage. Arch Neurol 8:644–661, 1963
52. Nelson JR, Johnston DH: Ocular bobbing. Arch Neurol 22:348–356, 1970
53. Norris JW, Eisen AA, Branch L: Problems in cerebellar hemorrhage and infarction. Neurology 19:1043–1050, 1969
54. Novak E. Quoted in Kornyey, S., Rapidly fatal pontile hemorrhage. Arch Neurol Psychiat (Chicago) 41:793–799, 1939
55. Obrador S, Dierssen G, Odoriz BJ: Surgical evacuation of a pontine-medullary hematoma: Case report. J Neurosurg 33:82–84, 1970
56. Odom GL, Tindall GT, Dukes HT: Cerebellar hematoma caused by angiomatous malformations. Report of four cases. J Neurosurg 18:777–782, 1961
57. Ojemann RG: Intracerebral and intracerebellar hemorrhage. In Youmans JR (ed.): Neurological Surgery, Vol 2. WB Saunders, Philadelphia, 1973, pp 844–851
58. Oppenheim H: Diseases of the Nervous System. Lippincott, Philadelphia, 1900
59. Ott KH, Kase CS, Ojemann RG, Mohr JP: Cerebellar hemorrhage: Diagnosis and treatment. A review of 56 cases. Arch Neurol 31:160–167, 1974
60. Papo I, Pasquini U, Salvolini U: Subendymal brain stem hematomas: A report of two cases. Neuroradiology 11:279–282, 1976

61. Payne HA, Maravilla KR, Levenstone A, Henter J, Tindall RSA: Recovery from primary pontine hemorrhage. Ann Neurol 4:557–558, 1978
62. Pressman BP, Kirkwood JR, Davis DO: Posterior fossa hemorrhage. Localization by computerized tomography. JAMA 232:932–933, 1975
63. Ray-Bellet J: Cerebellar hemorrhage: A clinicopathologic study. Neurology 10:217–222, 1960
64. Richardson AE: Spontaneous cerebellar hemorrhage. In Vinken PJ, Bruyn GW (eds.): Handbook of Clinical Neurology, Vol 12. North Holland Publishing, Amsterdam, 1972, pp 54–67
65. Rosenberg GA, Kaufman DM: Cerebellar hemorrhage: Reliability of clinical evaluation. Stroke 7:332–336, 1976
66. Russell DS: The pathology of spontaneous intracranial hemorrhages. Proc Roy Soc Med 4:689–704, 1954
67. Scott BB, Seeger JF, Schneider RC: Successful evacuation of a pontine hematoma secondary to rupture of a pathologically diagnosed "cryptic" vascular malformation: Case report. J Neurosurg 39:104–108, 1973
68. Scott M, Silverstein A: Intrapontine cyst verified by surgical drainage into the fourth ventricle: Report of a case with an unusual neurological syndrome. J Neurosurg 17:520–528, 1960
69. Scott WR, New PFJ, Davis KR, Schnur JA: Computerized axial tomography of intracerebral and intraventricular hemorrhage. Radiology 112:73–80, 1974
70. Scoville WB, Poppen JL: Intrapeduncular hemorrhage of the brain: Successful operative approach with evacuation of clot and a seven and one-fourth year observation period. Arch Neurol Psychiatry 61:688–694, 1949
71. Sedillot J: Epanchement de sang dans le lobe droit du cervelet suivi de la mort. J Gen Med Chir Pharm 47:375–379, 1813
72. Silverstein A: Primary pontine hemorrhage. Confin. Neurol (Basil) 29:33–46, 1967
73. Silverstein A: Primary pontine hemorrhage. In Vinken PJ, Bruyn GW (eds.): Handbook of Clinical Neurology, Vol 12. North Holland Publishing, Amsterdam, 1972, pp 37–53
74. Siris H, Beller J: Spontaneous intracerebellar hemorrhage: Surgical treatment. Surg Clin North Am 28:412–415, 1948
75. Steegman AT: Primary pontile hemorrhage. J Neur Ment Dis 14:35–65, 1951
76. Susac JO, Hoyt WF, Duroff RB, Lawrence WF: Clinical spectrum of ocular bobbing. J Neurol Neurosurg Psychiatry 33:771–775, 1970
77. Sypert GW: Cerebellar hemorrhage and infarction. Compr Ther 3:42–47, 1977
78. Sypert GW, Alvord EC Jr: Cerebellar infarction. A clinicopathological study. Arch Neurol 32:357–363, 1975
79. Webster SJ: The diagnosis and etiology of apoplexy. Ohio St Med J 25:871–878, 1929
80. Wilson G, Winkelman NW: Gross pontile bleeding in traumatic and non-traumatic cerebral lesions. Arch Neurol Psychiatry 15:455–469, 1926
81. Wilson SAK, Bruce AN: Neurology, Vol 3. Williams and Wilkens, Baltimore, 1955
82. Yoshida S, Sasaki M, Oka H, Gotoh O, Yamada R, Sano K: Acute hypertensive cerebellar hemorrhage with signs of lower brain stem compression. Surg Neurol 10:79–83, 1978

11

Cerebellar Infarction

George W. Sypert

Introduction

Despite recent advances in the diagnosis and treatment of neurologic diseases, acute vascular mass lesions of the cerebellum often remain undiagnosed during life and are not recognized as potentially treatable neurologic emergencies in patients with stroke syndromes.[32] Acute massive cerebellar infarction is thought to be rare compared with hemorrhage and infarction elsewhere in the brain. In addition, early attempts at recognizing a reliable syndrome have been unsuccessful because the signs and syndromes are too protean. Cerebellar infarction often occurs in patients having evidence of brainstem infarction. Large cerebellar infarctions may also present clinically and radiologically as rapidly progressing posterior fossa mass lesions and may be mistaken for hemorrhage or tumor. However, recent clinical[5,9,20,23,24,36] and clinicopathologic studies[34] demonstrate that infarction of a cerebellar hemisphere is not rare and that early diagnosis and prompt neurosurgical attention are mandatory.

The prognosis and treatment of cerebellar infarction depend on rapid and exacting diagnosis and a clear knowledge of the natural history of the lesion. Although diagnosis can be made on clinical evaluation, it is exceedingly difficult. The recent development of computed tomography (CT) scanning continues to be an invaluable tool for accurate diagnosis.[2,9]

Incidence and Mortality

Acute massive cerebellar hemorrhage as a cause of death was first reported by Schwartz.[30] Although numerous cases of massive infarction of the cerebellum have since been reported at autopsy[1,7,8,10,16,17,19,29] only in recent years has there been an extensive clinicopathologic study of them.[34] Recent clinical case reports have begun to establish a clinical syndrome related to massive cerebellar infarction and swelling.* It is apparent from these studies that diagnosis is all too frequently made at postmortem.

The true incidence of infarction of a cerebellar hemisphere is unknown and difficult to ascertain. In an early clinical series, four cases were observed over a 10-year period in a 1,000-bed general hospital.[20] A more recent clinicopathologic study in three university-affiliated general hospitals during a similar time interval found 28 cases of acute fatal cerebellar infarctions uncomplicated by massive brainstem or cerebral infarction—an adult autopsy incidence of 0.5%.[34] Acute cerebellar hemorrhage was found to occur with a similar incidence in that same autopsy population. Acute cerebellar infarction is therefore not rare, but remains largely unrecognized clinically. An estimate of the clinical incidence of cerebellar infarction will probably only be ascertained at a center

* References 5, 6, 9, 20, 21, 23, 24, 26, 27, 36.

where a large number of CT scans are aggressively performed in evaluating cerebrovascular disease.

The importance of acute massive cerebellar infarction is emphasized by its high mortality. Although it is not possible to exactly determine, available data suggest that the mortality rate of large cerebellar infarctions may approach 50%.[34] Certainly the mortality of smaller cerebellar infarctions is lower, with most patients recovering spontaneously (Duncan et al, 1975) if there is no associated brainstem infarction. Careful clinical evaluation combined with CT scanning will hopefully permit more accurate estimates of mortality risks for individual patients in the future.

Etiology and Pathology

As with most occlusive cerebrovascular diseases, acute cerebellar infarction is a disease of later life (fifth through eight decades), predominating in males.[34] Cerebellar infarction with brainstem compression has been reported in an infant[23] and in an adolescent.[10]

Preexisting artherosclerotic cardiovascular disease appears to be the most important predisposing factor.[34] Hypertension, usually of 5 or more years duration, has also been found to be an important predisposing condition. Additional predisposing factors include recent myocardial infarction, diabetes mellitus, polycythemia, and contraceptive agents.

Many patients have a history suggestive of previous neurologic disturbances, and vertebral insufficiency is not an infrequent clinical diagnosis. Patients may also have a history of previous occlusive-type cerebrovascular accident.

The neuropathologic observations of Sypert and Alvord[34] suggest that the majority of cases of cerebellar infarction are secondary to atherosclerotic arterial occlusion. As many as 25% of cases may appear to be embolic in nature.

Although vertebral artery occlusion is frequently asymptomatic, in 65% of cases the most common cause of massive cerebellar infarction was an acute ipsilateral vertebral artery occlusion.[34] A similar high incidence of vertebral artery occlusion has been shown to be etiologic in patients with lateral medullary (Wallenberg) syndrome.[26] Occlusion of either a posterior inferior cerebellar artery or a superior cerebellar artery is also a frequent cause of cerebellar infarction, with ipsilateral vertebral or posterior inferior cerebellar artery occlusion accounting for approximately 90% of cases.

The cerebellum has a rich collateral circulation, possibly explaining the observation that cerebellar infarction may be less common than brainstem infarction.[22] However, recent angiographic studies[35] show a high incidence of anatomic variations in arterial supply, and this may be of paramount importance in patients who sustain massive cerebellar infarctions.

The most common site of massive cerebellar infarction is the posterior-inferior half of a cerebellar hemisphere.[34] This site represents that portion of the cerebellum predominantly supplied directly from the ipsilateral vertebral artery via the posterior-inferior cerebellar artery. Bilateral infarction with extensive destruction of both cerebellar hemispheres is not common.

Postmortem examination of fatal cases of acute cerebellar infarction reveals massive softening and swelling of the affected cerebellum. The infarction is hemorrhagic (Fig. 11.1) in one-quarter of cases[34] and involves greater than one-third of the affected hemisphere. Autopsy examination of patients who survived a cerebellar infarction and did not develop brainstem compression reveals that the volume of the infarction is considerably smaller than in acutely fatal cases. An example of a large old cerebellar infarction is illustrated in Fig. 11.2.

Marked molding with compression of the medulla and pons is present at autopsy in fatal cases (Fig.11.3) and is the probable cause of death.[34] Obliteration and/or shift of the fourth ventricle is observed in almost all fatal cases, frequently accompanied by secondary obstructive hydrocephalus. Most fatal cases show herniation of necrotic cerebellar tonsil through the foramen magnum (Fig.11.1). Upward transtentorial herniation of the anterior cerebellum may also occur after massive superior cerebellar infarctions.

In fatal cases the microscopic appearance is that of ischemic or hemorrhagic infarction (necrosis), varying from hours to as much as two weeks' duration. The majority of cases examined at autopsy revealed microscopic changes consistent with an infarction of three to six days' duration, with substantial pallor and

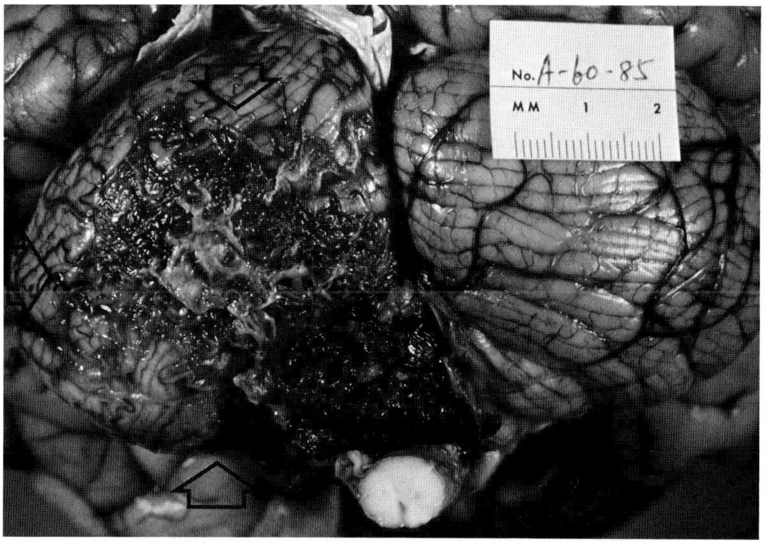

Fig. 11.1. Posterior view of uncut brain showing a hemorrhagic infarct of the posterior left cerebellar hemisphere. Necrotic friable cerebellar tonsil sloughed at autopsy.

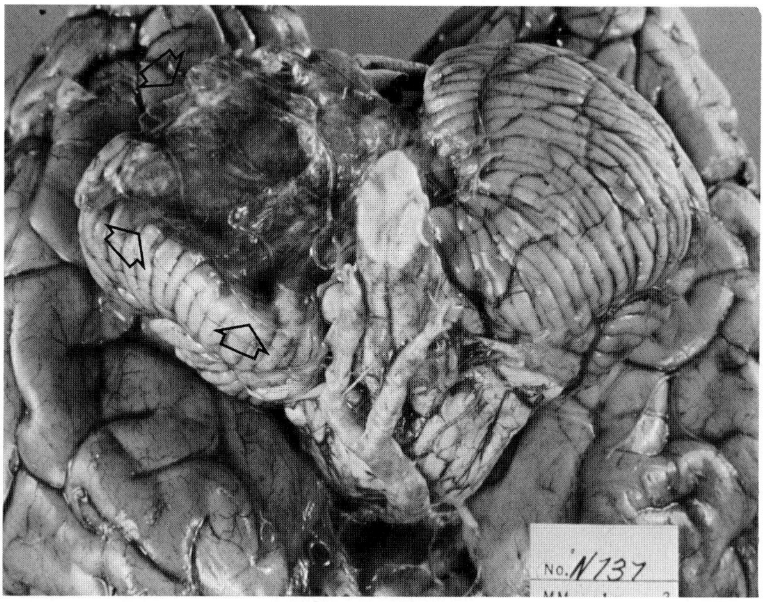

Fig. 11.2. Inferior view of uncut brain showing an old cystic ischemic infarct of posterior half of left cerebellar hemisphere (*arrows*).

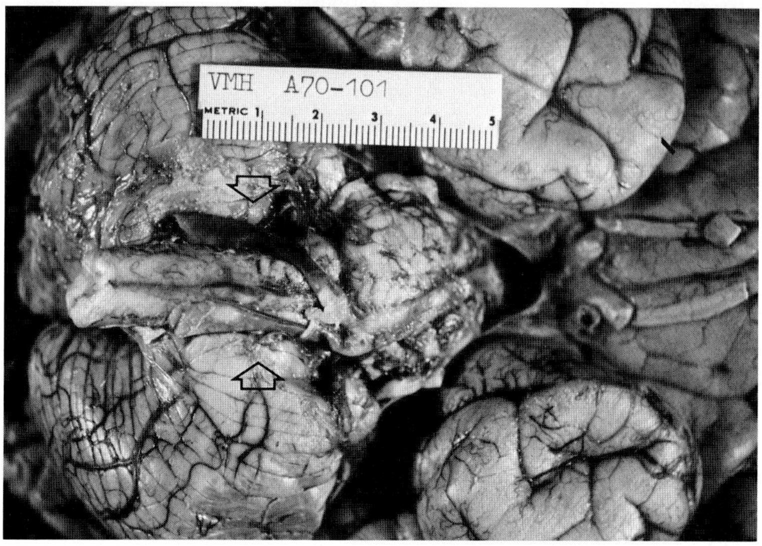

Fig. 11.3. Inferior view of uncut brain showing large ischemic infarct of posterior left cerebellar hemisphere with marked molding about the hindbrain (*arrows*).

edema, loss of neurons, ischemic neuronal change, invasion of polymorphonuclear and mononuclear cells, astrocytic swelling, and the early appearance of gitter cells.[34] Gross and microscopic examination of the brainstem in cases of massive cerebellar infarction uncomplicated by a concurrent brainstem infarction failed to show any substantial abnormality.

The pathogenesis of the massive swelling that accompanies large cerebellar infarctions is not known. Available evidence, although partly inferential and incomplete, indicates that the initial abnormality leading to swelling is an ischemic defect in the capillary and/or an ischemic derangement of glial cell metabolism, resulting in progressive intracellular and extracellular fluid accumulation.[26] The size of the infarct is important, as massive fatal cerebellar swelling has not been observed with infarcts affecting less than one-third of a cerebellar hemisphere. Additional factors need to be resolved, including the role of embolization in the vertebrobasilar system. Embolization appears to occur with a high incidence in acutely fatal cases (at least 25%), possibly a reflection of the sudden occlusion associated with an embolus that does not permit time for collateral formation or induces spasm in the collaterals already present and therefore results in large symptomatic cerebellar infarctions.

Massive cerebellar swelling becomes symptomatic by direct compression of the brainstem. In some patients, upward and downward transtentorial herniations may also be significant. The effect of such compression and/or herniation is to directly damage the neural tissue and distort the vessels of the brainstem, ultimately resulting in necrosis of both neural and vascular elements. The incidence of symptomatic brainstem compression is greater with large cerebellar infarcts (approximately 75%)[34] than with large supratentorial infarcts (approximately 25%).[31] This is probably related to the smaller size of the posterior fossa, with less ability of neural elements, cerebrospinal fluid, and blood to compensate for the rapidly expanding mass lesion.

Clinical Presentation

The onset of symptoms is usually sudden without any immediately premonitory symptoms or precipitating factors.[5,9,23,34] In most patients the initial symptom is a fall with the inability to stand and ataxia of gait. Vomiting, dizziness or vertigo, dysarthria, and ataxia of the extremities are common at onset. Transient loss of consciousness or confusion with clouding of consciousness may occur in some patients. Headache is rare. An acute cerebellar infarction may be clinically silent at onset in some patients, particularly if the infarct is small.

On admission to the hospital, most patients are hypertensive, with an altered state of consciousness (confusion, drowsiness, or stupor). Some patients may be comatose when first examined. In noncomatose patients, cerebellar-type signs are usually prominent, including gait ataxia, ipsilateral extremity dysmetria, and dysarthria. The pupils are usually small and reactive. Cranial nerve findings often include an ipsilateral gaze paresis, ipsilateral peripheral facial palsy, nystagmus, and depressed corneal reflex. Findings consistent with a classic lateral medullary (Wallenberg) syndrome may be present in one-fifth of patients. Motor system disturbances such as hemiparesis, quadriparesis, or Babinski sign may be observed in one-third of patients. A few may exhibit some degree of respiratory disturbance, pupillary abnormalities, and sensory systems involvement. A patient may occasionally have a normal neurologic examination on admission.

Clinical Course

The clinical course of massive cerebellar infarction generally follows two basic patterns[5,9,34]:

1. Cerebellar infarction may resemble an acute benign labyrinthine disorder, with the sudden onset of vertigo, ataxia, vomiting, and nystagmus. Brainstem compression does not occur, and complete recovery is usually achieved (case 1).
2. Some patients have a rapid course of brainstem compression resembling the acute course often seen in acute cerebellar hemorrhage[34], with loss of consciousness and rapid, progressive deterioration of brainstem function that begins within 24 hours of onset of symptoms (case 2).

Case 1

This 65-year-old man was admitted to the University of Florida Shands Teaching Hospital because of the sudden development of vertigo after arising and going to the bathroom early on the day of admission. The vertigo was aggravated by movement, and the patient noted difficulty in maintaining a steady upright posture. Vomiting occurred twice. He had a history of mild hypertension for which he was treated with hydrochlorothiazide. Four years earlier he had a mild myocardial infarction.

On examination in the emergency room, the patient was uncomfortable from persistent vertigo and occasional vomiting, but alert and oriented. His extraocular movements were full, but he exhibited rotating nystagmus on left lateral gaze, which increased when lying supine with the left ear down. He had a mild dysarthria. Motor power and sensory function were intact. The patient was unable to stand unsupported and on attempting to walk, fell backward and to the left. There was no extremity dysmetria or intention tremor. The tendon reflexes were symmetrical, and there were no pathologic reflexes.

The diagnosis of acute labyrinthitis was considered, and the patient was treated with bedrest, antimetics, and antivertiginous agents. A CT scan obtained the day following admission demonstrated a large low-density area in the left cerebellar hemisphere (Fig. 11.4). The diagnosis of acute cerebellar infarction was made. Over the next three weeks, the patient made a gradual, uneventful recovery.

Case 2

This 56-year-old man had suffered a myocardial infarction eight months before admission to the Gainesville Veterans Administration Center. Since the myocardial infarction, atrial fibrillation had been very difficult to control. On the afternoon of admission the patient suddenly developed vertigo and fell, unable to stand or walk. There was no headache, but he experienced multiple episodes of vomiting. Over the next two hours he noted progressive slurring of speech and was admitted to the hospital three hours after onset of symptoms.

On admission the patient was alert, oriented, and cooperative. Blood pressure was 170/110 mm Hg. Coarse horizontal nystagmus was elicited on right lateral gaze. Moderate dysarthria was present. Motor power was excellent and sensory function was intact. Moderate cerebellar dysmetria and intention tremor were present in the right upper and lower extremities. The patient was unable to sit or stand unsupported. The tendon reflexes were symmetrical, and there were no pathologic reflexes. An ECG demonstrated atrial fibrillation. A lumbar puncture was performed and showed pink fluid (RBC, 4,700/μL; WBC, 7/μL; protein 47 mg/100 mL) that did not clear. The opening pressure was 160 mm of cerebrospinal fluid.

Sixteen hours later the patient became drowsy, with paralysis of conjugate gaze to the right and a peripheral right facial paresis. An emergency four-vessel cerebral angiogram was performed (Fig. 11.5). The diagnosis of massive cerebellar infarction was made. Over the next

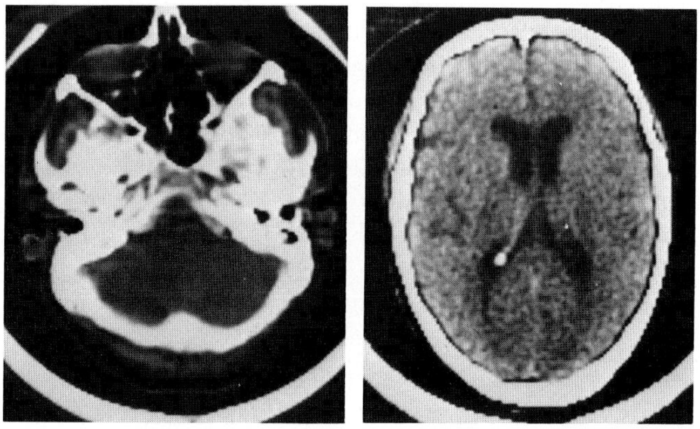

Fig. 11.4. Case 1. CT scan showing large left cerebellar infarction. Comparison between left and right cerebellar hemispheres shows a large, low-density area in the left cerebellar hemisphere **(A).** Higher cut shows minimal evidence of hydrocephalus **(B).**

A B

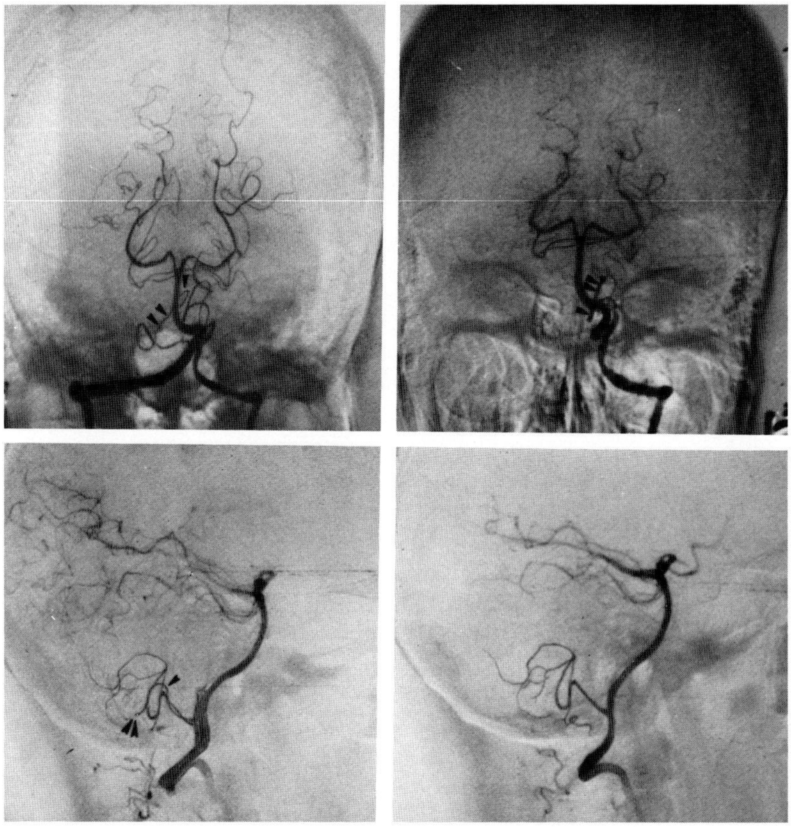

Fig. 11.5. Case 2. Bilateral vertebral angiograms showing an avascular mass in right cerebellar hemisphere pushing left posterior inferior cerebellar artery from right to left (*upper arrows*). In this patient with a massive cerebellar infarction, there is an occluded right posterior inferior cerebellar artery (*lower left, arrows*).

two hours the patient ceased to follow commands and became stuporous, with a left hemiparesis.

An emergency suboccipital craniectomy was performed. The right cerebellar hemisphere was necrotic, swollen, friable, and avascular. The right cerebellar tonsil was herniated to the level of the arch of the axis. A complete resection of the necrotic cerebellar tissue was accomplished. Histologic examination of the resected tissue confirmed the diagnosis of cerebellar infarction.

Postoperatively, the patient made an uneventful recovery. Three months later he returned to work and his neurologic examination was normal.

In the majority of patients suffering brainstem compression from cerebellar swelling secondary to massive cerebellar infarction, the course is generally slower and more predictable than that of cerebellar hemorrhage.[32,33] There is usually an interval of 60 hours or more between the onset of symptoms and death.[34] The subsequent course following onset of symptoms is usually characterized by a latent interval of 24 to 96 hours, followed by a progressive neurologic deterioration, including impairment of consciousness, ipsilateral facial paresis, ipsilateral gaze paresis, and motor (pyramidal-type) dysfunction. Once these symptoms and signs appear, a relentless progression to quadriplegia, coma, and death over a few hours or days is the usual course. Less than 20% of patients developing these signs of progressive brainstem dysfunction survive without decompressive therapy.[34] Normally there are approximately six hours between the onset of drowsiness or stupor and the onset of coma. A similar time interval usually exists between the onset of coma

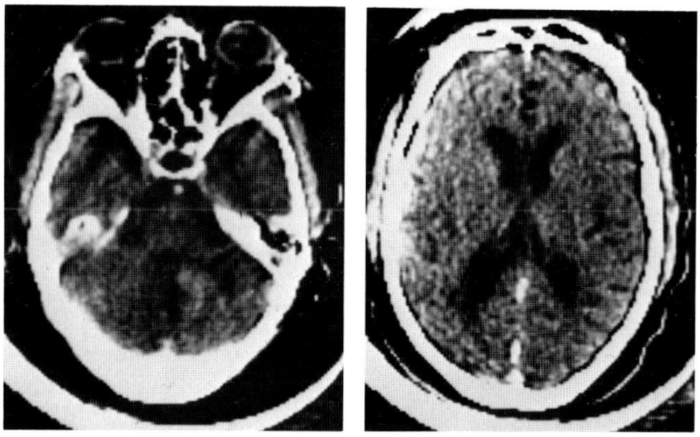

A B

Fig. 11.6. Case 3. CT scan showing large right cerebellar infarction. Comparison between right and left cerebellar hemispheres shows a large, diffusely high-density area in the right cerebellar hemisphere **(A).** Higher cut shows moderately severe hydrocephalus **(B).**

and death. Death is due to a sudden arrest of cardiorespiratory function following a brief period of ataxic respirations. The orderly and predictable pattern of respiratory failure usually seen in transtentorial herniation is rarely observed in these patients.

Case 3

This 61-year-old man who was in good health suddenly developed light-headedness, vertigo, and difficulty walking without assistance three days before his admission to the University of Florida Shands Teaching Hospital. During the preceding three weeks, he had experienced repeated transient episodes of mild headache and dizziness. On the day of admission he vomited and became drowsy.

On examination the patient was drowsy but oriented and able to follow commands. Blood pressure was 150/90 mm Hg. The pupils were small and reacted poorly to light. At rest, the eyes were conjugately deviated to the left. Right conjugate gaze paralysis was present. Dysarthria was marked. The face moved symmetrically. The patient was unable to sit or stand, falling to the right. Motor power and sensation were intact. There was a moderate generalized hyperreflexia of the tendon reflexes. Bilateral extensor plantar responses were present.

During the next five hours, the patient became stuporous and unable to follow commands. An emergency CT scan was performed, demonstrating a diffuse high-density area in the right cerebellar hemisphere (Fig. 11.6). The diagnosis of massive hemorrhagic cerebellar infarction with swelling and progressive brainstem compression was made.

An emergency suboccipital craniectomy was performed. The posterior fossa was tight. On opening the dura, soft, partially liquefied avascular cerebellar tissue exuded out under pressure. The entire inferior half of the right cerebellum was hemorrhagic, swollen, avascular, and necrotic. The necrotic tissue was radically excised. Histologic examination was consistent with hemorrhagic infarction.

Postoperatively, recovery was rapid, with complete resolution of pathologic neurologic signs over seven days. Two months later the patient had returned to full activities with a normal neurologic examination.

In patients sustaining a large cerebellar infarction, most of the early symptoms and signs can be explained on the basis of destruction of cerebellar tissue. All of the later developing symptoms and signs plus the clinical progression point directly to brainstem compression. Since no anatomic changes are found at autopsy in the medulla, pons, or midbrain on gross and microscopic evaluation,[34] it is reasonable to assume that the progressive brainstem dysfunction is due to mechanical compression by the massive cerebellar swelling that is found at autopsy or surgery. The frequent, complete resolution of brainstem symptoms and signs after emergency decompressive surgery further supports this postulate.* The time course of the development of maximal symptoms, signs, and death also lends support to such a model. Medullary failure and death occurred in most patients three to five days after the onset of symptoms. This time interval is similar to that noted

* References 3, 6, 9, 20, 21, 23, 24, 27, 32, 26.

for maximal swelling following sudden, massive cerebral encephalomalacia due to occlusion of a major supratentorial artery.[26,31] Thus, each acutely fatal case of massive cerebellar infarction presents clinically as an expanding posterior fossa mass with progressive mechanical compression of the brainstem.

Diagnosis

The clinical diagnosis of massive cerebellar infarction can be made if the clinician has a high index of suspicion and an accurate clinical evaluation. Essentially, the patient presents with dizziness and ataxia and a course consistent with an expanding posterior fossa mass lesion resembling acute cerebellar hemorrhage.* Posterior fossa subdural and epidural hematoma or rapidly expanding cerebellar neoplasms or abcesses may also present similar clinical pictures. However, the initial clinical differentiation of these various clinical entities may not be necessary, as they all all represent neurosurgically treatable, expanding posterior fossa mass lesions.

Fisher et al (1965, 1967), Loeb and Meyer, (1965), and Plum and Posner (1972)[11,14,22,26] have clearly described the differentiating features of the various other stroke syndromes, and in most cases these should not offer difficulties with the differential diagnosis. Certain cases of progressive brainstem infarction or hemorrhage and subarachnoid hemorrhage from a ruptured aneurysm remain difficult diagnostic problems. The diagnosis may be especially difficult with those patients in a stuporous state who have no history, limiting the clinical examination.

Clinicians must immediately and accurately distinguish treatable posterior fossa mass lesions from brainstem infarction. In a patient demonstrating progressive brainstem dysfunction, a delay will usually result in irreversible brainstem damage and death. A lumbar puncture may be hazardous, needlessly delaying and frequently confusing the clinician. In contrast to the more fulminating course of cerebellar hemorrhage, the syndrome of cerebellar infarction usually evolves more slowly, and there is sufficient time to permit accurate neuroradiologic studies. The diagnostic procedure of choice is the CT scan.[2,9] In centers without CT scan facilities, the procedure of choice appears to be combined carotid and vertebral angiography.[23,34] This latter approach implies that angiography will be performed on some patients whose primary lesion is a brainstem infarction; however, the risks of modern contrast media and neuroradiologic techniques are sufficiently low to be justified.[35] If these signs of brainstem compression are critical and the diagnosis of a posterior fossa mass lesion is suspected, the clinician should not wait for neuroradiologic confirmation but should procede to emergency posterior fossa decompression, even if the patient is in extremis.

CT scanning has proved to be a rapid and accurate method for the diagnosis and localization of massive cerebellar infarction.[2,9] A CT scan should be performed immediately whenever there is a suspicion of cerebellar infarction. Typical CT scans of acute cerebellar infarction are illustrated in Fig. 11.4 and 11.6. In the early stages (24 to 48 hours after onset), the CT scan ordinarily reveals a diffuse low-density (+2 to +8 Hounsfield units) parenchymal process of variable size, with or without evidence of mass effect. Speckled hemorrhagic changes may be prominent in some cases (Fig. 11.6). If the infarction is large with marked swelling, shift and/or obliteration of the fourth ventricle may be evident. Moderate to severe hydrocephalus may be present with obliteration. In patients who do not develop brainstem compression, these changes gradually subside over a few months and resolve ultimately into a residual lacunae or porencephalic cyst.

In patients with a massive cerebellar infarction with swelling and brainstem compression, the vertebral angiogram should show an avascular cerebellar mass and the presence of tonsillar herniation[23] and may demonstrate the site of arterial occlusion (Fig. 11.5). In two-thirds of patients, vertebral angiography shows an occluded ipsilateral vertebral artery.[34] The carotid angiogram may demonstrate hydrocephalus (Fig. 11.7). Reflux filling of the basilar artery from the carotid artery via the posterior communicating artery may occur owing to poor circulation in the posterior fossa.

* References 3–5, 9, 14, 20, 23, 24, 26, 28, 32–34, 36.

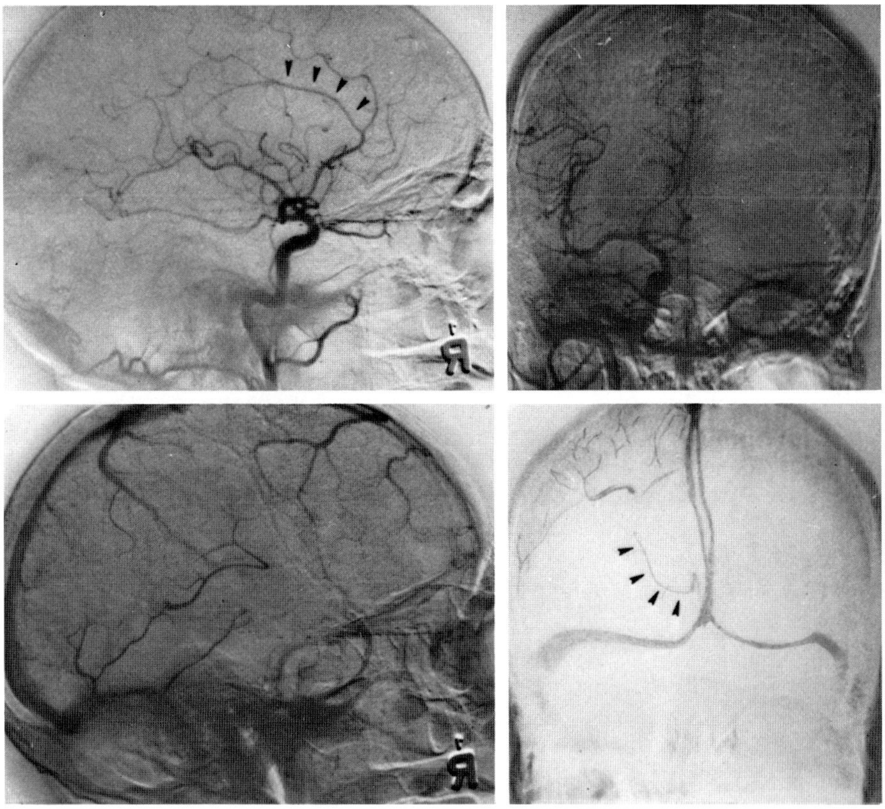

Fig. 11.7. Case 2. Right carotid angiogram shows changes of hydrocephalus (*arrows*) in a case of massive cerebellar infarction.

Treatment

Patients with acute cerebellar infarction should be observed closely for signs of brainstem compression. If these signs develop, consideration should be given to immediate suboccipital decompression with resection of all necrotic cerebellar tissue, since the mortality approximates 80% for unoperated patients.[9,34] Although some patients survive spontaneously without substantial neurologic morbidity, despite the development of apparent brainstem compression, the probability of a worthwhile survival is greatest with surgery. Table 11.1 lists the outcome of cases available in the literature of massive cerebellar infarction with brainstem compression and includes our recent experience with six patients.

It has been suggested that nonsurgical means of therapy, e.g., steroid, diuretic agents, and hyperventilation, may have a place in the treatment of acute cerebellar infarction associated

Table 11.1. Results of treatment in cases of cerebellar infarction with brainstem compression.

Treatment	No. of cases	Full recovery	Partial recovery	Mortality
Nonsurgical	42	6	1	35 (83%)
Surgical[a]	34	20	7	7 (20%)

[a] Surgical treatment refers to suboccipital craniectomy and resection of necrotic cerebellar tissue.

with massive swelling.[9,34] If instituted early in the course, it is possible that this form of therapy will be beneficial. However, if brainstem compression occurs, it is exceedingly unlikely that a significant decompression of the brainstem can be achieved by these nonsurgical methods. Despite multiple laboratory and clinical trials, there is no conclusive evidence to suggest that glucocorticoids will have any significant effect on the swelling associated with either cerebellar or cerebral infarction. The small confines of the posterior cranial fossa make diuretic agents and hyperventilation somewhat ineffective as modes of therapy because they seem to work primarily on normal cerebral structures. In the case of acute massive cerebellar infarction, a major portion of the posterior fossa cerebral tissue has been infarcted and thus is unlikely to respond to these modes of management. Therefore, it is most probable that in patients with evidence of brainstem compression, prompt neurosurgical decompression is required, and any delay for other modes of management will result unsatisfactorily for the patient.

References

1. Adams RD. Occlusion of the anterior inferior cerebellar artery. Arch Neurol Psychiat 49:765–770, 1943
2. Baker HL, Houser OW: Computed tomography in the diagnosis of posterior fossa lesions. Radiol Clin North Am 14:129–147, 1976
3. Cohadon F, Guerin A, Castel JP, et al: Le ramollissement psuedo-tumoral du cervelet. Bordeuax Med 3:385–397, 1970
4. Dinsdale HB: Spontaneous hemorrhage in the posterior fossa. Arch Neurol 10:98–115, 1964
5. Ducan GW, Parker SW, Fisher CM: Acute cerebellar infarction in the PICA territory. Arch Neurol 32:364–368, 1975
6. Fairburn D, Oliver LC: Cerebellar softening: A surgical emergency. Br Med J 1:1335–1336, 1956
7. Fang HCH, Palmer JJ: Vascular phenomena involving brainstem structures: A clinical and pathological correlation study. Neurology 6: 402–419, 1956
8. Fattovich G: Sui rammolliment cerebelli. Cervello 26:48–64, 1950
9. Feely MP: Cerebellar infarction. Neurosurgery 4:7–11, 1979
10. Fischer EG, Strand RD, Gilles FH: Cerebellar necrosis simulating tumor in infancy. J Pediat 81:98–100, 1972
11. Fisher CM: Some neuro-ophthalmological observations. J Neurol Neurosurg Psychiat 30: 383–392, 1967
12. Fisher CM: Occlusion of the vertebral arteries. Arch Neurol 22:13–19, 1970
13. Fisher CM, Karnes WE, Kubik CS: Lateral medullary infarction: The pattern of vascular occlusion. J Neuropath Exp Neurol 20:323–379, 1961
14. Fisher DM, Picard EH, Polak A, Dalal P, Ojemann R: Acute hypertensive cerebellar hemorrhage: Diagnosis and surgical treatment. J Nerv Ment Dis 140:38–57, 1965
15. Ford FR, Clark D: Thrombosis of the basilar artery with softenings in the cerebellum and brainstem due to manipulation of the neck. Bull Johns Hopkins Hospl 98:37–42, 1954
16. German A, Morran A: Ramollissement cerebelleux pseudotumoral. Bull Soc Med Hop Paris 54:1695–1700, 1938
17. Goodhart SP, Davidson C: Syndrome of the posterior inferior and anterior inferior cerebellar arteries and their branches. Arch Neurol Psychiat 35:501–524, 1936
18. Graham DI, Adams RD: "Idiopathic thrombosis" in the vertebrobasilar arterial system in young men. Br Med J 1:26–28, 1972
19. Kubik CS, Adams SD: Occlusion of the basilar artery: A clinical and pathological study. Brain 69:6–121, 1946
20. Lehrich JR, Winckler GF, Ojemann RG: Cerebellar infarction with brainstem compression: Diagnosis and treatment. Arch Neurol 22:490–498, 1970
21. Lindgren SO: Infarctions simulating brain tumors in the posterior fossa. J Neurosurg 13:575–581, 1956
22. Loch C, Meyers JS: Strokes Due to Vertebro-Basilar Disease. Charles C Thomas, Springfield, 1965
23. Momosa KJ, Lehrich JR: Acute cerebellar infarction presenting as a posterior fossa mass. Radiology 109:343–352, 1973
24. Norris JW, Eisen AA, Branch CL: Problems in cerebellar hemorrhage and infarction. Neurology 19:1043–1050, 1969
25. Plum F: Barin swelling and edema in cerebral vascular diseases. Res Publ Assoc Res Nerv Ment Dis 41:318–348, 1966
26. Plum F, Posner JP: Diagnosis of stupor and coma, ed 2. FA Davis Co, Philadelphia, 1972
27. Pomme B, Terrasse P, Janny H, et al: Le ramollissement pseudotumoral du cervelet: A propos de deux observations. Sem Hop Paris 35:791–793, 1969

28. Rey-Bellet J: Cerebellar hemorrhage: A clinicopathologic study. Neurology 10:217–222, 1960
29. Schaffer K: Uber einige Bahnen des menschlichen rhombencephalons. Z Neurol Psychiatr 46:60–94, 1919
30. Schwartz E: Uber den anatomischen und klinischen befund bei verschluss der arteria cerebelli posterior inferior. Monatsschr Psychiatr Neurol 32:132–159, 1912
31. Shaw CM, Alvord EC Jr, Berry RG: Swelling of the brain following ischemic infarction with arterial occlusion. Arch Neurol 1:161–177, 1959
32. Sypert GW: Cerebellar hemorrhage and infarction. Compr Ther 4:42–47, 1977
33. Sypert GW: Cerebellar and brain stem hematoma. In: Fein JM, Flamm E (eds.): Textbook of Cerebrovascular Surgery. Springer-Verlag, New York, 1979
34. Sypert GW, Alvord EC Jr: Cerebellar infarction: A clinico-pathological study. Arch Neurol 32:357–363, 1975
35. Takahashi M: Atlas of Vertebral Angiography. University Park Press, Baltimore, 1974
36. Wood MW, Murphey F: Obstructive hydrocephalus due to infarction of a cerebellar hemisphere. J Neurosurg 30:260–263, 1969

12

Surgery of the Dural Sinuses

R.M. Peardon Donaghy

Introduction

The adult human is commonly considered to have six systems of veins:[41] (1) the pulmonary system, (2) the cardiac system, (3) the superior caval system, (4) the azygos system, (5) the inferior caval system, and (6) the portal system. The venous structures about which we are here concerned are parts of the superior caval and cardiac systems, which have developed from the cardinal system of the embryo.

In the early embryo, mesodermal cells give rise to angioblasts, which, by a process of proliferation or sprouting, coalescence, and vacuole formation, fashion a syncitial capillary mesh that covers the developing brain.[44,52,53] In turn this mesh divides into a deeper layer, which will eventually extend and coalesce to form the venous channels of the brain, and a more superficial layer, which runs in the adult dura (Fig. 12.1).

In the primitive dura these coalescing channels first form relatively sizeable venous lakes, which, by connecting and by becoming directionally oriented, form the long tubes known as the dural sinuses. These sinuses have certain characteristics that make them unique, and it behooves those who would perform surgery upon them to take these characteristics into consideration.

The sinuses are lined by endothelium that is continuous with and similar to that of the extracranial veins. The sinus walls have no elastic tissue and are relatively rigid, for they are actually endothelial-lined clefts in the dura. There are no valves, but they are traversed by fibrous trabeculae, sometimes called the chordae Willisii.[4,21] These are rather firm in some areas such as the superior sagittal sinus, and somewhat softer, we are told, in the cavernous sinus. The interior of the cavernous sinus, however, has mostly been viewed at autopsy and in cadavers, and knowledgeable descriptions in living subjects have only recently been given.[9,21,22,37,55]

Some venous lakes may persist along the sinuses.[7,18,19] It is not unusual on skull x-ray films to see an area of thinning along the side of the superior sagittal sinus, even in the adult where constant mild pressure of a lake has supposedly caused a mild erosion of bone. Radiologists frequently point these out. They are not of great importance to the surgeon except that it would be preferable to avoid them when operating, and they must not be confused with other lesions that cause bone erosion in the same area. Pacchionian bodies are frequently found in these areas.

Sinus surgeons must bear in mind that thrombosis readily occurs after injury or surgery for several reasons:[1,12,29,42,50,59]

1. The sinuses do not have the brisk flow of an artery.

2. The flow is under less pressure than in an artery.
3. The flow may be reduced by numerous trabeculae.
4. Tributary veins not uncommonly enter the sinus in such a manner that flow in the sinus and in the tributary is almost in opposite directions.

Moreover, different sinuses, in addition to sharing hemodynamic problems in general, have different problems of their own. Hence it is probably better to consider them individually (Fig. 12.2).

The Superior Sagittal Sinus or Superior Longitudinal Sinus

The superior longitudinal sinus begins anteriorly at the foramen cecum between the ethmoid and frontal bones where it was in communication with veins of the nasal cavity in fetal life. This communication rarely continues into adult life. The sinus is at first small, 1.1 mm at the crista galli, but quickly enlarges until it attains a width of 10 to 12 mm at its termination into the torcular Herophili, usually immediately subjacent to the external occipital protuberance. Along its way it receives as tributaries (1)

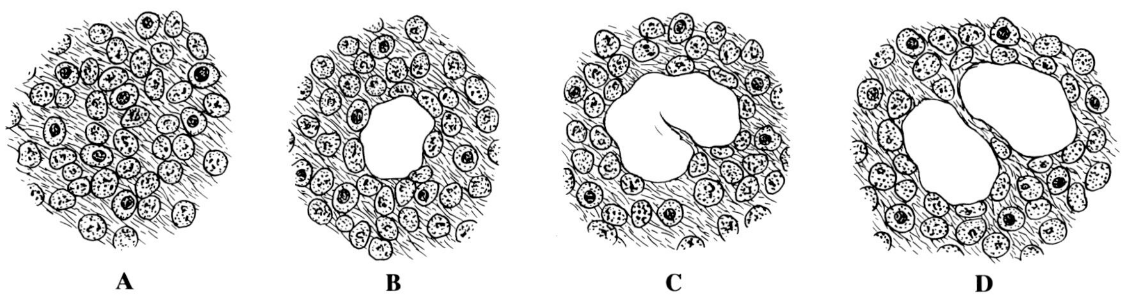

Fig. 12.1. A. Primitive angioblasts, **B,** vacuole formation, **C,** sprout dividing a vacuole, **D,** completed division of vacuole.

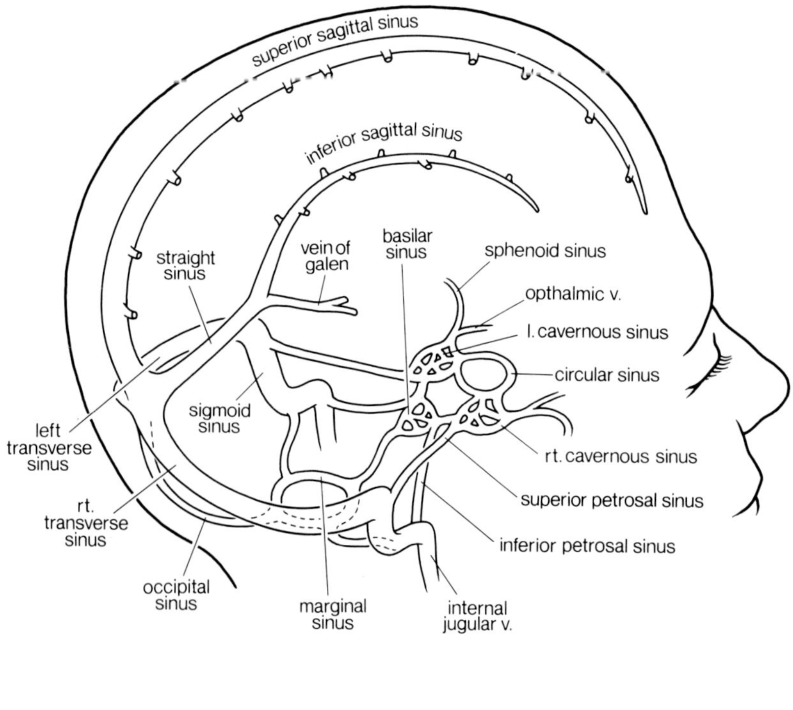

Fig. 12.2. The intracranial venous sinuses.

branches from meningeal veins and adjacent dura; (2) the superior cerebral veins from the cerebral hemispheres, 10 to 15 in number on each side; and (3) diploetic veins from the diploe. It also communicates with an emissary vein that may traverse the parietal bone.

Deviations from the Anatomic Norm

Very rarely the superior longitudinal sinus may be markedly undersized, in which case most of the tributaries that commonly flow into it will flow into the inferior longitudinal sinus.

The superior longitudinal sinus may divide into two channels, most commonly at the caudal end, but it has been known to divide into two or three channels for a short distance and then rejoin to end in one. Rarely it may divide into two channels, one of which goes to each transverse or lateral sinus, thus avoiding the torcular Herophili altogether.

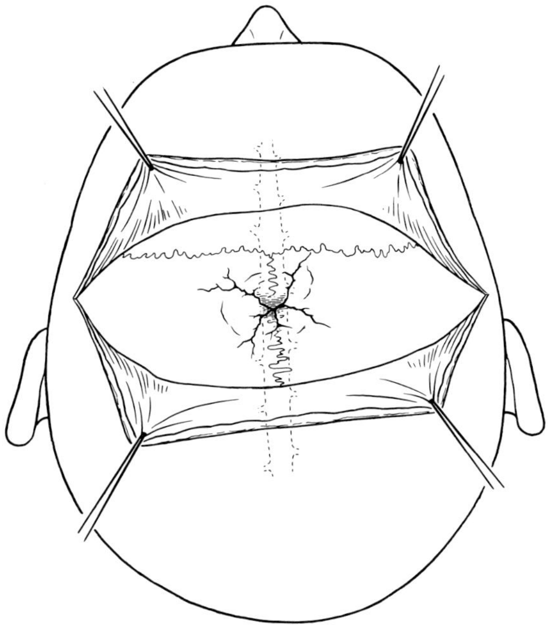

Fig. 12.3. Depressed fracture covering small dural tear.

Types of Trauma

Laceration of Sinus by Depressed Bone or Penetrating Sharp Object Without Loss of Tissue

Lacerations caused by bone or sharp objects may clot by themselves and give no further trouble, but exploration is mandatory, of course, for the compounded wounds, and the surgeon should be prepared to deal early with signs of increasing intracranial pressure.[43] Such wounds, however, may be simply sutured once exposed (Figs. 12.3 and 12.4).

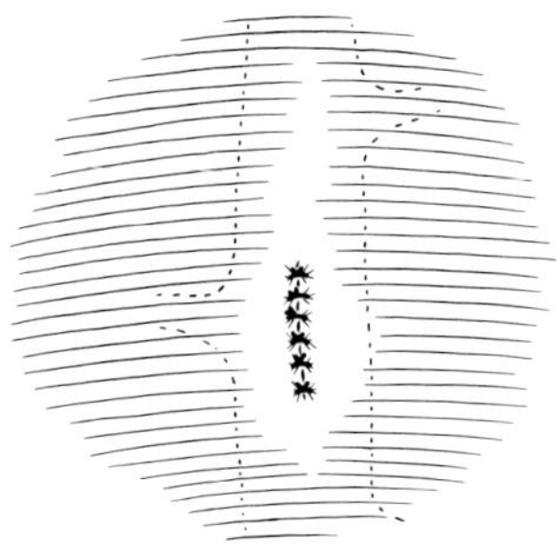

Fig. 12.4. Sutured linear tear in sinus.

Although laceration of the superior longitudinal sinus in its anterior one-third may create a fairly serious problem because of the extent of bleeding, an injury at this level is likely to thrombose on its own, and thrombosis of the sinus at this level may be compensated for by collaterals so that the sudden thrombosis may be well tolerated.[5,23] This is far less likely to be true in the posterior two-thirds of the sinus, where acute thrombosis may give rise to an early marked increase in intracranial pressure with deterioration of the clinical state of the patient.[15,16]

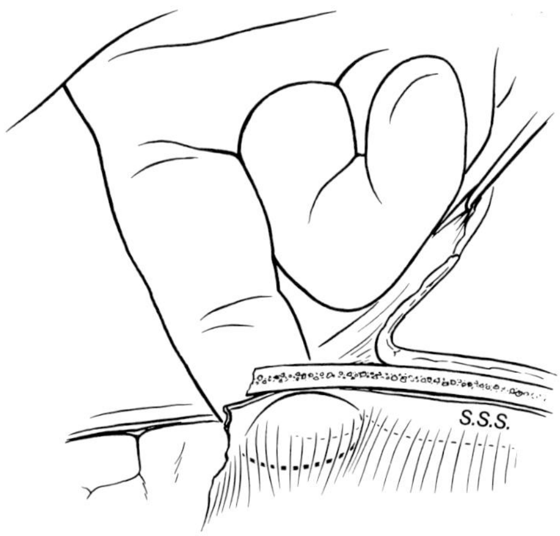

Fig. 12.5. Method of quickly controlling exsanguinating hemorrhage from superior sagittal or lateral sinus in case of partial avulsion.

If during the initial exploration, bleeding from the sinus is so profuse as to portend disaster unless it can be readily controlled, control may be quickly gained by simply enlarging any opening in the skull, either the opening from the initial injury or a burr hole placed lateral to the sinus. Rapidly increase the size to make an opening in the dura lateral to the sinus until a finger can be placed underneath the sinus and pressure exerted upward against the skull while an assistant does the same thing at the other extremity of the wound (Fig. 12.5). The bleeding is then brought under control in a very short period of time. Care must be exercised so that any bridging veins are not injured in this process; therefore the finger should not be inserted blindly except in the greatest emergency.

Loss of Sufficient Surface of the Sinus So That Simple Suturing Cannot Be Employed

Sinus wounds may be closed by elevating a piece of dura to form a patch or by fashioning a patch from some other material such as vein (Fig. 12.6). In the instance where there is extensive loss of the sinus, the situation can be brought under control rapidly by inserting a siliconized T tube into the remaining sinus and placing a ligature about the sinus to hold the T tube in place, both rostrally and caudally, thus reinstituting flow in the sinus immediately. Suctioning may take place through this tubing as it is inserted to remove any clot, and dilute heparin solution may be introduced from time to time through the T, which is brought out through the skin. If the patient's condition is critical, one may elect to wait several days before doing any actual sinus repair, and flow will be maintained through the tube during this period of time. A sinogram may be obtained at any time through the T of the tube. Restoring flow allows the surgeon time to plan a strategy so that the delicate surgery of sinus repair does not have to take place under suboptimal conditions[10] (Fig. 12.7).

Vein Graft

A section of vein removed from the lower extremity may be used to graft a sizable area of the sinus either as an on-surface graft, or, if the entire sinus has been sectioned and a portion lost, the vein may be implanted in its place. The vein has an advantage in that it is a venous structure and is lined by endothelium. It has the disadvantage of having valves within it, which either must be removed or the graft must be oriented in such a way that the flow of blood is not impaired by the valves. Another disadvantage is that since the wall of the vein graft is not stiff, it may well collapse when the patient is in certain positions, particularly in the erect position in the adult as pressure within the sinus falls. Bonnal and Brotchi[2] have suggested that vein collapse may be avoided by suturing the adventitia of the vein graft to the scalp or to superficial tissue to hold the vein open in this position.

Technique for Vein Grafting. If the patient is in excellent condition, reconstruction of the sinus may be done acutely. However, the patient's condition is usually precarious with an injury of a magnitude that totally destroys or removes the sinus for some distance (over 1–1.5 cm). It is probably best to reinstitute flow in the sinus via a T tube and then wait three or

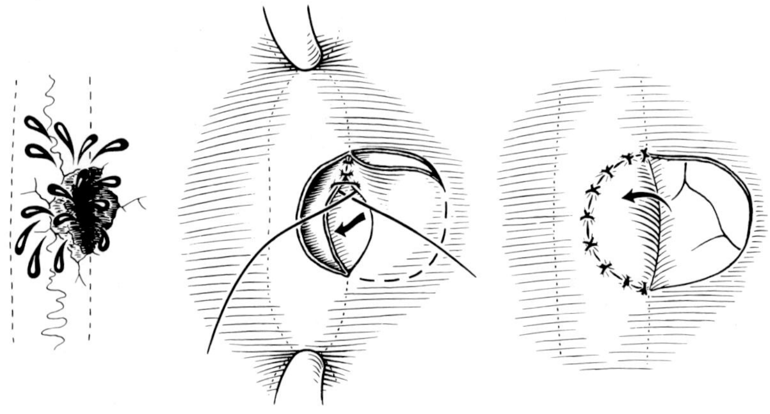

A B C

Fig. 12.6. **A.** Bleeding sinus; **B,** attachment of dural patch (note suture knots lie outside the sinus); **C,** attached dural patch.

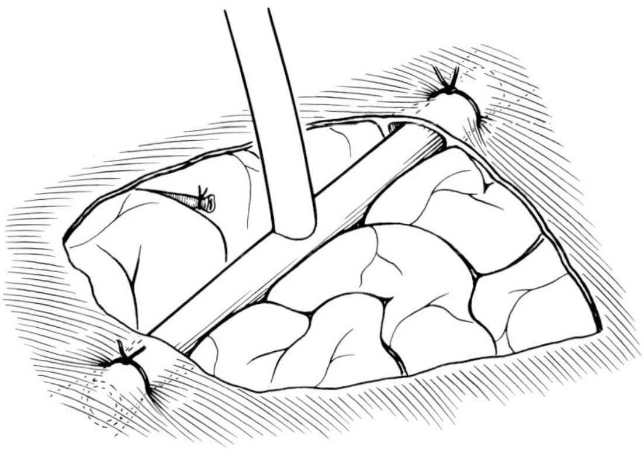

Fig. 12.7. A T tube in place in sinus.

four days before grafting. During this period of time one may plan a strategy and construct an appropriate graft.

The length of vein necessary for grafting should be determined at the time of initial surgery and of insertion of the T tube. Angiograms or sinograms obtained in preparation for grafting will acquaint one with the status of clot in the sinus and the status of the local cerebral veins. A length of vein somewhat longer than the sinus defect is removed from any upper or lower extremity together with any branch that matches any cerebral vein one is interested in repairing. The vein is thoroughly washed in heparinized saline and then either the valves are resected or the orientation of the vein is marked so that when it is substituted for the segment of sinus, blood will flow in the proper direction past the valves.[10,26]

When the sinus ends have been prepared for suture, the vein is distended with heparinized saline and closed lightly to hold the saline in place; the vein is then brought to the edge of the wound. The T of the tube is now cut out (Fig. 12.8). Suctioning of one end of the sinus through the sectioned tube is now done while the other tube is held closed (Fig. 12.9). Then the process is reversed so that clots visible on the angiograms or sinograms have been removed from both ends of the sinus. Both cut ends of the T tube are then removed from the sinus. The sinus is temporarily closed by clip or ligature at either end at this time, and each end of the vein graft is anastomosed end-to-end to the sinus with sutures (Fig. 12.10). As soon as this is completed, the sinus is opened. When it is clear that a good flow through the graft has been obtained, any cerebral vein that has been severed during trauma may be anastomosed to the branch of the vein graft. Anastomosis in a vessel of this size is stil unpredictable and should only be done if it will not prolong the operation unduly. The sinus should not be kept closed during this small vein anastomosis, as anastomosis can be done between gentle clips on the cerebral vein and on the graft branch after flow has been restored to the sinus.

The advantages of the vein graft method are the following:

1. There is an opportunity to plan the procedure while the T tube is in place.
2. The sinus has been replaced with a venous structure that is lined with its own intima.
3. Cerebral veins can be repaired simultaneously.
4. Flow may be checked by sinography immediately if it be deemed necessary.

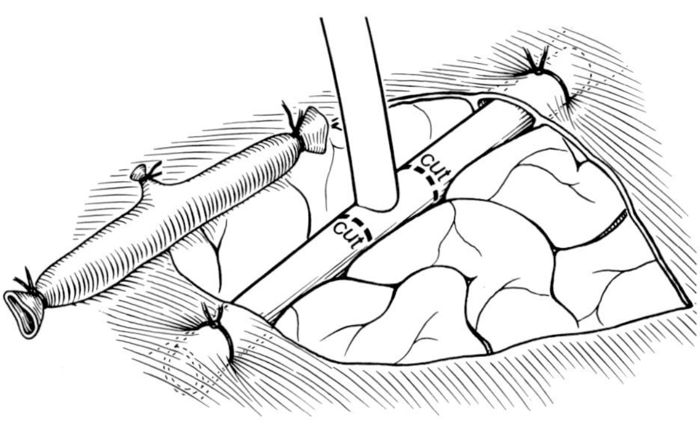

Fig. 12.8. Vein graft at edge of wound. T tube is cut as indicated.

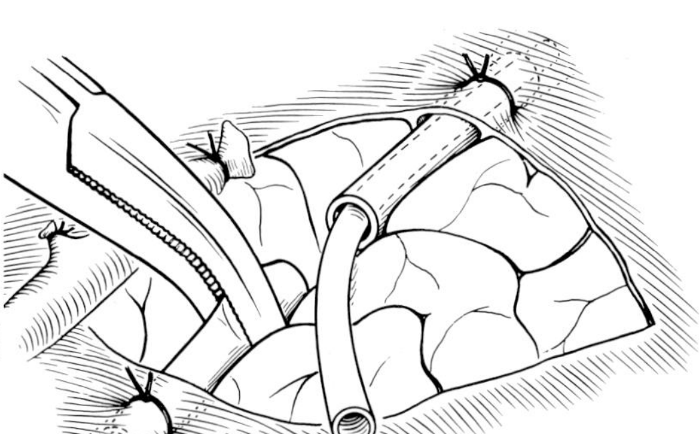

Fig. 12.9. Suctioning through cut T tube.

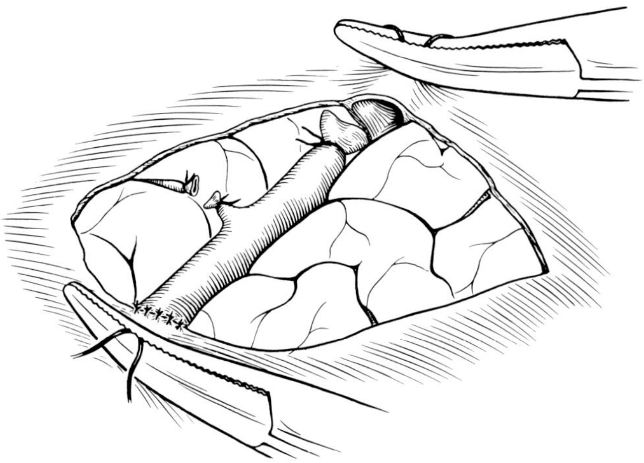

Fig. 12.10. One end of the graft has been sutured.

The disadvantages are

1. The presence of valves in the vein graft narrows the sinus somewhat whereas removal of the valves leaves areas denuded of intima.
2. The vein is thin walled rather than rigid like the sinus, and with reduced pressure in the sinus the graft may tend to collapse under certain conditions unless it is held open by sutures to the adventitia by the method of Bonnal and Brotchi.[2]
3. The double end-to-end anastomosis is time-consuming, and flow through the sinus must be interrupted during that period or carried over a temporary shunt during anastomosis.

Based on the observations of Sawyer et al,[45–47] who noted that a positive electrical charge on the intima of a blood vessel promoted clotting whereas a negative charge discouraged clotting; the experience of Mullan,[33] who utilized positive current to cause clotting in aneurysms; and the experience of Seymour Schwartz (personal communication), who used negative current in the walls of small anastomosed blood vessels to diminish clotting, the following technique has been employed in sinus repair by either vein graft or by the use of intimal-lined stents, as noted later in this chapter.

Following the insertion of either a venous sinus graft or an intima-lined stent, fine platinum wire is passed through the sinus at the suture lines or at either end of the stent or graft (Fig. 12.11). One wire is passed into the lumen of the graft near its midpoint. The platinum wires are insulated by threading them through small polyethylene tubes. The ends of the wires are placed around the negative terminal of a 9-V battery. A similarly insulated wire is passed from the positive terminal of the battery to the chest wall. The wire is soldered to a 25-cent piece, and this is placed on the chest with a suitable EEG gel or ointment between the 25-cent piece and the chest wall. The position of the 25-cent piece is changed daily to prevent skin reaction beneath it.

When all the wires have been connected, a negative current flows into the bloodstream, and a positive current develops on the chest wall for as long as the equipment is left in place (5–7 days). The wires are then cut and removed at the sinus by open incision.

Sindou et al[51] have presented an interesting and original idea—a bypass in cases where the sinus must be resected, as in invasion by tumor. They performed venous and arterial bypasses in dog using end-to-end anastomoses. They preferred vein as the bypass conduit, as arterial bypasses have sometimes lost patency because of continued fibrosis of the wall.

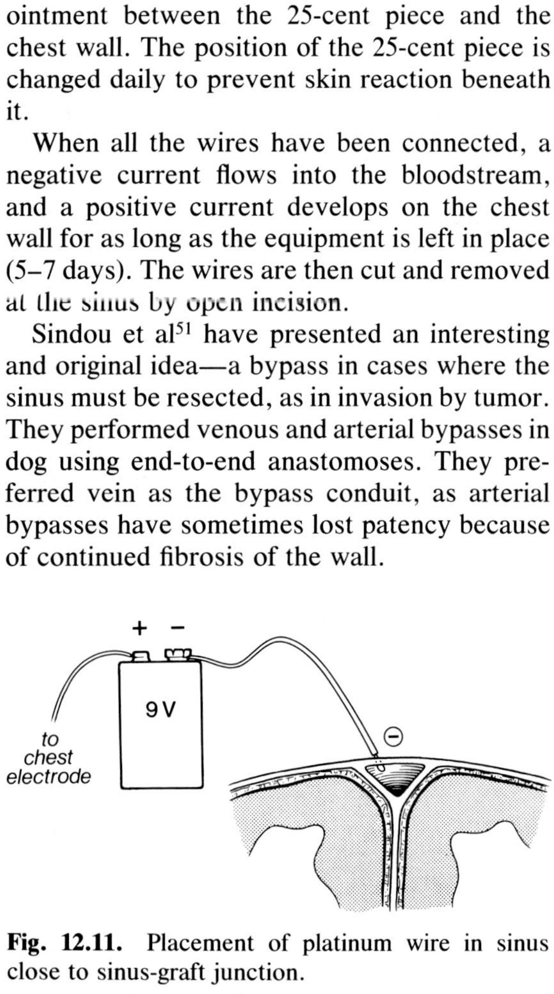

Fig. 12.11. Placement of platinum wire in sinus close to sinus-graft junction.

(NB: The occlusion time necessary in performing this type of bypass could be diminished by utilizing a temporary bypass as used by Kapp et al[24] at the expense of creating two small linear incisions in the sinus for the Sindou bypass. These incisions could be closed by simple sutures at the end of the operation.)

Intima-Lined Stent

An alternative form of sinus reconstruction is by use of an intima-lined stent.[10] In this procedure the T tube is introduced at the primary operation; the interim angiogram or sinogram is likewise done. At the time of secondary surgery a section of a siliconized T tube that is slightly longer than the defect in the sinus and of a circumference that would just fit within the sinus is cut. Small holes are made around the circumference of this tube.

A vein graft considerably longer than the cut tubing is now removed, and the valves are either removed or the orientation of the vein marked so that when inserted into the sinus, flow will readily pass the valves.

The vein segment is thoroughly washed inside and out with heparinized saline solution and then passed through the tubing. The vein ends are now folded back over the tube and held by a ligature at either end.

Fine silk sutures are now passed from hole to hole of the silicon tube and into the adventitia of the vein so that when tightened, the vein will be held open and will not collapse.[10]

When this stent has been prepared and flushed with heparinized saline, it is ready for introduction into the sinus. The T of the T tube is now removed, and the T tube transected as in the procedure for vein graft. Clots are suctioned from the sinus through the cut ends of the T tube. When brisk blood flow is obtained from each end of the sinus, the T tube segments are removed and the intima-lined stent is introduced—first into one end of the sinus and then into the other. It is held in place by single silk ligatures at either end placed circumferentially about the sinus and the stent. The advantages of this method are

1. Long gaps can be bridged.
2. The vein segment does not collapse.
3. Most important, blood flow is interrupted in the sinus for only two to five minutes.

The disadvantages are

1. The technique requires the sacrifice of an extremity vein.
2. A foreign body is introduced, but that body is not in contact with blood flow.

Postoperatively, flow may be checked by angiograms or sinograms. Some attempts also have been made to monitor flow with Doppler ultrasound techniques.[3,22]

Invasion of Sinus by Tumor

In those rare instances when the superior sagittal sinus is invaded by tumor, one may wish to resect only a portion of the sinus if the tumor does not occlude the entire sinus. Such a sinus may be repaired with a dural graft, or, in cases where the sinus is totally occluded, a vein graft or an intima-lined stent may be required. Either of these procedures, however, would be necessary only in those instances where flow through the superior sagittal sinus must be maintained. In addition, since the occlusion by tumor growth was gradual rather than acute as in trauma, an adequate collateral venous flow may already have developed, and the sinus may not be required at all. It is important, therefore, that the collateral venous flow and the necessity for patency in the sinus be established as clearly as possible by clinical signs, angiograms, and sinograms before surgery.[4,11,32]

The Inferior Longitudinal Sinus

The inferior longitudinal sinus is an unpaired sinus that lies in the free edge of the falx cerebri beginning at about the midpoint of the border of the falx and passing backward, gradually increasing in size, until it reaches the junction of the falx cerebri and the tentorium cerebelli, where it opens into the straight sinus. It receives small tributaries from the falx and sometimes also from the corups callosum.[17] Knowledge of sinus anatomy is important to the surgeon working in the area of the corpus callosum and tentorium, but the sinus can be occluded if the remainder of the venous anatomy is normal. No restorative surgery on the sinus has been reported. In those cases of a diminished superior sagittal sinus where the inferior sagittal sinus is very large, the inferior sagittal sinus would have to be treated as a superior sagittal sinus, but these cases are extremely rare. This author has never seen one.

The Straight Sinus

The straight sinus lies along the junction of the tentorium cerebelli and the falx cerebri. It is formed at the anterior border of the tentorium cerebelli by the junction of the inferior longitudinal sinus and the great cerebral vein (vein of Galen) and is directed backward to open into the torcular Herophili or commonly into the left lateral sinus. It receives in its course a number of small branches from the tentorium and branches from the posterior portion of the medial surface of the cerebral hemispheres and sometimes from one of the superior cerebellar veins. This sinus may be displaced or distorted or invaded by neoplasms in the region of the tentorium. Restoration or repair seems feasible under certain conditions, but no one has accumulated much experience in this area. A number of reports of successfully handling aneurysms of the great vein of Galen are readily available. There has been some difference of opinion as to whether or not the great vein or the straight sinus ordinarily may be sacrificed.[8,14,60] As far as trauma to the straight sinus is concerned, minor bleeding from the area will very likely arrest itself. An injury of a severity to cause major bleeding is very likely lethal. These have been poorly recognized in the past, however, and it may be that in the future, with better angiographic and scanning techniques, bleeding from this source may be picked up at a much earlier period and be successfully combatted.

The Occipital Sinus

This is an unpaired or occasionally paired sinus running from the torcular Herophili along the line of attachment of the falx cerebelli to the occipital bone and the posterior border of the foramen magnum. At the foramen magnum it divides into two trunks, which become the marginal sinuses that pass around the foramen magnum to eventually open into the superior bulb of the corresponding internal jugular vein.[41] Tributaries of the occipital sinus include branches from the falx cerebelli and local dura and veins from the inferior surface of the cerebellum. At the posterior border of the foramen magnum near its bifurcation into the marginal sinuses, it communicates with the posterior spinal plexus.

Deviations from the Anatomic Norm

The occipital sinus may occasionally be absent. Frequently it extends only as far as the posterior border of the foramen magnum, in which case the marginal sinuses are usually undeveloped. Also, occasionally at its upper end it may enter into either the right or left lateral sinus or into the straight sinus. Surgery on the occipital sinus has been performed mostly to arrest hemorrhage underneath a fracture at this point. Meningeal tumors may be found along its course, but these pose no unusual problem in this area unless they involve the torcular Herophili at the upper end of the sinus.

Occasionally on operating in the vicinity of the occipital sinus, particularly in children, large venous lakes are found in the bone just lateral to the sinus.[7] In these cases the sinus is likely to be quite limited in its formation, a situation that has caused some to consider the situation as one where the embryonal venous lakes have not completely joined in sinus formation. The surgical importance of the lake, of course, is the likelihood of hemorrhage. If one cannot tell from looking at the area whether a venous lake is present or not, it has been recommended that jugular compression be performed. This will distend the area if, indeed, it is a venous lake.[6] (One should be certain, however, that there is no contraindication to jugular compression in that particular instance since jugular compression in individuals with increased pressure within the posterior fossa would not be indicated unless the area is already well decompressed.)

Torcular Herophili and Transverse or Lateral Sinuses

The torcular Herophili (confluens sinuum) usually lies subjacent to the external occipital protuberance and is the meeting point of five different sinuses: the right transverse or lateral sinus, the left transverse or lateral sinus, the superior longitudinal sinus, the straight sinus, and the occipital sinus. Leading into the lateral sinus from above is the superior sagittal sinus and from in front, the straight sinus. Draining from the area laterally along the attachment of the tentorium cerebelli and over the squamous portions of the occipital bone are the lateral or transverse sinuses, one on the left and one on the right, each continuing on the inner surface of the temporal bone and the jugular process of the occipital bone to reach the jugular foramen, where the sinus opens into the internal jugular vein. As it leaves the point of attachment of the tentorium cerebelli, it passes downward and then inward to follow the line of junction between the petrous and mastoid portions of the temporal bone in a configuration suggesting the letter "S." For this reason this portion of the sinus has been called the sigmoid sinus.

Deviations from the Anatomic Norm

Variations in the configuration of the torcular area and the lateral sinuses are so common that they probably should not be considered as abnormalities but merely normal variations. The large number of these has led to investigation and a number of excellent summaries.[4,20,32,56] The lateral sinuses are frequently quite different in size. When this occurs, the right is usually but not always, the larger. The relative size often depends on venous flow into the region of the torcular. The superior longitudinal sinus most frequently empties into the right transverse sinus and the straight sinus most commonly into the left. Occasionally the right lateral sinus is practically the continuation of the superior longitudinal sinus and the left lateral a continuation of the straight sinus. There may or may not remain a small connecting channel as a vestigial torcular Herophili in those instances.

In a series of 100 autopsies, Rudinger found that the right lateral sinus was larger in 70, the left was larger in 27, and both were equal in size in 3. Occasionally the left lateral sinus was extremely small or even absent. This fact is of great surgical importance as thrombosis of the lateral sinus may be well tolerated if the other lateral sinus is widely open. If thrombosis occurs, however, in the one functioning sinus the patient may develop severe intracranial pressure very rapidly. Rarely the lateral sinus connects to the posterior auricular vein by an unusually large emissary vein. When this is found to be the case the sigmoid sinus is usually small. Occasionally the petrous squamosal sinus opens into the lateral sinus as it travels down and in on the mastoid portion of the temporal bone. Tributaries of the lateral sinuses include:

1. The superior sagittal sinus, the straight sinus, and a number of the posterior inferior cerebral veins, which pass from the temporal areas of the cerebral hemisphere.
2. The superior petrosal sinus, which communicates with the lateral sinus as it leaves the attachment of the tentorium cerebelli.

The sigmoid sinus receives the internal auditory vein, which exits from the internal auditory meatus. In addition, it receives a mastoid emissary vein and veins from the pons and medulla, which may enter beyond the inferior petrosal sinus into the region of the jugular bulb.

Surgery of the Lateral Sinuses

Trauma

The most highly emergent indication for surgery of this sinus would be, of course, a compounded wound with sinus tear and hemorrhage. Such a situation is usually apparent, and the hemorrhage must be stemmed by aseptic packing until the patient can be transferred to an operating facility, the fracture opening enlarged, and the sinus directly repaired or a T tube bypass inserted to provide a temporary sinus flow until a repair plan can be formulated.

Occasionally a much more subtle danger develops, that is, where a very narrow linear fracture has occurred over the lateral sinus, inducing a small tear in the posterior sinus wall so that the blood lodges between the bone and the sinus in sufficient quantities to compress the sinus. Whereas this may produce no problem or very little problem in an individual who has two equally functioning lateral sinuses, in that individual who has but one lateral sinus and that one on the side of the injury, the patient may worsen with explosive suddenness; in such an individual simple decompression of the area with control of the sinus would be a life-saving procedure.

Thrombosis

Surgery on the lateral sinus for removal of a thrombus has been quite common in the past because of the number of cases noted in mastoiditis. The introduction of antibiotic therapy and the use of anticoagulants has very greatly decreased the incidence of this complication. When it does occur, the situation usually will respond to antibiotics and sometimes to anticoagulation therapy, but when it occurs in a patient with an inadequate collateral drainage system, a surgical approach must be considered so that the patient may survive for a long enough period to allow his or her medical therapy to function. In those cases an approach directly to the sinus with removal of the thrombus and closure of the sinus walls, preserving an intact lumen, is indicated. If the condition of the patient permits, considerable knowledge may be gained from angiograms or sinograms before the surgery.

A rarity

The author has known of two cases of reversal of the direction of flow in the sagittal sinus. One of these was secondary to an AV malformation in the region of the torcular that obstructed both lateral sinuses to some degree. It had been in the surgical plan to run a venous graft from the superior sagittal sinus to a jugular vein since the patient was steadily worsening from increasing intracranial pressure. It is uncertain if this measure would have been helpful, but no other solution was apparent. Surgery was refused in this instance, and the patient succumbed to her problem within a relatively short time. One should be aware of this possibility, however, as it seems quite certain similar cases will be seen in the future.

If the surgery on the neck is being performed, particularly for a local malignancy and the internal jugular vein is involved, one should refrain from sacrificing the jugular vein if it is not certain that there is functioning internal jugular system on the opposite side. Therefore, it would appear that angiograms before surgery for a radical neck dissection should be considered.[13,54]

It has been suggested that x-ray films of the jugular foramina on both sides be taken in instances where it is thought necessary to know whether the patient has two good jugular operating systems, as in the congenital absence of a jugular system, one jugular foramen is likely to be much smaller than the other.[13] The use of such a noninvasive simple procedure has its appeal.

The Cavernous Sinus

This is a paired sinus lying along the sides of the body of the sphenoid bone from the sphenoidal fissure anteriorly to the apex of the petrous portion of the temporal bone posteriorly. It is approximatly 2 cm in length, with a diameter of 1 cm, and is roughly quadrilateral to triangular in shape on cross-section.[41] In the past it has been described as an area of dura, with arterial channels and free-flowing venous blood in the sinus surrounding the arterial channels. Some recent workers,[9,30,36–38,55] however, have described numerous venous channels that are separate from one another, although they communicate, surrounding the arterial components within the sinus. On cross-section, the appearance of the cavenous sinus is said to be not unlike that of the corpus cavernosum penis from which the sinus derives its name (given by Winslow)[55a]. Many structures lie within the sinus. The internal carotid artery and the abducens nerve travel in the sinus; in the outer wall from above the oculo motor nerve, the ophthalmic nerve and the maxillary divisions of the trigeminal nerve are included.[9,55]

At the level of the sphenoidal fissure the cavernous sinus receives the ophthalmic vein. A small venous channel passes from one cavernous sinus to the other in front of the sella and another posterior to it. These have been named the anterior intercavernous sinus and the posterior intercavernous sinus; the name circular sinus is sometimes seen referring to these two venous channels and to the area of the cavernous sinus, which connects them on either side.[22]

Besides these tributary vessels are emissary vessels, i.e., those leading blood away from the sinus. The superior petrosal sinus and the inferior petrosal sinus in which the cavernous sinus terminates are two of these. The superior petrosal sinus is the smaller of the two posterior branches into which the cavernous sinus drains. It passes outward and backward along the superior border of the petrous portion of the temporal bone and empties into the lateral sinus as this leaves the attachment of the tentorium cerebelli to become the sigmoid sinus. On its way it receives small tympanic veins and small branches from the cerebellum and the cerebrum. This sinus may be encountered in performing transtentorial procedures or in combined operations in the region of the internal acoustic meatus. It may be divided to provide improved visibility.

The inferior petrosal sinus is the larger terminal branch of the cavernous sinus and travels along the petro-occipital suture line to the jugular foramen where it opens into the jugular bulb or into the jugular vein. Tributaries of the inferior petrosal sinus include branches from the dura, branches from the medulla and pons, veins from the internal auditory meatus, and a vein communicating with a small plexus surrounding the hypoglossal nerve in the condyloid foramen and named an anterior condyloid vein.

Anteriorly the inferior petrosal sinus communicates with the basilar sinus or what is sometimes known as the basilar plexus, a vein or veins running on the clival portion of the occipital bone. The cavernous sinus, in addition, communicates with:

1. A plexus of veins—the carotid plexus—which invests the internal carotid artery through the carotid canal, where they communicate with the internal jugular vein.
2. Veins that accompany the mandibular division of the trigeminal nerve through the foramen ovale into the pterygoid plexus.
3. A vein that passes through the foramen of Vesalius when this foramen is present.
4. A vein that accompanies the maxillary division of the trigeminal nerve through the foramen rotundum into the veins of the pharynx and neck.

The sphenoparietal sinus, also known as the sinus alae parvae because of its position, arises at the outer extremity of the lesser wing of the sphenoid bone from the meningeal veins and then passes under the cover of the posterior border of the lesser wing of the sphenoid bone to reach the cavernous sinus near its anterior end. It receives tributaries from the dura and diploe. It is frequently encountered in meningiomas of this area.

Surgical Considerations

Acute Trauma

Acute intervention following direct trauma of the cavernous sinus is very infrequent. Usually direct injury will produce bleeding from the sinus that will either stop by itself or be fatal. In those rare instances where bleeding from the sinus is found when exploration is being carried out in the middle fossa in a case of trauma, the sinus may be repaired by sealing it with Gelfoam or by attaching a dural patch if the sinus cannot be sutured directly.

AV Communication

The most common indication for surgery of the cavernous sinus is that of the communication between the carotid artery and venous structures of the cavernous sinus, commonly known as the carotid-cavernous AV communication. Although there are, on record, cases of spontaneous sealing of AV communications, these are indeed rare, and, by far, the most common course of events is a gradual increasing proptosis of the ipsilateral eye with chemosis and swelling of the conjunctiva, local pain, and a bruit that is audible to patient and examiner. Such patients develop ophthalmoplegia and may go on to blindness in the affected eye.

Surgical Procedures

An early form of treatment was ligation of the ipsilateral carotid artery in the neck. There are advocates of occlusion of the ipsilateral internal carotid artery and advocates of ipsilateral ligation of the common carotid artery. The former was alleged to have had a higher incidence of complications such as hemiplegia, the latter a higher failure rate. Actually, both procedures have a high failure rate, and this procedure is rarely done at the present time.

Entrapment

In this procedure the leak from the carotid artery into the venous channels of the cavernous sinus is trapped by occluding the carotid artery in the neck and intracranially. When such entrapment is done, care should be taken to place the clip on the internal intracranial carotid artery proximal to the posterior communicating artery so that the posterior communicating artery may remain functional in supplying blood from the vertebral system to the middle cerebral system. Some have advocated attempting to place a clip proximal to the ophthalmic artery, but in an AV communication where there is marked pressure within the sinus, this is difficult and may not be possible. Some surgeons have preferred to occlude the carotid artery in the neck first, others intracranially first. More recently, individuals have been attracted to clipping the intracranial portion first because it has a lesser risk of embolism. Some surgeons have attempted gradual occlusion of the cervical portion by means of Selverstone or Crutchfield clamp. This does not eliminate risk, however, in that occasionally, following the application of the clamp, a clot may occur within the cervical vessel and an embolism may be sustained.

Although these procedures carry a definite risk of hemiplegia, particularly in older individuals, because they involve the sacrifice of a carotid artery, they are standard procedures with an outcome relatively favorable and have to be considered.

Embolization

Emboli of various types have been used in occluding the aperture from the artery into the vein. These have consisted of Gelfoam or muscle,[25,27,31,35] and, more recently, Serbinenko[48] and others have perfected small balloons that can be detached from their carriers once they have reached the site of pathologic communication.[40] Serbinenko's approach has been through the arterial system. Others have included a venous approach.[34,58] All of these procedures have a record of some success, but are formidable procedures none the less. More recently, a form of therapy considered has been the use of entrapment with carotid bypass utilizing an arterial or venous graft from the carotid artery in the neck to the carotid artery intracranially beyond the site of clipping.[26,28,49,57] This, again, is a complex procedure. It has a better chance of success than a similar bypass in cases of spontaneous occlusions in the elderly because most of the AV communications of this type are secondary to trauma in the young, and the parent blood vessel has a better wall than is likely to be true in the individual who suffers from atherosclerosis. Enough procedures have yet to be performed, however, so that a respectable success rate has been achieved. This has been due to technical factors, it is believed, i.e., tendency to thrombosis in venous grafts, tendency to contraction of arterial grafts, or necessity for sacrifice of an artery of some importance if an artery is chosen.

Recently Parkinson[37–39] has used the direct approach. This is a physiologic approach that includes performing a craniotomy, directly opening the sinus, and repairing the rent in the carotid artery under direct vision. It is a procedure, however, that to this date has required hypothermia and cardiac arrest, and, although Parkinson has achieved a laudable success record, it is not a procedure to be undertaken lightly by those without experience and without the utmost in sophisticated operating equipment and competent support teams.

Dr. Vinko Dolenc of Ljubljana, Yugoslavia has recently reported his experience on approaching A.V. communications in the cavernous sinus by using a slightly more lateral approach[9a]. He has been able to control arterial hemorrhage by temporarily clipping the internal carotid artery extradurally as it enters the skull and again intradurally either above or below the ophthalmic artery and has controlled venous hemorrhage in the sinus by compression. The major problem has been to avoid injury to branches of the nerves to the extraocular muscles and the divisions of the trigeminal nerves. This interesting technique is one more step toward control of this very difficult problem.

Lesions of the many other veins within the cranium have no special problems but share the problems of all other venous structures, and these will not be dealt with in this chapter.

References

1. Bedford THB: The effect of variations in the subarachnoid pressure on the venous pressure in the superior longitudinal sinus and in the torcular of the dog. J Physiol 101:362–368, 1942
2. Bonnal J, Brotchi J: Surgery of the superior sagittal sinus in parasagittal meningiomas. J Neurosurg 48:935–945, 1978
3. Brisman R, Hilal SK, Tenner M: Doppler ultrasound measurements of the superior sagittal sinus blood velocity. J Neurosurg 37:312–315, 1972

4. Browder J, Browder A, Kaplan HA: The venous sinuses of the cerebral dura mater. Arch Neurol 26:175–180, 1972
5. Browder J, Kaplan HA: Venous drainage following ablation or occlusive isolation of the rostral superior sagittal sinus. Surg Neurol 1:249–251, 1973
6. Browder J, Kaplan HA, Krieger AJ: Venous channels in the tentorium cerebelli: Surgical significance. Surg Neurol 3:37–39, 1975
7. Browder J, Kaplan HA, Krieger AJ: Venous lakes in the suboccipital dura mater and falx cerebri of infants: Surgical significance. Surg Neurol 4:53–55, 1975
8. Browder J, Kaplan HA, Krieger AJ: Anatomical features of the straight sinus and its tributaries. J Neurosurg 44:55–61, 1976
9. Day AL, Rhoton AL Jr: Aneurysms and arteriovenous fistulae of the intracavernous carotid artery and its branches. In Youmans JR (ed.): Neurological Surgery. WB Saunders, Philadelphia, 1982, pp 1764–1785
9a. Dolenc, V: Direct Microsurgical Repair of Intracavernous Vascular Lesions Journal of Neurosurgery 58:824–831, 1983
10. Donaghy RMP, Wallman LJ, Flanagan ME, Numoto M: Sagittal sinus repair. Technical note. J Neurosurg 38:244–248, 1973
11. Eades JW, Dugger GS: Carcinoma of the scalp treated by resection of the sagittal sinus. Arch Surg 93:507–510, 1966
12. Ekstedt J: CSF hydrodynamic studies in man. 2. Normal hydrodynamic variables related to CSF pressure and flow J Neurol Neurosurg Psychiatry 41:345–353, 1978
13. Fitz-Hugh GS, Robins RB, Craddock WD: Increased intracranial pressure complicating unilateral neck dissection. Laryngoscope 76:893–906, 1966
14. Hammock MK, Milhorat TH, Earle K, DiChiro G: Vein of Galen ligation in the primate. J Neurosurg 34:77–83, 1971
15. Kalbag RM, Woolf AL: Thrombosis and thrombophlebitis of cerebral veins and dural sinuses. In Winken PJ, Bruyn GW (eds.): Handbook of Clinical Neurology, Vol 12. North Holland Publishing Co, Amsterdam, 1972
16. Kaplan HA, Browder J: Atresia of the rostral superior sagittal sinus: substitute parasagittal venous channels. J Neurosurg 38:602–607, 1973
17. Kaplan HA, Browder J: Venous aneurysm of the inferior sagittal sinus. J Neurosurg 39:537–539, 1973
18. Kaplan HA, Browder J: Neurosurgical consideration of some features of the cerebral dural sinuses and their tributaries. In Congress of Neurological Surgeons: Clinical Neurosurgery. Williams & Wilkins, Baltimore, 1976, pp 155–169
19. Kaplan HA, Browder J, Howard EM, Browder A: Vascular spaces of the middorsal dura mater. Arch Pathol 97:173–177, 1974
20. Kaplan HA, Browder J, Knightly JJ, Rush BF Jr, Browder A: Variations of the cerebral dural sinuses at the torcular Herophili. Am J Surg 124:456–461, 1972
21. Kaplan HA, Browder J, Krieger AJ: Venous channels within the intracranial dural partitions. Radiology 115:641–645, 1975
22. Kaplan HA, Browder J, Krieger AJ: Intercavernous connections of the cavernous sinuses. J Neurosurg 45:166–168, 1976
23. Kapp JP, Alfred HC, Jones T: Isotope sinograms. Technical note. J Neurosurg 44:393–394, 1976
24. Kapp JP, Geilchimsky I, Deardourff SL: Operative techniques for management of lesions involving the dural venous sinuses. Surg Neurol 7:339–342, 1977
25. Krayenbühl H: Treatment of carotid-cavernous fistula consisting of one operation by muscle embolization of the fistulous carotid segment. In Donahgy RMP, Yasargil MG (eds.): Micro-Vascular Surgery. Georg Thieme Verlag, Stuttgart, 1967, pp 151–167
26. Lougheed WM, Marshall BM, Hunter M, Michel ER, Sandwith-Smyth H: Common carotid to intracranial internal carotid bypass venous graft: Technical note. J Neurosurg 34:114–118, 1971
27. Luessenhop AJ, Presper JH: Surgical embolization of cerebral arteriovenous malformations through internal carotid and vertebral arteries. Long-term results. J Neurosurg 42:443–451, 1975
28. Maroon J, Donaghy RMP: Experimental cerebral revascularization with autogenous grafts. J Neurosurg 38:172–179, 1973
29. Martins AN, Kobrine AI, Larsen DF: Pressure in the sagittal sinus during intracranial hypertension in man. J Neurosurg 40:603–608, 1974
30. McGrath P: The Cavernous sinus: An anatomical survey. Aust NZ J Surg 47:601–613, 1977
31. Mixter J: Personal communication, 1940
32. Morris L: Angiography of the superior sagittal and transverse sinuses. Br J Radiol 33:606–613, 1960
33. Mullan S: Experiences with surgical thrombosis of intracranial berry aneurysms and carotid cavernous fistulas. J Neurosurg 41:657–670, 1974
34. Mullan S: Treatment of carotid-cavernous fistulas by cavernous sinus occlusion. J Neurosurg 50:131–144, 1979
35. Ohta T, Nishimura S, Kikuchi H, Toyama M:

Closure of carotid-cavernous fistula with polyurethane foam embolus. Technical note. J Neurosurg 38:107–112, 1973
36. Parkinson D: Collateral circulation of cavernous carotid artery: Anatomy. Can J Surg 7:251–268, 1964
37. Parkinson D: A surgical approach to the cavernous portion of the carotid artery. Anatomical studies and case report. J Neurosurg 23:474–483, 1965
38. Parkinson D: Transcavernous repair of carotid cavernous fistula. Case report. J Neurosurg 26:420–424, 1967
39. Parkinson D: Carotid-cavernous fistula: direct repair with preservation of the carotid artery. Technical note. J Neurosurg 38:99–106, 1973
40. Picard L, Lepoire J, Montant J, Hepner H, Roland J, Guyonnaud JC, Jacob F, Andre JM: Endarterial occlusion of carotid-cavernous sinus fistulas using a balloon-tipped catheter. Neuroradiology 8:5-10, 1974
41. Piersal G (ed.): Human Anatomy. JB Lippincott, Philadelphia, 1923
42. Potts DG, Deonarine V: Effect of positional changes and jugular vein compression on the pressure graident across the arachnoid villi and granulations of the dog. J Neurosurg 38:722–728, 1973
43. Reilly HF Jr, Erbengi A, Sachs E, Dyke JR: Penetration of the sagittal sinus by a depressed skull fracture. Roentgenographic diagnosis in an asymptomatic boy. JAMA 202:841–842, 1967
44. Sabin FR: Origin and development of the primitive vessels of the chick and of the pig. Contrib Embryology 6:61–124, 1917
45. Sawyer PN, Pate JW: Bio-electric phenomena as an etiologic factor in intravascular thrombosis. Am J Physiol 175:103–107, 1953
46. Sawyer PN, Pate JW: Electric potential differences across the normal aorta and aortic grafts of dogs. Am J Physiol 175:113–117, 1953
47. Sawyer PN, Pate JW, Weldon CS: Relations of abnormal and injury electric potential differences to intravascular thrombosis. Am J Physiol 175:108–112, 1953
47a. Schwartz S, Personal communication, 1962.
48. Serbinenko FA: Balloon catheterization and occlusion of major cerebral vessels. J Neurosurg 41:125–145, 1974
49. Shields C: Autogenous artery and vein grafts in common carotid-supraclinoid carotid anastomoses. J Microsurg 1:114–119, 1974
50. Shulman K, Ransohoff J: Sagittal sinus venous pressure in hydrocephalus. J Neurosurg 23:169–173, 1965
51. Sindou M, Mazoyer J-F, Fischer G, Pialat J, Fourcade C: Experimental bypass for sagittal sinus repair. J Neurosurg 44:325–330, 1976
52. Streeter GL: The development of the venous sinuses of the dura mater in the human embryo. Am J Anat 18:145–178, 1915
53. Streeter GL: The development of alterations in the vascular system of the brain of the human embryo. Contrib Embryology 7:5–38, 1918
54. Troupp H, Tarkkanen J: Continuous recording of the sigmoid sinus pressure after radical neck dissection. J Laryngol Otol 82:1013–1016, 1968
55. Umansky F, Nathan H: The lateral wall of the cavernous sinus. With special reference to the nerves related to it. J Neurosurg 56:228–234, 1982
55a. Winslow: Human anatomy, George A. Peirsol Ed, 86h Edition p. 872. J.B. Lippincott Co, Philadelphia/London 1923
56. Woodhall B: Variations of the cranial venous sinuses in the region of the torcular Herophili. Arch Surg 33:297–314, 1936
57. Woringer E, Kunlin J: Anastomose entre la carotide primitive et la carotide intra-cranienne ou la sylvienne par greffon selon la technique de la suture suspendue. Neurochirurgia 9:181–188, 1963
58. Wright S, Donahgy RMP, Unpublished case.
59. Yada K, Nakagawa Y, Tsuru M: Circulatory disturbance of the venous system during experimental intracranial hypertension. J Neurosurg 39:723–729, 1973
60. Yasargil MG: Microsurgery Applied to Neurosurgery George Thieme Verlag, Stuttgart, 1969

Index to Volume I–IV

Abdominal aorta, and IVC, separation of, 291
Abscess
  epidural, 321
  intracerebral, 321
Accelerators, linear, 1163
Acetylsalicylic acid (ASA), *see* Aspirin
Acidosis, brain tissue, CBF in, 79–80
Acromegaly, 598
Activated partial thromboplastin time test (APTT), 97
Acute infantile hemiplegia (AIH), Moyamoya disease and, 569–570
Acute stroke, 404–405
Acute stroke patient
  hemispheric CBF values in, 196
  regional CBF values in, 196–197
Adhesive
  cyanoacrylate, characteristics and toxicity of, 503–505
  plastic, *see* Plastic adhesive
  tissue, 503–515
ADP (Adenosine diphosphate), platelet aggregation and, 91
Adson cerebellar retractor, 258
Age, risk of stroke and, 360
Age distribution, multiple aneurysms and, 983–984
Air embolism, during surgery, 223
AITIA study, 370
Albin's monitoring retractor, 259
Alcohol intoxication, and risk of aneurysmal hemorrhage, 1062
Alligator applier, 257
Alpha type clips, 1001–1002
  force exerted by, equation for, 1023–1024
Alpha-adrenergic blocking agents, for CVS, 778
Amaurosis fugax, 139, 162
  DIVA for, 351
Amines, sympathomimetic, for CVS, 777–778
Aminophylline, for CVS, 765, 779
Amnesia
  psychologic, 534
  transient global, 534
Amorphosynthesis, 162
Amyloid angiopathy, 598
Amyloidosis, 98
Anastomosis
  of diseased artery, 388
  lymph vessel, 388–389
  of normal artery, 387–388
  STA-MCA, 294–295
  technique of
    in end-to-end, 288
    in end-to-end vein, 290
    in end-to-side, 288, 290
  vascular, technique of, 386–389
Anatomy
  of ACA aneurysms, 881–882
  of AComA aneurysms, 881–882
  of aneurysm sites, 617–625
  of carotid-ophthalmic aneurysm, 808–816
  microsurgical, of intracranial aneurysm, 607–663
  of saccular aneurysm, 607–617
  surgical
    of carotid-ophthalmic aneurysm, 816
    of MCA aneurysm, 861–862
  vascular
    of cerebral hemispheres, 11–46
    of posterior fossa, 49–73
  vertebrobasilar, *see* Vertebrobasilar anatomy
Anesthesia
  for balloon catheterization, 1248
  for carotid endarterectomy, 408–409
  for frontotemporal approach to basilar aneurysm, 928
  for intracranial surgery, 847
  for MCA aneurysms, 863–864
    induction of, 863–864
    maintenance of, 864
    preoperative medication prior to, 863
  for neurovascular surgery, 122, 213–228
Anesthetic technique, in EC-IC bypass surgery, 473

Aneurysm, *see also specific types* eg Carotid-ophthalmic aneurysm
 angiography of, special projection for, 713–714, 717
 of anterior circulation, carotid ligation for, 785–801
 asymptomatic, management of, 983–994
 atherosclerotic, 738
 bacterial, *see* Bacterial aneurysm
 berry, congenital, 679–682
 bifurcation, anatomic considerations of, 842
 bulbous, surgery for, 827–828, 831, 834–835
 as cause of SAH, in children, 943
 cerebral, *see* Cerebral aneurysm
 and circle of Willis, 617, 625, 629
 circulation, *see* Circulation aneurysm, posterior
 direct visualization of, 700–701
 dissecting, 743
 extravasation of contrast medium from, 725, 727
 false, 738, 743
 giant, *see* Giant aneurysm
 "global", 816
 incidental, diagnosis of, 756
 infectious, 737–738, 1047–1059
 intracranial, *see* Intracranial aneurysm
 late morbidity after, 676–677
 late mortality after, 677
 Moyamoya disease and, 565
 multiple, *see* Multiple aneurysm
 multiplicity of, 984
 mycotic, 585
  in children, 953–954
 plastic adhesive treatment of, 505–508
 plastic monomers and, 599–600
 pyogenic, 737–738
 rebleeding of
  in first six months, 669–671
  after six months, 671
 ruptured
  angiographic identification of, 722–730
   accuracy of, 733
  arteriography for, 987
  carotid-cavernous fistula due to, 735
   case histories, 975–976
  clip placement and, 936–937
  complications of, 733–735
  CT scanning of, 986–987
  electrocephalogram of, 986
  electrothrombosis for, 979–980
  ischemia due to, 733
  natural history of, 987–988
  patterns of cisternal blood in, 694
  predicting site of, 694
  space occupying lesion due to, 735
  treatment of, 989
  vasospasm as complication of, 707
  ventricular dilatation after, 729–730, 735
 saccular, *see* Saccular aneurysm
 with SAH, in children, 949, 951–954
 sites of
  anatomy of, 617–625
  rate of rebleeding at, 673–674
 size of, 674–675
 traumatic, 738–743
  in children, 953
  of carotid artery, 792
 unruptured
  natural history of, 988–989
  nonsurgical treatment of, 989
  surgical treatment of, 989–990
Aneurysm surgery, *see* Surgery
Aneurysmal subarachnoid hemorrhage, *see* subarachnoid hemorrhage (SAH), aneurysmal
Angiitis, 581
 granulomatous, 594
Angina pectoris, preoperative considerations, 118–119
Angioendotheliosis, 599
Angiography, *see also specific types*
 of AICA, 63
 of anterior spinal artery, 59
 of AVM, 1102, 1121–1122
 of bacterial endocarditis, 1052–1053
 of basilar artery, 59, 61, 63
 carotid, 717, 722
 of carotid-ophthalmic aneurysm, 821–822
 cerebral, *see* Cerebral angiography
 of CVS, 775–776, 845
 of cerebrovascular disease, 297–303
 complications of, 303–306
 after EC-IC bypass surgery, 479
 and identification of ruptured aneurysm, 722–730
 intraoperative, for electrothrombosis, 971–973
 of IVV, 69
 of LMV, 69
 of Moyamoya disease, 562–565
  operative treatment of, 573–575
 of PCV, 68
 of PICA, 55–59
 of PMV, 68
 posterior circulation, for multiple aneurysms, 985
 of posterior fossa, 49–55
 of SCA, 63–68
 of SCV, 69
 in stereotactic surgery, 902
 of vein of Galen, 68–69
 of venous angiomas, 1141–1145
 vertebral
  of carotid cavernous fistula, 1233–1235
  of cerebellar infarction, 1306
 of vertebral artery, 55
Angioma, *see also individual types*; Arteriovenous malformations (AVM)
 classification and descriptions of, 1073–1088
 "cryptic", 1088–1089
 gliomas and, 1091
 growth of, 1091–1092
 introduction, 1073
 location of, 1090–1091
 multiple, 1090
 natural history of, 1091–1093
 pathology of, 1073–1093
 prevalence of, 1089–1090
 rupture of, 1092
 and saccular aneurysms, 1091
 scalp cirsoid, case histories, 973–975
 spontaneous thrombosis of, 1093
 transitional forms of, 1085, 1088
 venous, *see* Venous angioma
Angioma steal, 1092–1093
Angiopathy, amyloid, 598
Angular gyrus artery, 23–24

Animals, in microvascular neurosurgery, 284
Anosognosia, 162
Anterior cerebral artery (ACA), 17, 19, 28–29
  aneurysm of, 609, 611
  AVM involving, embolization of, 1152–1154
  cortical branches of, 19
  horizontal segment of, 30–31
  microsurgical anatomy of, 629–631
  recurrent branch of, 641–644
Anterior cerebral artery aneurysm, 879–895
  anatomy of, 881–882
  distal, CT scanning of, 699
  results of surgery for, 892–893
    problems affecting, 893–895
  surgical approach to, 885
  surgical techniques for, 885–892
Anterior cerebral artery syndrome, 163–164
Anterior cerebral-anterior communicating aneurysm, 633, 639
Anterior cerebral-anterior communicating-recurrent artery complex, 625–645
Anterior choroidal artery, 14, 33
  microsurgical anatomy of, 622–625
  organs supplied by, 625
Anterior choroidal artery aneurysm, anatomic considerations of, 841–842
Anterior choroidal artery syndrome, 163
Anterior communicating artery (AComA)
  angiographic definition of, 639
  anomalies of, 641
  approach to, 639–641
  basal perforating branches of, 644–645
  microsurgical anatomy of, 629–631
Anterior communicating artery aneurysm
  anatomy of, 881–882
  angiography of, 713–714
  carotid ligation of, 791–792
  CT scanning of, 694, 699
  diagnosis of, 883–884
  incidence of, 881
  after ligation, 798–799
    anatomic changes, 799
  long term outcome after, 671–677
  short term outcome after, 669–671
  surgical approach to, 884–885
  surgical management of, 884
  surgical results in, 892–893
    problems affecting, 893–895
  surgical techniques in, 885–892
Anterior inferior cerebellar artery (AICA), 61–63
Anterior inferior cerebellar artery syndrome, 167–168
Antiarrhythmic therapy, 120
Anticoagulant therapy
  in cardiogenic cerebral embolus, 371–372
  in completed stroke, 371
  and coagulation system, 367–368
  and fibrinolysins, 390–391
  major groups of, 367–368
  in progressing stroke, 370–371
  side effects of, 368
  for TIA, 369–370
Anticubital vein, contrast injection into, 345
Antidiuretic hormone, syndrome of inappropriate release of and aneurysms, 893–894
Antifibrinolytic therapy, for SAH, 761–763
  mechanism of action, 762
Antihypertension therapy, 120–122
Antiplatelet therapy
  and arachidonic acid cascade, 368–369
  in cardiogenic cerebral embolus, 372
  in completed stroke, 371
  in progressing stroke, 371
  for TIA, 370
Antithrombin, 99–100
Antithrombotic therapy
  in asymptomatic patients, 369
  general considerations, 367–369
  in ischemic cerebrovascular disease, 359–374
  specific indications for, 369–372
  summary of recommendations, 372–374
Anti-VIII:C antibody, 100
Anton's syndome, 169
Aorta, coarctation of, SAH and, 1062–1063
Aortic arch
  occlusive disease of, 429–444
  study of, in extracranial vascular disease, 297–298
  visualization of, 301
Aortic arch syndrome, 592
Apophyseal osteoarthrosis, 530
Aprotinin, for carotid-ophthalmic aneurysm, 823
Aquamephyton (vitamin K), 105
Arachidonic acid, platelet aggregation and, 92
Arachidonic acid cascade, antiplatelet drugs and, 368–369
Arachnoiditis, ascending, 599
Archimedes's law, 1019
Aron Alpha A Sankyo, 504
Arrhythmia
  cerebral embolus and, 366
  preoperative considerations, 120
Arteria termatica of Wilder, 641
Arterial angiography, 470
Arterial blood gas levels, in carotid endarterectomy, 409
Arterial embolectomy, 391–393
Arterial lesions, and EC-IC bypass surgery, 471–472
Arterial structures, DIVA visualization of, 347
Arteriography, 401–404
  bilateral carotid, for multiple aneurysms, 985
  cerebral, in carotid ligation, 789–790
  for ruptured aneurysms, 987
  transbrachial retrograde, 538
Arterionecrosis, plasmatic, and microaneurysms, 1261
Arteriosclerotic disease, preoperative considerations, 117–118
Arteriotomy, technique of, 286
Arteriovenous malformations (AVM)
  blood supply of, 1099
  as cause of SAH, in children, 943
  and cerebellar hematomas, 1284
  cerebral
    embolization of, 1151–1160, *see also* Embolization
    introduction, 1151
    radiosurgery for, 1161–1211, *see also* Radiosurgery

Arteriovenous malformations (AVM) (*cont.*)
  in children, 954–962
    diagnosis of, 955
    natural history of, 954–955
    treatment of, 958–961
      results of, 961–962
  deep-seated, case histories, 977, 979
  description of, 1073–1079
  dural, 1128–1133
    anatomic considerations in, 1130–1131
    pathophysiology of, 1131
    symptoms of, 1132
    treatment of, 1132–1133
  histologic evaluation of, 1099
  infratentorial, 1117–1134
    incidence of, 1119–1120
    introduction, 1117
    pathology of, 1117–1119
    results of, 1133–1134
  intracranial, embolization of, 1152–1159
  obliteration of, by radiation, 1209, 1211
  plastic adhesive treatment of, 508–511
  and pontine hematomas, 1290
  spinal cord, 1217–1228
    clinical diagnosis of, 1219–1222
    incidence of, 1218
    introduction, 1217
    microsurgical technique for excision of, 1226–1228
    pathogenesis of, 1218–1219
    radiologic diagnosis of, 1222–1223
    surgical treatment and results of, 1223–1226
    terminology and classification of, 1217–1218
  superficial large, 976
  supratentorial, 1097–1113
    anatomic considerations in, 1097, 1099
    diagnosis of, 1102
    introduction, 1097
    natural history of, 1099, 1101–1102
    treatment of, 1102–1113
Arteritis
  acute necrotizing, 585–586
  carotid, 585–586
  cerebral, 581–601
  cranial, neuroradiology in, 321–322
  definition of, 581
  diagnosis of, 582
  drug, 600–601
  giant-cell, 592–593
  hypertensive fibrinoid, 597
  infectious, 583–587
  Takayasu's, 333
  temporal, 592–593
Artery(ies)
  anatomic correlation of, 581–582
  angiographic correlation of, 582
  bacterial and fungal infection of, 583–587
  clinical correlation of, 582–583
  diseased, anastomosis of, 388
  normal, 387–388
  physical damage to, 367
Arthritis, rheumatoid, 593
Ascending arachnoiditis, 599
Aspergillus, and fungal intracranial aneurysm, 1059
Aspirin, 368–369
  platelet disorders and, 94
  after STA bypass, 476
Asymptomatic aneurysm, management of, 983–994
Asymptomatic bruit, DIVA for, 351
Asymptomatic lesions, management of, 408
Ataxia, 138–139
  homolateral, 171
Ataxic hemiparesis, 171
Ataxic hemiparesis syndrome, lacunes and, 366
Ateriosclerotic vascular disease, extracranial, as contraindication for ligation, 793
Atherogenesis, hypotheses of, 361
Atheroma, in carotid arteries, 399
Atheromatous debris embolus, 363–364
Atherosclerosis, 361–362
  in carotid arteries, 399–400
  complicated plaque in, 361
  fibrous plaque in, 361
  general management of, 394
  segmental tertiary, 596
  stages of, 361
Atherosclerotic aneurysm, 738
Atherosclerotic cerebrovascular disease, 306–314
Atherosclerotic index, 362
Atherosclerotic occlusive disease, Moyamoya disease and, 568–569
Atherosclerotic plaque, 297
Atom, 1162
Atrial myxoma, 151, 366
Atrial vein, medial, 45
Audio-visual equipment, 276–277
Auditory loss, vascular insufficiency and, 534
Auscultation, for bruits, 153–156
Autoimmune diseases, SAH and, 1065
Axillo-axillary bypass graft, in subclavian steal, 448
Axillo-axillary bypass, in subclavian steal, 448

Bacterial aneurysm
  associated with meningitis, 1055
  of internal carotid artery, with cavernous sinus thrombophlebitis, 1055
Bacterial endocarditis
  angiography for, 1052–1053
  cerebral ischemia and, 1052
  CT scanning for, 1052
  intracranial aneurysm associated with, 1047–1055
  SAH and, 1052
  subacute, 150–151
Bacteriology, of aneurysms associated with endocarditis, 1048
Balint's syndome, 169
Ball dissectors, 284
Balloon,
  detachable
    Becton-Dickinson, 1247–1248
    Debrun's latex, 1240–1245
    Heyer-Schulte, 1248
    Taki's, 1248
  detachment of, 1251
  iodine-filled, 1243–1244
  penetration of cavernous sinus with, 1250–1251
  silicon-filled, 1244–1245
Balloon catheter, *see also* Catheter
  introducer of, 1245–1246
  type 1, 1240
  type 2, 1243
Balloon catheterization, *see also* Catheterization
  anesthesia for, 1248

- of AVM, 1107
- of carotid cavernous fistula
  - through internal carotid artery, 1237, 1240
  - through ophthalmic vein, 1236–1237
- radiologic equipment for, 1248–1250

Barbiturates, in carotid endarterectomy, 408–409
Basal ganglia, 29–33
- nuclei of, 29–30
- vascular supply to, 30–33
- venous drainage from, 41, 44

Basal vein, 44
Basilar artery, 59, 61, 63
- microsurgical anatomy of, 647
- transclivial approach to, in cat, 292
- upper
  - anomalies of, 645, 647
  - and circle of Willis, 645–657
  - bifurcation of, 647
  - neural relationships of, 647

Basilar artery aneurysm, 611–617
- angiography of, 714
- common sites of, 611, 617
- CT scanning of, 694
- detection of, 694
- frontotemporal approach to, 925–938
  - anesthetic considerations in, 928
  - applications and contra-indications, 926–928
  - clip reapplication in, 937–938
  - inadequate exposure, 935–936
  - intraoperative complications in, 935–938
  - patient positioning in, 928–929
  - results of, 938
  - rupture in, 936–937
  - surgical technique in, 929–935
- pterional exposure of, 926–927
- transclivial approach to, 911
- vertebral artery ligation of, 910–911

Basilar artery syndrome, 166–167
Basilar branch syndrome, 167–170
Battered child syndrome, and SAH, 943
Bayonet clip of Sugita, for aneurysm surgery, 912
Bayonet forceps, 248
Becton-Dickinson balloon, 1247–1248
Behcet's disease, 595
Bench surgery, 389
Benedict's syndrome, 169
Bernard-Soulier syndrome, 93
Berry aneurysm, congenital, 679–682
Betatron, 1164
Bifurcation aneurysm, anatomic considerations of, 842
Binocular diploscope, 241
Binocular head assembly, of operating microscope, 236
Binocular prism, of operating microscope, 236–237
Biobond (EDH-adhesive), 505
Biocompatibility, of vascular clips, 1028
- laboratory evidence of, 1029–1030

Biologic factors, of clip-function dynamics, 1006–1014
Bipolar cautery, for aneurysm surgery, 912
Bipolar coagulating forceps, 281
Birth trauma, as cause of SAH, 942–943
Blades, separation of, affecting clip closing force, 1019
Blalock-Taussig procedure, 445
Bleeding
- mechanism of, in hypertensive intracerebral hemorrhage, 1261
- surgical, treatment of, 106–108

Bleeding time, 93–94
Blood
- cisternal, in ruptured aneurysm, 694
- dextran and, 391

Blood clotting factors, 95
Blood coagulation mechanism, 94–102
Blood dyscrasias, as cause of SAH, in children, 944
Blood gas levels, arterial, in carotid endarterectomy, 409
Blood pressure
- control of, in SAH, 761
- multiple aneurysms and, 984
- systemic, in carotid endarterectomy, 409

Blood supply
- of AVM, 1099
- of visual system, 156–157

Blood vessel
- depth of insertion of, affecting clip closing force, 1015, 1019
- radiation pathology of, 1166–1167
- radiobiology of, 1165–1167

Blood vessel clamps, 390
Blood vessel graft, infected, 393
Blood viscosity, 89
Blurring, bilateral, vascular insufficiency and, 535
Bonnet's syndrome, 170
Bony erosion, local, x-ray of, 686, 690
Botterell classification, of SAH, 757
Brachial angiography, retrograde, 51
Brachial-basilar insufficiency syndrome, *see* Subclavian steal syndrome
Bragg peak, 1165
Brain
- anterior circulation to, 161–165
- central region of, 21–22
  - external surface of, 21–22
  - internal surface of, 22
- deep areas of, 27–36
- frontal region of, 15–21
- occipital region of, 24–25
  - external surface of, 24
  - inferior aspect of, 24–25
  - internal surface of, 24
- parietal region of, 22–24
  - external surface of, 23–24
  - internal surface of, 24
- posterior circulation to, 165–170
- rate of blood flow to, 486
- sinuses of, 38–39
- temporal region of, 25–27
  - external surface of, 25–26
  - inferior aspect of, 26–27
  - superior surface of, 27
- vascular topography of, 14–36
- veins of, 36–46
- venous angiomas of, 1139–1148

Brain stem, malformations of, 1120–1128
- clinical syndromes of, 1120–1121
- diagnostic tests for, 1121–1122
- natural history of, 1120
- treatment of, 1126–1128

Brain tissue acidosis, CBF in, 79–80

Brain-volume reduction, in neurovascular surgery, 218–219
Bretylium tosylate (Bretylol), 123
Bridge graft, interposition, with shunt, 290–291
"Bright" plaques, 401
Bruit
  asymptomatic, DIVA for, 351
  auscultation for, 153–156
  craniocervical, 155
  diastolic, 155
  orbital, 155
  subclavian, 154
  systolic, 155
  vertebral artery, 154
Bruit analysis, 183–184
B-scanner device, 183
Bucrylate, embolization of cavernous sinus with, 1247
Bulbous aneurysm, surgery for, 827–828, 831, 834–835
Bypass graft, for occlusive disease, 434–442

Calcarine artery, 24–25
Calcification, intracranial, x-ray of, 690
Calcium, in extracranial vascular disease, 306
Calcium (Factor IV), 95
Candelabra artery, 16
Capillary angioma
  description of, 1081, 1085
  SAH and, 1063
Carbon dioxide, effect on CBF, 77–78
Cardiac arrhythmias, 151
Cardiac auscultation, 153–154
Cardiac complications, after carotid endarterectomy, 420
Cardiac disease
  risk of stroke and, 360
  valvular, cerebral embolus and, 366
Cardiac function, effect of CNS pathology on, 124–125
Cardiac output, suboptimal DIVA studies and, 349
Cardiogenic cerebral embolus
  anticoagulants in, 371–372
  antiplatelet drugs in, 372
Cardiovascular consideration, during surgery 117–125
Cardiovascular instability, during surgery, 222–223
Caroticotympanic artery, 12–13
Carotid angiography, 717, 722
  anteroposterior views for, 713
  external, 717, 722
Carotid arteritis, 585–586
Carotid artery
  adjacent infection and, 586
  adventitial stripping of, 285–286
  atheroma in, 399
  atherosclerotic lesions in, 399–400
  cavernous, 13
  cross compression of, 717
  exposing, 285
  internal, 11–14, *see also* Internal carotid artery
  occlusive disease of, 429–444
  traumatic aneurysm of, ligation for, 792
  visualization of, 301
Carotid artery aneurysm
  giant, ligation for, 791
  ruptured internal, 790–791
Carotid artery disease
  direct tests for, 182–185
  indirect tests for, 185–188
  noninvasive studies of, 181–190
    indications for, 189–190
Carotid bruit, 154
Carotid-cavernous AV communications, of cavernous sinus, 1321
Carotid cavernous fistula (CCF)
  case histories, 975–976
  etiology of, 1229–1232
  introduction, 1229
  plastic adhesive treatment of, 511–512
  radiologic evaluation of, 1233–1235
  due to ruptured aneurysm, 735
  spontaneous, 1229–1230
    clinical presentation of, 1232–1233
    treatment of, 1252–1253
  traumatic, 1229
    clinical presentation of, 1232
    results of treatment of, 1251–1252
    treatment of, 1235–1251
  treatment of, 1229–1253
Carotid endarterectomy, 399–421
  angiographic indications for, 406–408
  barbiturates and, 408–409
  clinical indications for, 404–406
  complications after
    local, 420
    neurovascular, 420–421
  and coronary artery disease, 118
  EEG during, 417–418
  halothane and, 409
  healing after, 420
  intraoperative monitoring, 417–419
  patient selection for, 404–408
  physiologic and anesthetic consideration in, 408–409
  plaque removal in, 413
  postoperative considerations, 419–421
  regional anesthesia for, 408
  regional CBF during, 419
  stump pressure measurements during, 418–419
  surgical technique, 410–417
  systemic complications after, 420
  use of shunt in, 413
  vein patch graft in, 417
Carotid lesions, in TIA, 400–401
Carotid ligation
  for aneurysms of anterior circulation, 785–801
    choice of vessel, 795–796
    clinical improvement after, 800
    contraindications for, 792–793
    favorable anatomic changes after, 799
    historical aspects, 785–787
    indications for, 790–792
    management of complications of, 797–798
    Matas test in, 794
    physiologic studies, 787–790
    postoperative closure of occlusive clamp in, 795–796
    pressure measurements at surgery, 800
    results of, 798–799
    surgical procedure in, 794–795
    technique of, 794–797
    timing of surgery, 793–794
  for AVM, 1103
  for carotid cavernous fistula, 1235
  for internal carotid aneurysms, 857
    technique of, 858

at neck, for carotid-ophthalmic aneurysm, 825–826
Carotid occlusive disease
diagnosis of, 401
internal, 407–408
pathophysiology of, 399–401
Carotid-ophthalmic aneurysm, 609, 805–836
age of onset of, 806
anatomy of, 808–816
general points, 808–809
surgical, 809–816
first form, 809
second form, 809
third form, 816
fourth form, 816
clinical features of, 816–819
giant, surgery for, 827–828
incidence of, 805
laterochiasmal, with superior development, 818
management and results of, 822–828
and multiple aneurysm, 823–824
origins of, 807
preoperative care for, 822–823
radiological diagnosis of, 819–822
sex predilection of, 805–806
subchiasmal, 818–819
suprachiasmal, 818
surgery for
direct, 826–827
indirect, 825–826
surgical technique, 828–836
Carotid siphon, 12
occlusion of, 1235
Carotid stenosis
bilateral, 406–407
and contralateral carotid occlusion, 407
unilateral, 406
Carotid subclavian bypass graft
failure of, 447–448
in subclavian steal, 447
variations on, 448
Carotid system, distal, reduced intravascular pressure in, 800
Carotidynia, 153
Cat, basilar artery of, transclivial approach to, 292
Catheter
balloon, *see* Balloon catheter
double-lumen, 1243
single-lumen, 1243
Catheterization
balloon, *see* Balloon catheterization
selective, 49–51
technique of, 50–51
Caudate vein, 45
Caudato-putaminal hemorrhage, 173
Cautery, bipolar, for aneurysm surgery, 912
Cavernous angioma, description of, 1081
Cavernous carotid artery
lateral main stem trunk of, 13
meningohypophyseal trunk of, 13
Cavernous sinus, 14, 1320–1322
AV communication of, 1321
embolization of, 1322
with isobutyl 2-cyanoacrylate, 1247
entrapment of, 1321–1322
penetration of, with balloon catheter, 1250–1251
surgical considerations for, 1321
surgical procedures for, 1321–1322
trauma to, 1321
Cavernous sinus thrombophlebitis, bacterial aneurysms of internal carotid artery and, 1055
Central lobe
external surface of, 20–21, 21–22
internal surface of, 21
venous drainage from, 40
Central nervous system
pathology of, effect on cardiac function, 124–125
punctures of, and risk of hemorrhage, 1062
Central retinal artery occlusion, 160
Cerebellar fossa, meninges of, 72–73
Cerebellar hematoma
acute onset of, 1285
chronic onset of, 1286
clinical course of, 1285–1286
clinical presentation of, 1285
diagnosis of, 1286–1287
etiology and pathology of, 1284–1285
incidence and mortality of, 1283–1284
subacute onset of, 1285–1286
treatment of, 1287–1289
Cerebellar hemorrhage, 173–174
hematoma expansion from, 1265, 1267
Cerebellar infarction, 1299–1308
case histories, 1303–1305
clinical course of, 1302–1306
clinical presentation of, 1302
common site of, 1300
diagnosis of, 1306
etiology and pathology of, 1300–1302
incidence and mortality of, 1299–1300
introduction, 1299
massive swelling accompanying, 1302
treatment of, 1307–1308
Cerebellum, malformations of, 1120–1128
clinical syndromes of, 1120–1121
diagnostic tests for, 1121–1122
natural history of, 1120
treatment of, 1122–1126
Cerebral aneurysm
hypoplasia and, 633
SAH from, incidence of, 841
Cerebral angiography
of anterior communicating artery area, 713–714
of basilar artery, 714
cross-compression technique, 717
equipment for, 708
extravasation of contrast medium during, 725, 727
of inferior cerebellar artery, 714, 717
of internal carotid artery, 714
intraoperative, 737
investigative, 708
magnification technique in, 711–712
of MCA bifurcation area, 714
of ophthalmic artery, 714
of posterior communicating artery, 714
postoperative, 737
quantity of contrast medium in, 711
radiographic projections of, 713
selection of side in, 709–711
sequences of, 711
subtraction technique in, 712–713

Cerebral angiography (*cont.*)
  TIA and, 310–314
  timing of, 708–709
Cerebral arteriography, in carotid ligation, 789–790
Cerebral arteriovenous malformations, *see* Arteriovenous malformations (AVM)
Cerebral arteritis, 581–601
  differential diagnosis, 595–601
  inflammation of unknown cause, 587–595
Cerebral artery
  anterior, *see* Anterior cerebral artery
  middle, 294–295
  posterior, *see* Posterior cerebral artery
Cerebral vein, internal, 46
Cerebral blood flow (CBF), 75
  anatomic considerations and, 485–486
  autoregulation of, 77
  in brain tissue acidosis, 79–80
  chemical control of, 77–78
  clinical application of data, 195–197
  clinical evaluation of, 190
  conducting vessels in, 485–486
  in disease states, 79–82
  and EC-IC bypass surgery, 469, 788–789
  and electroencephalographic determinations, in carotid ligation, 788
  and EC-IC bypass, 788–789
  indicator techniques
    diffusable, 193–195
    nondiffusable, 192–193
  in ischemia, 80–81
  localized derangement of, 315
  in mass lesions, 81
  metabolic control of, 75–77
  methods for estimating, 190–192
  methods for measuring, 82–85, 192
  in Moyamoya disease, 567
    operative treatment of, 575
  neurogenic control of, 78–79
  penetrating vessels in, 486
  pharmacology of, 79
  regional, during surgery, 192, 419
  regulation of, 75–79
  in stroke cases, 81–82
  studies of, in CVS, 775
  tomography of, 200–202
  total, 192
  Xe-133 inhalation and, 469
Cerebral blood flow values
  hemispheric and regional
    in normal patients, 195–196
    in stroke patients, 196
  regional, in stroke patients, 196–197
Cerebral circulation, monitoring of, 186
Cerebral dysfunction, vascular examination, 152–156
Cerebral embolus
  of cardiac origin, 371–372
  causes of, 366
  heart disease and, 365–366
Cerebral hemispheres, vascular anatomy of, 11–46
Cerebral hemorrhage, lobar, 174
Cerebral infarction, CT scanning of, 707
Cerebral ischemia
  due to ruptured aneurysm, 733
  "transient migrainous accompaniment" in, 364
  and bacterial endocarditis, 1052
  as complication of carotid ligation, 797
    management of, 797–798
  mimics of, 367
  primary orthostatic, 487
Cerebral parenchyma, disturbance of, and hypertensive ICH, 1261
Cerebral vasospasm (CVS)
  angiography in, 775–776, 845
  as complication of ruptured aneurysm, 707
  control of, 763–766
  CT scanning in, 774–775
  diagnosis and treatment of, 773–781
  diagnostic evaluation of, 774
  induced hypertension and, 780
  induced hypervolemia and, 780
  radionuclide brain scans in, 774
  regional CBF studies in, 775
  time course and frequency of, 773–774
  treatment of, 776–780
Cerebral vein
  deep, 44–45
  superficial middle, 39
Cerebral vessels, platelet interaction with endothelium of, 764
Cerebrovascular disease
  angiography of, 297–303
    complications of, 303–306
  atherosclerotic, 306–314
  contrast injections and, 298
  digital intravenous angiography of, 301–303
  DIVA in, 301–303
  DSA in, 343–357
  historical introduction, 1–7
  intracranial, 314–315
  ischemic, *see* Ischemic cerebrovascular disease
  neurological evaluation in, 129–174
  neuroradiology of, 297–340
    method of investigation, 297–303
  surgically related clinical findings in, 197–200
Cerebrovascular physiology, 75–85
  clinical evaluation of, 181–202
Cerebrovascular surgery
  cardiovascular considerations in, 117–125
  hematologic considerations in, 89–109
  thromboembolic complications of, 108–109
Cervical myelopathy, 535
Cervical radiculopathy, 535
Cervical spondylosis, vertebral artery insufficiency and, 529–553
Cervical spondylotic syndrome, 530
Cervical venous hum, 155
Children
  aneurysms in, with SAH, 949, 951–954
  AVM in, 954–962
    diagnosis of, 955
    natural history of, 954–955
    treatment of, 958–961
      results of, 961–962
  mycotic aneurysm in, 953–954
  posterior circulation aneurysms in, 952
  SAH in
    causes of, 941–944
      surgical, 944–949
    incidence of, 941
    miscellaneous surgical causes of, 962
    secondary to systemic disease, 944

traumatic aneurysm in, 953
vein of Galen malformations in, 944–949
clinical presentation of, 947
treatment of, 947–949
Cholesterol embolization, 596–597
Choroidal artery, anterior, *see* Anterior choroidal artery
Chronic completed stroke, 405–406
Cigarette smoking, risk of stroke and, 361
Ciliary circulation, posterior, occlusion of, 160
Cingulate sulcus, 19
Circle of Willis, 11
aneurysm sites near, 617
anterior
abnormalities of, 631–633
aneurysms arising on, 625, 629
communication patterns in, 333
posterior, 645–657
anomalies of, 645, 647
and basilar artery, 645–657
bifurcation of, 647
neural relationships of, 647
spontaneous occlusion of, *see* Moyamoya disease
subclavian steal and, 445
Circulation aneurysm, anterior, 671, 673
after aneurysm, 671, 673
carotid ligation for *see* Carotid ligation
posterior, 909–923
in children, 952
efficacy of surgery for, 909–910
history of surgical approaches to, 910–911
mortality after surgery for, 910
surgical adjuncts in, 911–912
surgical exposure of, 912–922
Circulation ischemia, posterior, occlusion of, 160
Cisternal blood, patterns of, in ruptured aneurysm, 694
Classical scattering, of radiation, 1164
Clinical stroke syndrome, classification of, 359–360
Clips, vascular, *see* Vascular clips
Clivial artery, lateral, 70
Clot retraction, 93
Clotting Factor VII, deficiency of, 95
Clotting Factor VIII, von Willebrand's disease and, 94
Clotting Factor X, deficiency of, 98
Clotting pathways
common, 97–102
inherited deficiencies in, 97–98
vitamin K deficiency in, 98–101
extrinsic, 94–95
intrinsic, 95–97
Coagulation system
anticoagulants and, 367–368
mechanism of, 94–102
Coating procedure, in treatment of aneurysm, 836
Cobalt-60 gamma unit, and radiosurgery, 1168–1171
Cogan syndrome, 593
Cold welding, and clip appliers, 1033–1035
Collagen, platelet aggregation and, 91
Collagen vascular disease, neuroradiology of, 322
Collateral channels, neuroradiology of, 333
Communicating artery
anterior, *see* Anterior communicating artery
posterior, 13–14
Completed stroke, 131–132
anticoagulant therapy in, 371
antiplatelet therapy in, 371
definition of, 360
Complicated plaque, in atherosclerosis, 361
Compton scattering, of radiation, 1164
Computed tomography (CT), 469
of AVM, 1102, 1121
of bacterial endocarditis, 1052
of carotid-ophthalmic aneurysm, 820–821
of cerebellar hematoma, 1286–1287
of cerebellar infarction, 1306
of CBF, 192, 200–202
of CVS, 759, 774–775
of head, 690, 693–722
of hypertensive ICH, 1260–1261
diagnosis of, 1270–1273
of ICA aneurysm, 842–845
of Moyamoya disease and, 577
role of, in postoperative care, 708
of ruptured aneurysms, 986–987
stroke detection and, 333–340
of venous angiomas, 1140–1141
Computed tomography radiation attenuation coefficients, 693
Confluens sinuum, 1318–1319
Congenital disorders, SAH and, 1062–1063
Congenital saccular (berry) aneurysm, 679–682
distribution of sites of, 681–682
portions of, 680
unruptured, 680–681
Congestive heart failure, preoperative considerations, 119
Conjugate gaze palsy, 158
Conn's syndrome, SAH and, 1065
Connective tissue disease, 587–594
Consciousness
impairment of, as contraindication for ligation, 792–793
levels of
and cerebellar hematomas, 1285
and pontine hematomas, 1290–1291
loss of, 134–136, 644
Contact activation co-factor (CAC), 96, 97
Contraceptive drugs, vascular abnormalities and, 329
Contralateral carotid occlusion, carotid stenosis and, 407
Contrast angiography, CBF and, 190–191
Contrast injections, cerebrovascular disease and, 298
Contrast medium
extravasation of, from aneurysm during angiography, 725, 727
quantity of, in cerebral angiography, 711
Cooperative study classification, of SAH, 757
Coronary artery disease, carotid endarterectomy and, 118
Corpus callosum, 28–29
malformations of, embolization of, 1156

Corpus callosum (*cont.*)
vascular supply to, 28
venous drainage from, 41
Corrosion, of vascular clips, 1028–1029
laboratory evidence of, 1029–1030
Cortical artery pressure, in EC-IC bypass surgery, 468
Cortical vein, superficial, 37–38
Coumarin, 367–368
Counterpressors, 282
Cranial arteritis, neuroradiology in, 321–322
Craniocervical bruit, 155
Craniopharyngioma, Moyamoya disease and, 570
Craniotomy
for ICH, 1277
types of, 663
Crural paresis syndrome, 171
Crutchfield clamp, for carotid ligation, 795
"Cryptic" angioma, 1088–1089
CSF cyanide, and SNP, 225–226
Curare, 221
Current passage, in electrothrombosis, 970–971
Cyanoacrylate adhesives, *see also* Plastic adhesive
characteristics and toxicity of, 503–505
types of, 505
Cyclotron, 1164

Dacron prosthesis, 384–385, 385
Dacron sutures, 390
Death, ICH and, 1267–1268
Debrun's latex balloon, 1240–1245
iodine-filled, 1243–1244
silicon-filled, 1244–1245
type 1, 1240
type 2, 1243
Degos' disease, 593
Depth dose, of radiation received, 1165
Dexamethasone, 538
prior to intracranial surgery, 846
Dextran (Rheomacrodex), 538
and blood, 391
after intracranial surgery, 853
after SAH bypass, 476
Diabetes mellitus, risk of stroke and, 360
Diagnostic radiology, therapeutic techniques in, 393–394
Diastolic bruit, 155
Diazepam (Valium), prior to intracranial surgery, 847
Diazoxide (Hyperstat), 121
Digital angiography, 55
Digital arch angiography (DAA), 354–357
selective, 357
Digital fluorography, 302
Digital intravenous angiography (DIVA)
of cerebrovascular disease, 301–303
complications of, 346–347
indications for, 351–354
results of, 347–351
suboptimal studies, 348–349
technique of, 345–346
Digital subtraction angiography (DSA), 401–404, 470
advantages of, 343–344
in cerebrovascular disease, 343–357
after EC-IC bypass surgery, 479
image quality of, 344
injection site of, 344–357
physical principles, 343–344
Digoxin (Lanoxin), 123
Dilatation, ventricular, after ruptured aneurysm, 729–730
Diploscope, binocular, 241
Dipyridamole (Persantine), 368–369
for TIA, 370
Disease states, CBF in, 79–82
Dissecting aneurysm, 743
Disseminated intravascular coagulation (DIC), 101–102
chronic, 102
induction of, 106
management of surgical bleeding in, 107–109
Diuretic therapy, 120–121
Dizziness, in vertebral artery insufficiency, 531, 534
Dog
microvascular neurosurgery in, 294–295
MCA operations in, 294–295
Doll's eye maneuver, 158
Doppler examination
direction of flow, 184
frequency content, 185
mean frequency, 184–185
Doppler imaging device, 182–183
Doppler shift, 184
Doppler sonography
in Moyamoya disease, 567–568
operative treatment of 576
Dosage, integral, of absorbed energy, 1165
Double-lumen catheter, 1243
Drake-Kees clip, for aneurysm surgery, 912
"Drop attack", in vertebral artery insufficiency, 534
Drug abuse, 148
Drug abuse patient, arterial changes in, 329
Drug arteriris, 600–601
d-tubocurarine, for intracranial surgery, 847
Duke test, 93
Dura mater, incision of, in ICH 1277
Duraencephalosynanjiosis, Moyamoya disease and, 572
Dural arteriovenous malformations, 1128–1133, *see also* Arteriovenous malformations, dural
Dural sinuses
introduction, 1311–1312
laceraction of, without tissue loss, 1313–1314
loss of surface of, suturing and, 1314
reconstruction of, intima-lined stent in, 1317
surgery of, 1311–1322
trauma to, 1313–1317
tumor invasion of, 1317
and vein grafting, 1314
technique for, 1314–1317
Durapexia, and Moyamoya disease, 572
Dynamic studies, in CVS, 774
Dysarthria-clumsy-hand syndrome, 171
lacunes and, 366
Dyscrasias, blood, as cause of SAH, 944
Dysfibrinogenemia, 98
Dysplasia, fibromuscular, 597–598

Eastman 910 (Methyl 2-cyanoacrylate), 503–504
Edema, pulmonary, preoperative conditions in, 119
EDH-adhesive (Biobond), 505

Ehlers-Danlos syndrome,
aneurysms associated with,
1063
Elderly patient, preoperative
considerations, 120
Electrodes, thrombogenic,
insertion of, 969–970
Electroencephalography (EEG)
CBF in carotid ligation, 788
in Moyamoya disease, 568
for ruptured aneurysms, 986
during surgery, 417–418
Electronic attenuation coefficient,
1164
Electrothrombosis, 967–982
clinical results of, 980–981
historic background to, 967–968
indication for, 968–969
insertion of electrodes for, 969–
970
intraoperative angiography for,
971–973
methods of, 969–973
representative cases of, 973–980
Embolectomy, arterial, 391–393
Embolic stroke, 132–133
Embolism, 148
multiple, 596
Embolization
of AVM, 1103–1105
of cavernous sinus, 1322
with isobutyl 2–cyano-
acrylate, 1247
of cerebral AVM, 1151–1160
complications of, 1159
conclusions of, 1159–1160
contraindications to, 1159
history of, 1151–1152
introduction, 1151
technical considerations in,
1152
new, 1159
for control of headache, 1159
of dural AVM, 1132
of intracranial AVM, 1152–
1159
for progressive neurologic
deficit, 1158–1159
for seizure control, 1158
of vein of Galen malformations,
1156–1158
Embolus
atheromatous debris, 363–364
cerebral, 365–366
cardiogenic, 371–372
intra-arterial, 363
platelet-fibrin, 363
retinal, 401
Encephalitis
herpes simplex, 586
neuroradiology in, 321
varicella-zoster, 586–587
viral, 586–587
Encephalomyosynangiosis (EMS),
and Moyamoya disease,
571
Endarterectomy, carotid, *see*
Carotid endarterectomy
Endocarditis
bacterial, *see* Bacterial
endocarditis
marantic, 151
nonbacterial, 151
Endothelium, platelet interaction
with, of cerebral vessels,
764
Energy, absorbed, integral dose
of, 1165
Energy absorption coefficient,
1164
Energy transfer coefficient, 1164
Enflurane, 122, 226–227
Entrapment, of cavernous sinus,
1321–1322
Ependymomas, SAH and, 1067
Epidural abscess, 321
Epilepsy, and vertebro-basilar
insufficiency, 534
Epinephrine, platelet aggregation
and, 91
Epsilon aminocaproic acid
(EACA)
prior to intracranial surgery,
846
for SAH, 762–763
Equipment, for cerebral
angiography, 708
Established stroke, definition of,
360
Etat lacunaire, 366
Ethanol intoxication, SAH and,
1062
Ethmoidal Moyamoya, 563
Ethyl 2–cyanoacrylate, 504
Etiology
of carotid cavernous fistulas,
1229–1232
of cerebellar hematomas, 1284
of cerebellar infarction, 1300
of pontine hematomas, 1290
Etiopathogenesis, of carotid-
ophthalmic aneurysm, 817
Euglobulin lysis time, 103
Evolution, of hypertensive ICH,
1261, 1264–1265
Excision, of dural AVM, 1132
Exposure
inadequate, for basilar
aneurysm surgery, 935–936
of MCA aneurysms, 864–866
aids to, 864
Extraanatomical blood vessel
graft, 391
Extracranial lesions, vs.
intracranial lesions, 362
Extracranial vascular disease
arch study of, 297–298
calcium in, 306
roentgenographic examination
of, 298–301
Extracranial-intracranial (EC-IC)
bypass surgery, 467–480
alternatives to, 476–478
arterial lesions and, 471–472
CBF and carotid ligation, 788–
789
clinical indications for, 470–471
clinical results of, 479
complications of, 479–480
contraindications, 472
DSA following, 479
future prospects, 480
hemodynamic basis for, 468–
469
for internal carotid aneurysms,
857–858
technique of, 858
introduction to, 467–468
other indications for, 472
postoperative angiography and,
479
preoperative evaluation, 469–
470
results of, 478–479
sequence of procedures, 473
technique of, 473–476
timing of, 472–473
Extrinsic clotting pathway, 94–95
Eye movements, abnormalities of,
and pontine hematomas,
1291
Eyepiece, of operating
microscope, 237

Facial palpation, in carotid artery
disease, 187
False aneurysm, 738, 743
Falx cerebelli, 70, 72
Fat embolism, 148
Fatty streak, in atherosclerosis, 361
Femoral artery
bypass in rabbit, 293–294
exercises on, 291–292

Femoro-femoral bypass graft, 385
Femoro-tibial bypass graft, 385
Ferromagnetic properties, of vascular clips, 1035
Fibrin degradation products (FDP), 102
Fibrin split products (FSP), 102–104
Fibrinogen (Factor I), 95
  deficiency of, 98
    management of surgical bleeding in, 107
Fibrinolysins, anticoagulant drugs and, 390–391
Fibrinolytic mechanism, 102–104
  inhibitors of, 102
Fibromuscular dysplasia (FMD), 329, 597–598
Fibrous plaque, in atherosclerosis, 361
Fick principle, 193
Film arch angiography (FAA), 354–356
  limitations of, 354–355
Film subtraction angiography (FSA), 343–344
  image quality of, 344
Final common clotting pathway, *see* Clotting pathways
Fistula
  carotid-cavernous sinus
    case histories of, 975–976
    due to ruptured aneurysm, 735
  vertebral, treatment of, 1253–1256
Fitzgerald-Reid-Washington-Fleaujeac factor, 96
Fletcher factor (Prekallikrein), 96
Flip-flop phenomenon, CBF and, 191
Fogarty balloon catheter, 391–393
Foix-Alajouanine syndrome, 1078
Foramen (Foramina), transverse, unroofing technique of, 542–543
Forceps, predecessors of vascular clip, 999
Fossa, posterior, draining from, 69
    meningeal arteries of, 70–72
    vascular anatomy of, 49–73
Fossa angiography, posterior, 49–55
Fossa hematoma, posterior, 1283–1295
Fossa vasculature, posterior, 49–55
Frenzel glass, nystagmus through, 535
Frequency, of MCA aneurysm, 862
Frontal approach, to putaminal hemorrhage, 1277
Frontal artery, internal, 19
Frontal lobe
  external surface of, 15–17
  inferior surface of, 19, 21
  internal surface of, 17, 19
  venous drainage from, 39–40
Frontopolar artery, 19
Frontotemporal approach, to basilar aneurysms *see* Basilar artery aneurysm
Funduscopic examination, 159–161
Fungal intracranial aneurysm, 737–738, 1055, 1059
Fungemia, 585
Furosemide
  for basilar aneurysm surgery, 928
  to expose MCA aneurysms, 864
  and IPC, 218

Ganglionic blocking drugs, 227
Geometry factors
  affecting clip closing force, 1015
    implications of, 1024–1027
Gerald-style forceps, 249
Giant aneurysm, 701, 703
  completely thrombosed, 703
  electrothrombosis for, 979–980
  partially thrombosed, 703
  surgery for, 827–828, 831, 834–835
  thin-walled nonthrombosed, 701, 703
Giant-cell arteritis, 592–593
  headache of, 140–141
Glanzmann's thrombasthenia, 93
Glioma
  SAH and, 1066
  vascular malformations and, 1091
Glues, surgical, used in vascular clips, 1036
Graft occlusion, in interposition vein graft, 499
Granulomatosis, Wegener's, 589–590
Granulomatous angiitis, 594
"Gray-out of vision", vascular insufficiency and, 535
Great vein of Galen, 46
  malformation of, in children, 944–949
    embolization of, 1156–1158
Growth, of angiomas, 1091–1092
Gyrus artery, angular, 23–24

Hagman factor (Factor XII), 96
Half value layer (HVL), of beam, 1164
Halothane, 122, 226–227
  in carotid endarterectomy, 409
Haptoglobin, for CVS, 779–780
Harrison and Smyth's syndrome, *see* Subclavian steal syndrome
Head, CT scanning of, 690, 693–722
Headache, *see also* Migraine
  arteritis, 140–141
  control of, embolization for, 1159
Healing, after carotid endarterectomy, 420
Heart
  neurogenic influences on, 123–125
  stroke and, 150–152
Heart disease
  cerebral embolus and, 365–366
  valvular, preoperative conditions, 119–120
Heifetz clips, stress-corrosion failure of, 1030–1033
Hematocrit values, risk of stroke and, 361
Hematologic disease, SAH and, 1064
Hematologic factors, in cerebral ischemic events, 365
Hematoma
  access to, 1277–1279
    Sylvian sulcus approach to, 1278
    transtemporal lobe approach, 1277
  angiographic identification of, 724–725
  cerebellar, *see* Cerebellar hematomas

destruction of pyramidal tract by, 1269–1270
intracerebral, CT scanning of, 697–698
intracranial, as contraindication for ligation, 793
large, formation of, 1261
pattern of expansion of, 1265–1267
pontine, *see* Pontine hematoma
of posterior cranial fossa, 1283–1295
introduction, 1283
removal of, 1278
wound closure following, 1278–1279
subdural
CT scanning of, 700
due to ruptured aneurysm, 735
surgical approaches to, 1276–1277
wound, 420
Hemianopia, 158
homonymous, in interposition vein graft, 499
Hemichorea-hemiballismus syndrome, 171–172
Hemiparesis, ataxic, 171
Hemiparesis syndrome, ataxic, lacunes and, 366
Hemiplegia
acute infantile, Moyamoya disease and, 569–570
development of, mechanism for, 1269–1270
infantile-childhood, 586
pure motor, 171
Hemispheric data, on CBF, 197–198
Hemoclip, 257
Hemoconia, 90
Hemodynamic assessment, of venous angiomas, 1146–1147
Hemodynamic factors, in cerebral ischemic attacks, 364
Hemophilia
associated with SAH, in children, 944
hemorrhage and, 1064
and management during surgery, 106–107
Hemorrhage, 160, *see also* Rebleeding
anatomic location of, 142
in angiomas, 1092
from AVM, 1099, 1101
caudato-putaminal, 173
cerebellar, 173–174
hematoma expansion from, 1265, 1267
cerebral, lobar, 174
evolution of, 1261, 1264–1265
vs. infarction, clinical differentiation, 141–142
intracerebral, *see* Intracerebral hemorrhage
intraparenchymal, 172–174
intraventricular, CT scanning of, 699
late, aneurysm size and, 674–675
pontine, hematoma expansion from, 1265
putaminal, *see* Putaminal hemorrhage
recurrent, after carotid ligation, 798–799
subarachnoid, *see* Subarachnoid hemorrhage (SAH)
subcortical, hematoma expansion from, 1265
thalamic, 173
CT scanning of, 1272–1273
hematoma expansion from, 1265
Hemostatic agents, 390
Hemostatic defect
preoperative recognition of, 104–105
recognition during surgery, 106
surgical bleeding treatment for, 106–108
Hemotoma, angiographic identification of, 724–725
Heparin, 367–368
following surgery, 123
Herniation, due to ruptured aneurysm, 735
Herophilus(i), trocular, 1318–1319
deviations from anatomic noem, 1319
Herpes simplex encephalitis, 586
Heubner's artery, recurrent, 641–644
Heyer-Schulte detachable balloon, 1248
High-energy machines, 1163–1164
Hippocampal vein, 45
Histology, of venous angiomas, 1147
Historic background, to electrothrombosis, 967–968
Historical aspects
of carotid ligation, 785–787
of cerebrovascular disease, 1–7
of embolization of AVM, 1151–1152
of hypertensive ICH, 1259–1260
of intracranial aneurysms, 667–677
of multiple aneurysms, 983
of radiosurgery, in AVM, 1167–1168
of stereotactic thrombosis of aneurysms, 889–900
in surgical approach to posterior circulation aneurysm, 910–911
of vascular clips, 997–1006
early, 997–999
modern era, 999–1006
Hollenhorst plaques, 159
Homocystinuria, 601
Homolateral ataxia, 171
Homonymous hemianopsia, in interposition vein graft, 499
Hooke's law, equation defining, 1010
Horner's syndrome, 153, 157
Human placenta, acquisition of skill using, 295
Hunt classification, of SAH, 756–757
Hunterian ligation, variation of, 445
Hurler's syndrome, 150
Hydralazine (Apresoline), 121
Hydrocephalus
communicating, 730
CT scanning of, 707–708
Hyperlipidemia, risk of stroke and, 360
Hyperperfusion stain, vs. neoplastic stain, in neuroradiology, 317
Hypertension
and cerebellar hematomas, 1284–1285
complications following, 322–326
induced, and CVS, 780
lenticulostriate arteries and, 322
neurogenic, 125
neuroradiology of, 322–326
rebound, and SNP, 225
risk of stroke and, 360
SAH and, 1063–1064
following surgery, 223

Hypertensive fibrinoid arteritis, 597
Hyperthermia
  and pontine hematomas, 1291
  following surgery, 224
Hyperviscosity syndrome, 365
Hypervolemia, induced, and CVS, 780
Hypofibrinogenemia, 98
Hypoglossal paralysis, after carotid endarterectomy, 420
Hypoglycemia, 135
Hypophyseal artery, superior, 13
Hypoplasia, and cerebral aneurysm, 633
Hypoproconvertinemia, 95
Hypoprothrombinemia, 98
Hypotension
  introperative-controlled, 224–228, 847, 911–912
    maintenance of, 864
  induced, cerebral effects of, 227–228
  orthostatic, vascular insufficiency and, 534
Hypothermia, 219
Hyrocephalus syndrome, 136
Hysteresis, degree of, affecting clip closing force, 1019

IAP measurement, treatment of Moyamoya disease and, 576
Immune complex necrotizing vasculitis, 590
Incidental aneurysm, diagnosis of, 756
Infant, *see also* Children
  vein of Galen malformations in, 946–947
Infantile-childhood hemiplegia, 586
Infantile hemiplegia, acute, Moyamoya disease and 569–570
Infarction
  anatomic location of, 142
  cerebellar, *see* Cerebellar infarction
  cerebral, CT scanning of, 707
  vs. hemorrhage, clinical differentiation, 141–142
Infection
  after carotid endarterectomy, 420
  wound, after carotid ligation, 797
    management of, 798
Infectious arteritis, 583–587
Infectious diseases, SAH and, 1065
Infectious intracranial aneurysm, 737–738, 1047–1059
Infectious lesions, 321–322
Inferior cerebellar artery aneurysm
  anterior, angiography of, 717
  posterior, 714, 717
    detection of, 694
Inferior vena cava, and abdominal aorta, separation of, 291
Inferior vermian vein (IVV), 68–69
Inflammatory cerebral vasculopathy, 367
Infratentorial arteriovenous malformations, 1117–1134, *see also* Arteriovenous malformations, infratentorial
Innominate artery, occlusive disease of, 429–444
Instrumentation
  for microsurgical laboratory, 277–278
  for microvascular neurosurgery, 245–260
Insula, 27–28
  venous drainage from, 41
Integral dose, of absorbed energy, 1165
Intellect, 136
Internal carotid artery, 11–14
  bacterial aneurysms of, with cavernous sinus thrombophlebitis, 1055
  branches of, 12–13
    aneurysms of, 617–625
  cavernous portion of, 12–13
  damage to, 326
  occlusion of, 486
    management of, 471–472
  petrous portion of, 11–12
  spontaneous dissection of, 521–525
    angiographic findings in, 523–524
    clinical course and treatment of, 524–525
    clinical manifestations of, 522–523
    pathogenesis of, 521–522
  supraclinoid portion of, 13–14
    aneurysm sites on, 609
Internal carotid artery aneurysm
  angiography of, 714
  bacterial, with cavernous sinus thrombophlebitis 1055
  carotid ligation of, 785–787
  clinical presentation of, 842
  common sites of, 609, 617–625
  contralateral, as contraindication for ligation, 793
  CT scanning of, 699
  detection of, 694
  after ligation, 798
    anatomic changes, 799
  and relationship to branch arteries, 841
Internal carotid artery syndrome, 161–163
Internal carotid-posterior communicating artery aneurysm, 841–858
  anatomic considerations in, 841–842
  carotid ligation for, 857–858
    technique of, 858
  clinical presentation of, 842
  diagnostic evaluation of, 842–846
  EC-IC bypass for, 857–858
    technique of, 858
  intracranial surgery for
    preparation for, 846–847
    results of, 856–857
    techniques used in, 847–856
    timing of, 846
Internuclear ophthalmoplegia, 158–159
Interposition vein graft
  case history, 490–491
  complications of, 498–499
  in EC-IC bypass surgery, 480
  operative results, 498
  surgical technique of, 493–498
Intima-lined stent, in sinus reconstruction, 1317
Intra-arterial embolus, 363
Intra-parenchymal hemorrhage, syndromes of, 172–174
Intracerebral abscess, 321
Intracerebral hematoma, CT scanning of, 697–698
Intracerebral hemorrhage (ICH)
  hypertensive, 172
    classification, of, 1274–1275
    clinical features of, 172–173

CT classification of, 1270–1273
historical review of, 1259–1260
introduction, 1259
location of, 1260–1261
operative procedures, 1276–1277
pathology of, 1261–1267
pathophysiology of, 1267–1270
prognosis of, 1274
surgical treatment of, 1273–1276
rationale for, 1279–1281
surgical vs. conservative treatment for, 1275
spontaneous, 172
Intracerebral squeeze concept, in ICH, 1279–1281
Intracerebral steal, reversal of, 469
Intracranial aneurysm
associated with bacterial endocarditis, 1047–1055
bacteriology of, 1048
case history, 1054–1055
clinical presentation of, 1048, 1052
diagnostic studies of, 1052–1053
pathology and pathogenesis of, 1048
treatment of, 1053–1054
bacterial, associated with meningitis, 1055
carotid ligation of, 785–801
classification of, 679
fungal, 1055, 1059
history of, 667–677
incidence of, 679
infectious, 737–738, 1047–1059
lucency within, 727
microsurgical anatomy of, 607–663
multiple, *see* Multiple aneurysm
natural history of, 667–677
neoplastic, 743
neuroradiology of, 679–743
radiologic investigation and diagnosis of, 686–737
size of, 727
stereotactic thrombosis of, 899–907
current status of, 900–904
historical perspective, 899–900
patient selection, 904–907
results of, 905, 907
surgical technique, 903–904
Intracranial arteriovenous malformations, embolization of, 1152–1159
Intracranial artery, dissection of, angiography of, 525
clinical manifestations of, 525
pathogenesis of, 525
treatment of, 525
Intracranial bypass graft, for vertebrobasilar ischemia, 485–500
Intracranial calcification, abnormal, 690
Intracranial cerebrovascular disease, 314–315
Intracranial disease, DIVA for, 353–354
Intracranial hematoma, as contraindication for ligation, 793
Intracranial hemorrhage, hypertensive, timing of operation for, 1275–1276
Intracranial lesions, vs. extracranial lesions, 362
Intracranial neoplasm, SAH and, 1066
Intracranial pressure, increased, bony erosion and, 735
due to ruptured aneurysm, 735
and SNP, 225
and NTG, 226
Intracranial pressure (ICP), and treatment of hypertensive ICH, 1268–1269
Intracranial surgery, for aneurysms, preparation for, 846–847
results of, 856–857
technique of, 847–856
timing of, 846
Intracranial vascular disease, neuroradiology of, 314–315
Intracranial vasospasm, as contraindication for ligation, 793
Intracranial vertebral endarterectomy, for ischemia, 500
Intracranial transposition procedures, for ischemia, 500
Intraluminal angioplasty, for ischemia, 500
Intraoperative angiography, for electrothrombosis, 971–973
Intraparenchymal hemorrhage, syndrome of, 172–174
Intraspinal neoplasm, SAH and, 1066–1067
Intravascular approach, in treatment of aneurysm, 836
Intravascular pressure, measurements of, in carotid ligation, 787–788
Intravascular thrombosis, of portions of AVM, 1103–1105
Intravascular thrombus, 297
Intraventricular hemorrhage, CT scanning of, 699
Intrinsic clotting pathway, 95–97
Iodine-filled balloon, 1243–1244
Iron-acrylic, for stereotactic surgery, 902–903
Irrigating syringe, 256
Ischemia
CBF in, 80–81
cerebral, *see* Cerebral ischemia
posterior circulation, procedures for, 500
vascular, syndromes of, 161–170
vertebrobasilar
intracranial bypass graft for, 485–500
surgical intervention in, 499–500
Ischemic cerebrovascular disease
antithrombotic therapy in, 359–374
hematologic factors in, 365
hemodynamic factors in, 364
pathogenesis of, 361–367
Ischemic infarction, of brain, and hypertensive ICH, 1261
Ischemic stroke
CBS in, 81–82
epidemiology of, 360–361
risk factors, 360–361
Ischemic symptomology, introduction, 485
Ischemic syndromes, 487–488
Isobutyl 2–cyanoacrylate, 504–505
embolization of cavernous sinus with, 1247
Isodose curve, 1165

Isoflurane, 226–227
Isoproterenol (Isuprel), for CVS, 765, 778
Ivy test, 93

Jeweler's forceps, 248

Kanamycin, for CVS, 780
Karnofsky scale, 560
Kartchner-McRae method, of DBA, 184
Keratin meningitis, 599
Kidney
  bench surgery of, 389
  polycystic, aneurysms associated with, 1063
Kininogen, 96
Klinefelter's syndrome, SAH and, 1063
Korsakoff's syndrome, and aneurysms, 894–895
Krypton-79, CBF measurement with, 193
Krypton-85, CBF measurement with, 193
Krypton-77 emission tomography, CBF measuring by, 83–84

Labile factor (Factor V), 94, 95, 97
  deficiency of, 98
Laceration, of dural sinus, without tissue loss, 1313–1314
Lacunar disease, 170–172
Lacunar stroke, 133
Lacunes, ataxic hemiparesis syndrome and, 366
Language, 136
Large-vessel occlusive disease, patterns of, 486–487
Lasax, prior to aneurysmal surgery, 885
Lateral mescencephalic vein (LMV), 69
Lateral osteophyte, *see* Uncovertebral osteophyte
Lateral (transverse) sinus, 39, 1318–1319
  deviations from anatomic norm, 1319
  surgery of, 1319–1320
  thrombosis of, 1320
  trauma of, 1319
Lateral vein, direct, 45–46
Lees-Duncan-Kistler method, of SBA, 184
Leksell rongeur, 245
Lens, objective, of operating microscope, 235
Lenticulostriate artery, hypertension and, 322
Leptomeningeal collateral channels, 333
Lesions
  extracranial vs. intracranial, 362
  infectious, 321–322
  space-occupying, due to ruptured aneurysm, 735
Leukemia, associated with SAH, in children, 944
Leukoencephalopathy, acute hemorrhagic, 595
Lidocaine (Xylocaine), 123
  for CVS, 778
  for intracranial surgery, 847
Ligaclip, 257
Ligation, carotid, *see* Carotid ligation
Linear attenuation coefficient, 1164
Linear energy transfer (LET), 1165
Liver disease, coagulation pathway and, 101
Lobar cerebral hemorrhage, 174
Locked-in syndrome, 167
Longitudinal sinus, inferior, 1317–1318
Longitudinal sinus, superior, 1312–1313
    deviations from anatomic norm, 1313
Low force clips, 1002
Lupus erythematosis, arterial changes in, 322
Luxury perfusion, 315–321
  concept of, 315
Lymph vessel anastomosis, 388–389
Lymphnodo-capsularvenous shunt, 388–389

Magnesium sulfate, for CVS, 779
Magnification changer, of operating microscope, 235–236
Malleable clips, 999–1000
Mammary souffle, 155
Mannitol
  for basilar aneurysm surgery, 928
  and brain-volume reduction, 218
  to expose MCA aneurysms, 864
  and IPC, 218
  prior to aneurysmal surgery, 886
Marantic endocarditis, 151
Marfan's syndrome, 150
Mass lesions, CBF in, 81
Matas test, in carotid ligation, 794
Mayfield clip, 257
Mayo stand, 259–260
Mechanical factors, of clip-function dynamics, 1014–1027
Medullary syndrome, lateral, 165
Meglumine diagrizoate (Angiografin), 538
Meningeal artery, of posterior fossa, 70–72
Meningeal vessels, 157
Meningiomas, SAH and, 1066
Meningitis, 583–584
  bacterial intracranial aneurysms and, 1055
  keratin, 599
  neoplastic, 598
  neuroradiology in, 321
  "red", 583
  tuberculous, 148–149
Menkes kinky-hair syndrome, SAH and, 1063
Mesencephalic vein
  lateral, 69
  posterior, 68
Metallurgic factors
  affecting clip closing force, 1015
  of clip-function dynamics, 1027–1035
  in clip production and use, 1027–1028
Methyl 2–cyanoacrylate (Eastman 910), 503–504
Methylprednisolone, for SAH, 763
Meyer's loop, 160
Microaneurysm, plasmatic arterionecrosis and, 1261
Microdissection techniques, for MCA aneurysms, 866–868

Microembolus, 391
Microligature carriers, 281–282
Microscope, operating, *see* Operating microscope
Microsurgical anatomy, of intracranial aneurysm, 607–663
Microsurgical irrigation, 281
Microsurgical laboratory, 273–278
  animal area in, 278
  current, 275–276
  equipment for, 276–278
    audiovisual, 276–277
  machine shop for, 278
  purpose of, 273
  staffing of, 274–275
  types of, 273–274
Microsurgical technique, for total excision, of spinal AVM, 1226–1228
Microvascular neurosurgery, *see also* Neurovascular surgery
  alligator instruments in, 253–254
  anastomoses, 288–290
  arm rest in, 259–260
  bipolar coagulator in, 255–257
  clips in, 257–258
  dissectors in, 253
  in dogs, 294–295
  forceps for, 248–249
  hemostatic clips in, 257
  instrumentation in, 245–260
    care of, 260
    principles of, 245–248
  knives in, 252–253
  microinstruments for, 280–284
  micropatch technique, 287
  needle holders in, 251–252
  nerve hooks in, 253
  operating microscope in, 233–242
  operating table and seating arrangements, 280
  photodocumentation in, 261–272
  retractors in, 258–259
  scissors in, 249–251
  specific laboratory exercises, 284–286
  suction devices in, 254–255
  suturing technique, 286–287
  technical skills in, acquisition of, 279–295
Middle cerebral artery (MCA), 15–17, 27
  AVM involving, embolization of, 1153–1155
  cortical branches of, 15–17
  course of, 15
  horizontal segment of, 31–33
  microsurgical anatomy of, 645
  occlusion of, 472
Middle cerebral artery aneurysm, 861–875
  alternative management of, 874–875
  anesthesia for, 863–864
  angiography of, 714
  clinical presentation of, 862
  common sites of, 609
  CT scanning of, 699
  detection of, 694
  distribution and frequency of, 862
  large, techniques for, 868–873
  ligation for, 792
    anatomic changes, 799
  location of, 645
  microdissection techniques for, 866–868
  positioning and exposure of, 864–866
  preoperative clinical grade of, 862–863
  results of treatment for, 873–874
  surgical anatomy of, 861–862
  surgical approaches to, 863
Middle cerebral artery syndrome, 164–165
Migraine, 141
  control of, embolization for, 1159
  ophthalmoplegic 158
Minimum occlusion force (MOF)
  clinical concerns, 1036
  quantification of, 1014
Minor stroke, antithrombotic therapy for, 369
Mitral valve prolapse, 150
  cerebral embolus and, 366
Mobile fulcrum type clip, 1002
  force exerted by, equation for, 1023–1024
Morbidity
  associated with AVM, 1101–1102
  associated with intracranial surgery, 857
  late, after aneurysm, 676–677
Morphine sulfate, as anesthetic, for MCA aneurysms, 863
Mortality
  associated with AVM, 1101–1102
  associated with intracranial surgery, 857
  of cerebellar hematomas, 1283–1284
  of cerebellar infarction, 1300
  in first six months after SAH, 671
  late, after aneurysm, 677
  of pontine hematomas, 1289
  after surgery, for posterior circulation aneurysm, 910
Moyamoya disease, 315, 322, 472, 557–577, 596
  AIH and, 569–570
  aneurysms and, 565
  angiography of, 562–565
  CBF measurement in, 567
  clinical examination in, 562–568
  clinical signs and symptoms of, 558–560
  CT scans in, 565–567
  diagnosis of, 568–570
  Doppler sonography in, 567–568
  duraencephalosynanjiosis and, 572
  durapexia and, 572
  EEG in, 568
  EMS and, 571
  epidemiology of, 558
  ethmoidal, 563
  etiology of, 558
  historical review, 557–558
  IPA measurement, 3376
  medical treatment of, 570
  omentum transplant and, 571–572
  operative treatment in
    results of, 572–577
  pathology of, 560–562
  SAH and, 1064
  STA-MCA bypass and, 570–571
  treatment of, 570–572
  vault, 563
Moyamoya vessels, 560
Mucin embolization, 599
Mucoraceae hyphae, 149
Mucormycosis, 149
Multiple aneurysm
  age distribution of, 983–984
  blood pressure and, 984
  case history of, 990–994

Multiple aneurysm (*cont.*)
clinical features of, 983–985
diagnosis of, 985–987
history of, 983
identification of, 985
incidence of, 983
location of, 984–985
management of, 983–994
pathogenesis of, 985
sex predilection of, 983
subarachnoid pressure and, 984
treatment of, 989–990
untreated, natural history of, 987–989
Multiple angioma, 1090
Multiple embolism, 596
Mycotic aneurysm, 585
in children, 953–954
Myelopathic syndrome, 530
Myelopathy, cervical, 535
Myleography, for spinal AVM, 1223
Myocardial infarction, perioperative risk of, 118
Myxoma, 598–599

Natural history
of AVM, 1099, 1101–1102
of intracranial aneurysm, 667–677
Neck, carotid ligation at, 825–826
Necrosis, radiation, and radiosurgery of AVM, 1203–1208
Neoplasm
intracranial, and SAH, 1066
intraspinal, 1066–1067
Neoplastic intracranial aneurysm, 743
Neoplastic meningitis, 598
Neoplastic stain, vs. hyperperfusion stain, in neuroradiology, 317
Neoplastic vasculopathy, 326–329
Nephritis, SAH and, 1065
Nerve root syndrome, 530
Neurogenic hypertension, 125
Neurogenic influence, on heart, 123–125
Neurologic abnormalities, ill-defined, DIVA for, 351
Neurologic deficit, progressive, embolization for, 1158–1159
Neurologic state, after SAH, 668
Neuro-ophthalmologic examination, 156–157
Neuro-ophthalmologic signs, 157–159
Neuroradiology
of cerebrovascular disease, 297–340
method of investigation, 297–303
of intracranial aneurysm, 679–743
Neurovascular examination, 142
Neurovascular surgery
anesthesia for, 213–228
anesthetic drugs and, 219–221
anesthetic technique in, 221–222
brain-volume reduction, 218–219
controlled hypotension and, 224–228
heparin following, 123
hypothermia and, 219
intraoperative considerations, 122–123
intraoperative problems, 222–223
monitoring, 216–217
patient assessment in, 117–123
patient positioning, 217–218
postoperative care, 123
postoperative problems, 223–224
preoperative considerations, 117–120
preoperative evaluation, 215–216
Newborn, *see also* Children
SAH, causes of, 941–943
vein of Galen malformations in, 945
surgical approach to, 945–946
Newtonian fluid, equation defining, 1011
Nifedipine, for CVS, 779
Nipride, 121, 224–226
Nitroglycerin (NTG), 226
Nitroprusside, for CVS, 778–779
Nitrous oxide, CBF measurement with, 193
Nonatherosclerotic vasculopathy, 366–367
Nonbacterial endocarditis, 151
Noninflammatory cerebral vasculopathy, 367
Nonradioactive xenon tomography, CBF measuring by, 84–85
Norepinephrine, for CVS, 780
Nuclear magnetic resonance (NMR), 470
CBF measuring by, 85
Nystagmus, 159
through Frenzel glass, 535
optokinetic (OKN), 161

Objective lens, of operating microscope, 235
Occipital arcade, 70
Occipital artery pedicle
to cerebellar artery bypass procedure,
case histories, 488–490
to PICA bypass procedure, 488–490
surgical technique of, 491–493
Occiptial artery pedicle-PICA bypass procedure
case histories, 488–490
complications of, 498
operative results, 498
surgical technique of, 491–493
Occipital lobe
external surface of, 24
inferior aspect of, 24–25
internal surface of, 24
venous drainage from, 40
Occipital sinus, 1318
deviations from anatomic norm, 1318
Occipitoparietal artery, 25
Occipitotemporal artery, 24
Occlusion
intolerance to, as contraindication for ligation, 793
thrombotic, 362–363
Occlusive disease
clinical manifestations of, 430–432
diagnosis of, 432–434
etiology and incidence of, 429–430
of great vessels, 429–444
large-vessel, patterns of, 486–487
percutaneous transluminal balloon angioplasty in, 442–443
surgical treatment of, 434–443
results of, 443–444
vertebrobasilar, 487–488
"Ocular bobbing", 159
and pontine hematomas, 1291

Ocular complex, 156–157
Ocular tube, of operating microscope, 237
Oculomotor nerve palsy, 157
Oculoplethysmography (OPG), in carotid artery disease, 187–188
Omentum transplant, and Moyamoya disease, 571–572
Operating microscope
  accessories for, 240–241
  advantages of, 234
  for aneurysm surgery, 912
  care of, 242
  components and functions of, 235–237
  field of vision of, 239
  focus adjustments for, 241–242
  focus of, 239
  history of, 233–234
  illumination systems of, 239–240
  light path of, 237–238
  magnification of, 238–239
  in microvascular surgery, 233–242
  modern features of, 234–235
  support and balance for, 241
  used in intracranial surgery, 848
Operative procedures, for hypertensive ICH, 1276–1277
Ophthalmic artery, 13, 163
  aneurysms of, 618, 622
  branches of, 156–157
Ophthalmic artery aneurysm, 618, 622
  angiography of, 714
Ophthalmodynamometry (ODM), in carotid artery disease, 188
Ophthalmoplegic migraine, 158
Optic stimuli, vascular insufficiency and, 534–535
Optical beam splitter, of operating microscope, 236
Optokinetic nystagmus (OKN), 161
Orbital bruit, 155
Orbital circulation
  monitoring of, 186–188
  superficial, tests of, 186–187
  tests of, deep, 187–188
Orbital vessels, 156
Orbitofrontal artery
  branch of ACA, 19
  branch of MCA, 16
Orthostatic cerebral ischemia, primary, 487
Orthostatic hypotension, vascular insufficiency and, 534
Osteoarthrosis, apophyseal, 530
Osteophytes
  producing vertebral artery compression, 530
  unconvertebral, 530
    removal of, 542
    roentogenographic investigation of, 535–538
Oxalosis, 601
Oxygen, effect on CBF, 78

Pacemaker, 122
  reduced surgical morbidity with, 120
Pair production, radiation and, 1164
Palsy, pseudobulbar, 171
Paradoxical embolism, 148
Parahemophilia, 98
Paralysis
  denial of, 162
  hypoglossal, after carotid endarterectomy, 420
Parietal artery, anterior, 26
Parietal lobe
  external surface of, 23–24
  internal surface of, 24
  venous drainage from, 40
Parietotemporal junction, venous drainage from, 40
Parietotemporal region, 22–24
  external surface of, 23–24
  internal surface of, 24
Partial nonprogressing stroke (PNS), definition of, 360
Partial thromboplastin, 96
Partial thromboplastin time (PTT), 96–97
Passovoy factor, 96
Pathogenesis
  of AVM effects on spinal cord, 1218–1219
  of bacterial intracranial aneurysms, 1048
Pathology
  of angiomas, 1073–1093
  of AVM, 1117–1119
  of bacterial intracranial aneurysms, 1048
  of cerebellar hematomas, 1284–1285
  of cerebellar infarction, 1300–1302
  of hypertensive ICH, 1261–1267
  of pontine hematomas, 1290
  radiation, of blood vessels, 1166–1167
Pathophysiology
  of dural AVM, 1131
  of hypertensive ICH, 1267–1270
Patient
  grading of, with SAH, 756–758
  with ICH
    preoperative classification of, 1273–1275
    surgical treatment of, 1276
  late rebleeding, characteristics of, 674
  positioning of
    in basilar aneurysm surgery, 928–929
  selection of, in stereotactic surgery, 904–907
    in stereotaxic radiosurgery, 1171, 1174
Pencil-style scissors, 250–251
Penicillium, and fungal intracranial aneurysm, 1059
Percutaneous transluminal balloon angioplasty, in occlusive disease, 442–443
Percutaneous vertebral angiography, direct, 51, 54
Perfusion, luxury, 315–321
    concept of, 315
Periarterial stripping, 543
Periarteritis nodosa, 587–589
  SAH and, 1065
Pericallosal artery aneurysm, CT scanning of, 694, 697
Pericallosal vein, 41
Periorbital directional Doppler ultrasonography (PDDU), in carotid artery disease, 186–187
Petrosal arcade, 70
Petrosal sinus
  inferior, 1321
  superior, 14
Pharmacological management, reduced surgical morbidity with, 120
Pharmacology, and SAH, 1067
Phenobarbital, for SAH, 761
Phenoxybenzamine, for CVS, 778
Phenytoin, prior to intracranial surgery, 846
Phonoangiography, 183–184

Phosphodiesterase inhibitors, for CVS, 779
Photodocumentation
 advanced video techniques, 271–272
 basic principles of, 261–264
 in microvascular neurosurgery, 261–272
 technique of, 267–271
 video equipment for, 264–265
 video recorders in, 265
 video theory and, 265–267
Photography systems, 276–277
Physics, radiologic, 1162–1165
Physiology, of carotid ligation, 787–790
PICA bypass procedure, *see* Occipital artery pedicle-PICA bypass procedure
Pineal gland, calcified, displaced or shifted, 686
Pivot type clips, 1002
 force exerted by, equation for, 1022–1023
Placenta, human, acquisition of skill using, 295
Plaque
 atherosclerotic, 297
 "bright", 401
 complicated, 361
 fibrous, 361
 ulcerated, 310
Plasma thromboplastin antecedent (PTA), 96
Plastic adhesive
 aneurysm treatment with, 505–508
 AVM treatment with, 508–511
 CCF treatment with, 511–512
 vascular reconstruction with, 512–515
Plastic monomer, aneurysms and, 599–600
Platelet adhesion, 92–94
 laboratory testing of, 92
 role of prostacyclin in, 764
Platelet aggregation, 90–92
 ADP and, 91
 arachidonic acid and, 92
 collagen and, 91
 epinephrine and, 91
 measurement of, 90
 role of thromboxane A_2 in, 764
 thrombin and, 92
Platelet disorders, 94
Platelet effects, and SNP, 226
Platelet factor 3 (PF-3), 93, 96
Platelet-fibrin embolus, 363
Platelet function, tests of, 93–94
Platelet functional disease, surgical bleeding in, 107
Platelet retention, 92
Platelets, 90–94
 interaction with endothelium, of cerebral vessels, 764
Pneumoencephalography, of carotid-ophthalmic aneurysm, 820
Polycystic kidney, aneurysms associated with, 1063
Polypropylene sutures, 390
Polytetrafluoroethylene graft, 385
Pontine hematomas, 1289–1295
 clinical course of, 1291
 clinical presentation of, 1290–1291
 diagnosis of, 1291, 1294
 etiology and pathology of, 1290
 incidence and mortality of, 1289
 treatment of, 1294–1295
Pontine hemorrhage, 174
 hematoma expansion from, 1265
Pontine syndrome
 lateral inferior, 167–168
 lateral superior, 168
 medial superior, 168
Positioning clip, 283
Positron emission tomography (PET), and CBF, 200–202
Posterior cerebral artery (PCA)
 AVM involving, embolization of, 1154–1156
 P-1 segment of, 655–656
Posterior cerebral artery syndrome, 168–170
Posterior circulation aneurysm, *see* Circulation aneurysm, posterior
Posterior communicating artery, 13–14
Posterior communicating artery aneurysm
 angiography of, 714
 clinical presentation of, 842
 long term outcome after, 671–677
 short term outcome after, 669–671
Posterior inferior cerebellar artery (PICA), 55–59
Posterior inferior cerebellar artery syndrome, 165–166
Posterior mesencephalic vein (PMV), 68
Posterior parietal artery, 23
Postishemic stroke, CBF in, 81–82
Postoperative care, role of CT in, 708
Precentral artery, 16–17
Precentral cerebellar vein (PCV), 68
Prefrontal artery, 16
Pregnancy, 148
 SAH and, 1065
Prekallikrein (Fletcher factor), 96
Preoperative management, of hypertensive ICH, 1276
Procainamide (Procan), 123
Progressing stroke, 131, 487
 anticoagulants in, 370–371
 antiplatelet drugs in, 371
 definition of, 359–360
 management of, 405
Propranolol (Inderal), 119, 123
Prostacyclin (PGI), 368–369
 role in platelet adhesion, 764
Protamine gel test, 103
Protein C, 100
Prothrombin (Factor II), 95, 97
 deficiency of, 98
Prothrombin time (PT), 96
Prothrombinase complex, 95, 96
Proximal dissection, of MCA aneurysms, 863
Pseudobulbar palsy, 171
Pseudodementia, 136
Pseudohemophilia, SAH and, 1064
Pseudoxanthoma elasticum, SAH, 1063
Psychologic amnesia, 534
Psychomotor seizure, 135–136
Psychoorganic syndrome, and AComA aneurysms, 894
Pterional approach, to aneurysm surgery, 919–920
 proponents of, 921–922
 to basilar aneurysm surgery, 926–927
Ptosis, 157
Pulmonary edema, preoperative considerations, 119
"Pulseless" disease, 429
Puncture, CNS, and risk of hemorrhage, 1062
Pupillary abnormality, 158
Pure sensory stroke, 171
Purpura, thrombocytopenic, 597

Putaminal hemorrhage
"vulnerable triangle" in, 1269
classification of, 1274–1275
CT scanning of
advanced type, 1271–1272
localized type, 1271
hematoma expansion from, 1265
surgical approaches to, 1277
surgical vs. conservative treatment for, 1275
Pyogenic aneurysm, 737–738
Pyramidal tract, destruction of, by expanding hematoma, 1269–1270

Rabbit, femoral artery bypass in, 293–294
Radiation
for AVM, 1102–1103
measurement of, 1164–1165
obliteration of AVM by, 1209, 1211
of pathologic vessels, vs. feeding arteries, 1202
X and Y, interaction of, 1164
Radiation necrosis, and radiosurgery of AVM, 1203–1208
Radiation pathology, of blood vessels, 1166–1167
Radiation vasculopathy, 329
Radiculopathy, cervical, 535
Radioactive substances, naturally occurring, 1163
Radioactivity, artificial, 1163
Radiobiology, of blood vessels, 1165–1167
Radiographic projection, of cerebral angiography, 713
Radiologic diagnosis
of carotid-ophthalmaic aneurysm, 819–822
of SAH, 758–760
therapeutic techniques in, 393–394
of venous angiomas, 1140–1167
Radiologic equipment, for balloon catheterization, 1248–1250
Radiologic evaluation, of carotid cavernous fistula, 1233–1235
Radiologic investigations, of intracranial aneurysms, 686–737
Radiologic physics, 1162–1165
Radionuclide angiography, CBF and, 190–192
Radionuclide brain scans, of CVS, 774
Radionuclide imaging, in stroke, 333–340
Radionuclide scintigraphy, of venous angiomas, 1145–1146
Radiosurgery
of cerebral AVM, 1161–1211
Co-60 gamma unit and, 1168–1171
conclusion, 1211
historical sketch, 1167–1168
introduction, 1161
radiobiology of vessels in, 1165–1167
radiologic physics in, 1162–1165
stereotaxic, 1168–1211
Radiotherapy, vs. radiosurgery, in AVM, 1168
Rads, as measure of radiation, 1165
Rebleeding, *see also* Hemorrhage; Subarachnoid hemorrhage
aneurysmal
in first six months, 669–671
after six months, 671
incidence of, EACA and, 763
late
and aneurysmal site, 674–675
characteristics of, 674
late morbidity and, 676–677
late mortality and, 677
and radiosurgery of AVM, 1208–1209
Recurrent artery complex, anterior cerebral-anterior communicating, 625–645
"Red" meningitis, 583
Regional anesthesia, for carotid endarterectomy, 408
Regional data, on CBF, 198–199
Reserpine, for CVS, 780
Respiratory distress syndrome, associated with SAH, 942
Respiratory disturbance, and pontine hematomas, 1291
Respiratory motion, suboptimal DIVA studies and, 349
"Rete mirabile", 563
Retinal artery, pressure determination of, in carotid ligation, 788
Retinal embolus, 160, 401
Retractors, in microvascular neurosurgery, 282
Retrograde brachial angiography, 51
Reversible ischemic neurologic deficit (RIND), 131, 487
antithrombotic therapy for, 369
definition of, 359
Rheology, 89–90
Rheomacrodex (dextran), 538
and blood, 391
after intracranial surgery, 853
after STA bypass, 476
Rheumatic heart disease, 150
Rheumatoid arthritis, 593
Ring scissors, 250
Roentgen, 1162–1163
as measure of radiation, 1164–1165
Roentgenography, of extracranial vascular disease, 298–301
Romberg's sign, 535
Roth's spot, 151, 160
Rubber dam platforms, in microvascular neurosurgery, 282
Rubeosis oculi, 159

Saccular aneurysm
angiomas and, 1091
basic anatomy of, 607–617
congenital (berry), 679–682
distribution of sites of, 681–682
portions of, 680
unruptured, 680–681
sites of, 607–617
distribution of, 681–682
unruptured, 680–681
Sagittal sinus
inferior, 39
superior, 38–39, 1312–1313
deviations from anatomic norm, 1313
Sarcoidosis, 594–595
Scalp cirsoid angioma, case histories of, 973–975
Scalp incision, to approach ICA aneurysm, 847–848
Schonlein-Henoch syndrome, SAH and, 1065
Scintigraphy, radionuclide, of venous angiomas, 1145–1146
Sedation, for SAH, 761
Segmental tertiary atherosclerosis, 596

Seizure
from AVM, 1101
contol of, embolization for, 1158
psychomotor, 135–136
Seldinger's technique, of evaluation of carotid cavernous fistula, 1233–1235
Selverstone clamp, used in carotid ligation, 858
Sensorimotor stroke, 171
Sensory symptoms, 137–138
Septal vein, posterior, 45
Septicemia, 584–585
Sex predilection
of carotid-ophthalmic aneurysms, 805–806
multiple aneurysms and, 983
Shake-whiplash syndrome, and SAH, 943–944
Sickle cell anemia, and SAH, 1064
Silicon-filled balloon, 1244–1245
Silicone tubes, in microvascular neurosurgery, 283–284
Silk sutures, 390
Single-lumen catheter, 1243
Single-photon emission computed tomography (SPECT), and CBF, 200
Sinus, *see individual types*
Sinus alae parvae, 1321
Sinus fistula, carotid-cavernous, due to ruptured aneurysm 735
case histories, 975–976
Skin, incision of, in treatment of ICII, 1277
Skull, plain x-ray of, 686, 690
"Slow stroke", 359
Sodium nitroprusside (SNP), 121, 224–226
Sonography, Doppler, in Moyamoya disease, 567–568
operative treatment of, 576
Space-occupying lesion, due to ruptured aneurysm, 735
Sparks Mandril graft, 385
Speech, 136–137
Sphenoparietal sinus, 1321
Spinal artery, anterior, 59
Spinal artery syndrome, 165
Spinal cord arteriovenous malformations, 1217–1228, *see also* Arteriovenous malformations, spinal cord
Spinal drainage
as adjunct, for aneurysm surgery, 912
to expose MCA aneurysms, 864
prior to aneurysmal surgery, 886
Splenial vein, 41
Spring clips, *see* Vascular clips
Spring scissors, 249
STA-MCA anastomosis, 468
surgical technique in, 473–476
STA-MCA bypass graft
Moyamoya disease and, 570–571
surgical technique in, 473–476
Staphylococcus
and bacterial aneurysms, 1048, 1055
Staphylococcus aureus, 151, 1054
Static scans, in CVS, 774
Steal, angioma, 1092–1093
"Steal" syndrome, *see* Subclavian steal syndrome
Stereotactic apparatus, 900–901
Stereotactic magnetic technique, 900–904
Stereotactic probe, 902
Stereotactic thrombosis, of aneurysms, 899–907
current status of, 900–904
historical perspective, 899–900
patient selection, 904–907
surgical technique, 903–904
Stereotaxic radiosurgery
for cerebral AVM, 1168–1211
Co-60 unit for, 1168–1171
latency and, 1202–1203
method and material, 1168–1187
neurologic condition and, 1203
patients and, 1171, 1174
procedure for, 1176–1187
radiation necrosis and, 1203–1208
rebleeding after, 1208–1209
results and discussion, 1187–1211
target for radiation, 1171
Stokes-Adams attack, 134–135
Straight sinus, 1318
Strain, equation defining, 1009–1010
Streptococcus, and bacterial aneurysms, 1048
Streptococcus viridans, 151
Stress, equation defining, 1009
Stress-corrosion failure, of Heifetz clips, 1030–1033
Striate vein, 41
"String sign" 301, 353, 523–525
Stroke, *see also specific types*
cardiac, causes of, 150–152
CBF in, 81–82
clinical history in, 129–131
contraceptive drugs and, 329
CT and radionuclide scanning in, 333–340
EC-IC bypass surgery for, 470
neurovascular examination, 142
risk factors, 141
symptom complexes of
analysis of, 133–134
features of, 134–141
terminology in 131–133
Stroke-in-evolution, 131
definition of 359–360
Stroke-prone patient, regional CBF values in, 196–197
Stump pressure measurements, during surgery, 418–419
Sturge-Weber syndrome, SAH and, 1063
Subarachnoid hemorrhage (SAH), *see also* Hemorrhage; Rebleeding
aneurysmal
classification of, 756–758
diagnosis of, 756–760
management of, 755–768
preoperative management of, 760–763
radiologic diagnosis of, 758–760
symptoms of, 758
and bacterial endocarditis, 1052
and carotid-ophthalmic aneurysm, 816–817
cause of, 679–680
from cerebral aneurysm, incidence of, 841
in children, 941–962
causes of, 941–944
incidence of, 941
secondary to systemic disease, 944
surgical causes of, 944–949, 962
long term outcome of, 671–677
multiple aneurysms and, 984
neoplasms associated with, 1066–1067

neurologic state of patient with, 668
pharmacology associated with, 1067
short term outcome of, 669–671
stages of, 667–668
timing of surgery in, 766–768
trauma associated with, 1061–1066
Subclavian artery, occlusive disease of, 429–444
Subclavian bruit, 154
Subclavian steal syndrome, 166, 430, 432, 445–462
bypass procedures in, 447–449
advantages of, 449
causes of, 445
circle of Willis and, 445
clinical course and manifestations of, 446
historical review, 445–446
preoperative evaluation of, 446–447
surgical procedures in, 447–461
vertebral artery ligation in, 449
vertebral to carotid transposition in, 451
case histories, 451–462
comment on, 461–462
Subclavian to subclavian bypass graft, 448
Subcortical hemorrhage, hematoma expansion from, 1265
Subdural hematoma
CT scanning of, 700
due to ruptured aneurysm, 735
Subdural hygroma, in interposition vein graft, 499
Subependymal vein, 41
lateral group of, 45–46
medial group of, 45
Suboccipital approach, to aneurysm surgery, 913–914
Subtemporal approach, to aneurysm surgery, 922
Subtemporal craniotomy, 633
Subtemporal technique, anterior, of aneurysm surgery, 916–9191
Subtraction technique, in cerebral angiography, 712–713
Suction tips, 281
Sulfinpyrazone (Anturane), 369
Superficial temporal artery (STA), bypass surgery on, 474–476
Superior cerebellar artery (SCA), 63–68
Superior cerebellar artery syndrome, 168
Superior cerebellar vein (SCV), 69
Supratentorial arteriovenous malformations, 1097–1113
see also Arteriovenous malformations, supratentorial
Supratentorial vein, 37–38, 44–45
Surgery
for ACA aneurysms, 885–892
for AComA aneurysms, 885–892
aneurysm, anatomic principles of, 657, 663
for AVM, 1107–113
suboccipital approach, 1122
subtemporal approach, 1126
for basilar aneurysm, 929–935
for carotid-cavernous fistula, 1235–1236
for carotid-ophthalmic aneurysm
direct, 826–827
indirect, 825–826
for giant aneurysm, 827–828
for hypertensive ICH, 1273–1277
intracranial, *see* Intracranial surgery
on lateral sinuses, 1319–1320
for MCA aneurysms, 863
for posterior circulation aneurysms, 912–922
efficacy of, 909–910
group 1, 913–914
group 2, 914–916
group 3, 916–922
history of, 910–911
for SAH, timing of, 766–768
for spinal AVM, 1223–1225
thromboembolic complications of, 108–109
vascular, *see* Vascular surgery
Surgical adjuncts, in posterior circulation aneurysm, 911–912
Surgical anatomy
of carotid-ophthalmic aneurysm, 816
of MCA aneurysm, 861–862
Surgical approach, to vein of Galen malformations in newborn, 945–946
Surgical bleeding, treatment of, 106–198
Surgical clips, *see* Vascular clips
Surgical glues, used in vascular clips, 1036
Surgical instruments, serrated blades on, 1021–1022
Sutures, 390
Suture tying forceps, 284
Swallowing, suboptimal DIVA studies and, 348
Sylvian fissure approach, to putaminal hemorrhage, 1277
Sylvian sulcus approach, to hematoma, 1278
Sylvian vein, 39
Sympathomimetic amines, for CVS, 777–778
Synchrocyclotron 1164
Syncope, 487
Syndrome of inappropriate release of antidiuretic hormone (SIADH), and aneurysms, 893–894
Systemic blood pressure, in carotid endarteretomy, 409
Systemic disease
and SAH, 1063–1066
SAH secondary to, in childhood, 944
Systemic lupus erythematosus (SLE), 590–592
SAH and, 1065

Tachyphylaxis, to SNP, 225
Takayasu's arteritis, 333, 429, 592
Taki's detachable balloon, 1248
Tansient ischemic attack (TIA), carotid lesions in, 400–401
Telangiectasis
description of, 1081, 1085
SAH and, 1063
Teletherapy machines, 1163–1164
Temporal approach, to putaminal hemorrhage, 1277
Temporal arteritis, 592–593
headache of, 140–141
Temporal artery, inferior, 26–27
Temporal lobe
external surface of, 25–26
inferior aspect of, 26–27
superior surface of, 27
venous drainage from, 40–41
Temporo-occipital artery, 24
Tentorium cerebelli, 70

Thalamic artery
  inferior group of, 35
  posterior group of, 35
  superior group of, 35–36
Thalamic hemorrhage, 173
  CT scanning of
    advanced type, 1273
    localized type, 1272–1273
  hematoma expansion from, 1265
Thalamo-perforating artery, 35, 656
Thalamostriate vein, 41, 45
Thalamus, 33–36
  destruction of, 1273
  nuclei of, 34
  vascular supply to, 34–36
  venous drainage from, 41, 44
Thermography, in carotid artery disease, 187
Thiopental
  as anesthetic, for MCA aneurysms, 863
  for intracranial surgery, 847
Thrombectomy, venous, 393
Thrombin, platelet aggregation and, 92
Thrombocytopenia, 93
  hemorrhage and, 1064
Thrombocytopenic purpura, 597
Thromboembolic complication, of surgery, 108–109
Thromboembolic disease, treatment of, 109
Thromboendarterectomy, 389–391
Thrombogenesis, 362
Thrombogenic electrodes, insertion of, 969–970
Thrombophlebitis, 148
Thromboplastin (Factor III), 95
Thrombosis
  after carotid endarterectomy, 421
  electrically-induced, *see* Electrothrombosis
  induced, in treatment of aneurysm, 836
  intravascular, of portions of AVM, 1103–1105
  of lateral sinuses, 1320
  spontaneous, of angiomas, 1093
  stereotactic, *see* Stereotactic thrombosis
  venous, 367
Thrombotic occlusions, 362–363
Thrombotic stroke, 132
Thromboxane A, 92, 368–369
  role in platelet aggregation, 764
Thrombus, intravascular, 297
Thromophlebitis, cavernous sinus, internal carotid artery aneurysm and, 1055
Thyrotoxicosis, SAH and, 1065–1066
Time/activity curves, carotid artery disease and, 191
Tinnitus, vascular insufficiency and, 534
Tissue adhesive, 503–515, *see also* Plastic adhesive
Tolosa-Hunt syndrome, 593–594
Tomography, CBF measuring by, 83–85
Top of the basilar syndrome, 168
Toxicity, of cyanoacrylate adhesives, 503–505
Tracheostomy, technique of, 284–285
Transbrachial retrograde arteriography, 538
Transclivial approach, to basilar aneurysm, 911
Transcortical exposure, of MCA aneurysms, 863
Transdural collateral channels, 333
Transexamic acid, for carotid-ophthalmic aneurysms, 823
Transfemoral catheterization, complications of, 303
Transient global amnesia (TGA), 151–152
Transient ischemic attack (TIA), 487
  anticoagulant therapy for, 369–370
  antiplatelet therapy for, 370
  antithrombotic therapy for, 369
  atypical, 406
  cerebral angiographic study of, 310–314
  definition of, 359
  dipyridamole for, 370
  DIVA for, 351–353
  EC-IC bypass surgery for, 470
  headache of, 140
  hemodynamic factors in, 364
  management of, 404
"Transient migrainous accompaniment", in cerebral ischemia, 364
Transitional forms, of angiomas, 1085, 1088
Transplant, omentum, and Moyamoya disease, 571–572
Transtemporal lobe approach, to hematoma, 1277
Transverse foramina, unroofing technique of, 542–543
Trauma, 143
  birth, as cause of SAH, 942–943
  as cause of SAH, in children, 943–944
  of cavernous sinus, 1321
  to dural sinuses, 1313–1317
  to lateral sinuses, 1319
  neuroradiology following, 326
  and SAH, 1061–1062
Traumatic aneurysm, 738, 743
  of carotid artery, ligation for, 792
  in children, 953
Traumatic dissection
  of blood vessels, pathogenesis of, 525–526
  of vessels
    angiography of, 526–527
    clinical course and treatment of, 527
    clinical manifestations in, 526
Trichopoliodystrophy, SAH and, 1063
Trigeminal artery, carotid cavernous fistula associated with, 1229
Trimethaphan (Arfonad), 121, 227
Trocular herophili, 1318–1319
  deviations from anatomic norm, 1319
Tuberculous meningitis, 148–149
Tumor
  focal encasement of, 598
  sinus invasion by, 1317
Twining's line, 59

Ulcerative plaque, 310
  management of, 406
Uncectomy, with removal of osteophyte, 542
Uncovertebral osteophyte, 530
  removal of, 542
  roentogenographic investigation of, 535–538

Valium (Diazepam), prior to intracranial surgery, 847
Valsalva maneuver, 1221
Valvular heart disease, preoperative considerations, 119–120
Varicella-zoster encephalitis, 586–587
Vascular abnormality, contraceptive drugs and, 329
Vascular anastomosis, technique of, 386–389
Vascular anatomy
  of cerebral hemispheres, 11–46
  of posterior fossa, 49–73
Vascular approximators, 1004–1005
Vascular clip appliers, 1003–1004
  clinical concerns of, 1036
  cold-welding and, 1033–1035
Vascular clip-force testing device, 1005–1006
Vascular clip-force values, 1027
Vascular clip-function dynamics, 1006–1035
  biological factors, 1006–1014
  mechanical factors, 1014–1027
  metallurgic factors, 1027–1035
Vascular clip-mediated damage, evidence of, 1006, 1008–1009
Vascular clip-reapplication, in aneurysm surgery, 937–938
Vascular clips, 283
  biocompatability of, 1028
    laboratory evidence of, 1029–1030
  classification criteria for, 1038
  color-coding system of, 1039
  corrosion of, 1028–1029
    laboratory evidence of, 1029–1030
  damage inflicted by, 1006, 1008–1009
  directions for future of, 1038–1040
  effective storage system for, 1039–1040
  force disclosure of, 1038–1039
  force values produced by, 1027
  historic and biomechanical perspective of, 997–1040
  improper selection of, 1036
  improvement of, 1037
  malleable, 999–1000
  materials of, 1039
  mechanical predecessors of, 999
  medical technology and clinical applications of, 1035–1038
  microstructure, homogeneity and magnetic interaction of, 1035
  in microvascular neurosurgery, 283
  modifications to, 1002–1003
  MOF of
    clinical concerns of, 1036
    quantification of, 1014
  placement of, aneurysmal rupture during, 936–937
  production and use of, metallurgic principles of concern in, 1027–1028
  quality control of, 1037–1038
  self-closing spring, 1000–1002
    alpha type, 1001–1002
    low force, 1002
    mobile fulcrum type, 1002
    Pivot type, 1002
  steel selection for, 1030–1033
  surgical cleaning agent for, 1040
  surgical glues used in, 1036
Vascular compression, 143
Vascular diagnostic laboratory, 393
Vascular disease
  causes of, 143, 148–152
  extracranial arteriosclerotic, as contraindication for ligation, 793
  neuro-ophthalmologic examination in, 156–157
  neuro-ophthalmologic signs in, 157–159
  SAH and, 1063–1064
Vascular examination, and cerebrovascular disease, 152–156
Vascular ischemia, syndromes of, 161–170
Vascular lesions, clip-mediated, 1006, 1008–1009
Vascular malformations, *see* Angioma
Vascular overlap, effect on DIVA studies, 349–351
Vascular pathology, DIVA visualization of, 347
Vascular reconstruction, with plastic adhesive, 512–515
Vascular rupture, and hypertensive ICH, 1261
Vascular surgery
  historical introduction, 383–385
  principles of, 383–394
  saphenous vein alternatives in, 385–386
Vascular sutures, 390
Vascular tissue
  mechanical properties of, current conceptual understanding of, 1009–1013
  properties of, 1009
Vascular topography, of brain, 14–36
Vasculitis, 367, 581
  immune complex necrotizing, 590
Vasculopathy
  inflammatory cerebral, 367
  neoplastic, 326–329
  nonatherosclerotic, 366–367
  noninflammatory cerebral, 367
  radiation, 329
Vasospasm
  angiographic identification of, 722–724
  cerebral, *see* Cerebral vasospasm
  intracranial, as contraindication for ligation, 793
Vault Moyamoya, 563
Vein grafting, in reconstruction of sinus, 1314
  technique for, 1314–1317
Vein of Galen, 46, 68
  malformation of, in children, 944–949
Vein patch graft, in carotid endarterectomy, 417
Vena cava, inferior, 291
Venous angioma
  of brain, 1139–1148
    clinical characteristics of, 1139–1140
    clinical outcome of, 1147–1148
    draining veins of, 1141
    hemodynamic assessments of, 1146–1147
    histology of, 1147
    introduction, 1139
    radiologic studies of, 1140–1146
    therapy for, 1147
  description of, 1079–1081

Venous thrombectomy, 393
Venous thrombosis, 367
Venticular dilatation, after ruptured aneurysm, 729–730, 735
Ventricular vein, inferior, 46
Verapamil (Calan), 123
Vermian vein, inferior, 69
Vertebral angiography
  for carotid cavernous fistula, 1233–1235
  for cerebellar infarction, 1306
Vertebral artery, 55–59
  occlusive disease of, 429–444, 486
  spontaneous dissection of
    angiography of, 525
    clinical manifestations of, 525
    pathogenesis of, 525
Vertebral artery aneurysm, common sites of, 611–617
Vertebral artery bruit, 154
Vertebral artery insufficiency
  auditory loss and, 534
  bilateral blurring and, 535
  case histories, 545–551
  cervical spondylosis and, 529–553
  criteria and indications for surgery in, 543–545
  dizziness and, 531, 534
  "drop attack" and, 534
  "gray out of vision" and, 535
  historical review, 529–530
  neurologic signs of, 535
  optic stimuli and, 534–535
  orthostatic hypotension and, 534
  osteophytes producing, 530
  postoperative care, 543
  roentgenographic investigation of, 535–539
  surgical results and postoperative management of, 552–553
  surgical technique in, 539–543
  symptoms and diagnosis of, 531–535
  TGA and, 534
  tinnitus and, 531, 534
Vertebral artery ligation
  of basilar aneurysm, 910–911
  in subclavian steal, 449
Vertebral fistula, treatment of, 1253–1256
Vertebral neurovascular syndrome, 530
Vertebral to carotid transposition, in subclavian steal, 451
  case histories, 451–461
  comment on, 461–462
Vertebrobasilar anatomy
  arterial angiography in, 55–68
  normal, 55–73
  venous angiography in, 68–73
Vertebrobasilar arterial system, arteroposterior views for 713
Vertebrobasilar insufficiency, 168
  epilepsy and, 534
Vertebrobasilar ischemia
  intracranial bypass graft for, 485–500
  surgical intervention in, 499–500
Vertebrobasilar occlusive disease, 487–488
Vertigo, 138–139
  in vertebral artery insufficiency, 531, 534
Video equipment, 264–265
Video recorders, 265
Video techniques, 271–272
Video theory, 265–267
Viral encephalitis, 586–587
Viscosity, of blood, 89
Vision, 139–140
Visualization, direct, of aneurysms, 700–701
Visual symptoms, and carotid-ophthalmic aneurysm, 817
Visual system, blood supply of, 156–157
Vitamin K_1 (Aquamephyton), 105
  deficiency of, in clotting pathway, 98–101
Vocal cord paralysis, after carotid endarterectomy, 420
Von Willebrand's disease, 94
  management of surgical bleeding in, 107
  SAH and, 1064

Wallenberg's syndrome, 165
Weber's syndrome, 169
Wegener's granulomatosis, 589–590
Weitlaner retractor, 258
Welding, cold, and clip appliers, 1033–1035
Wells stereotactic device, advantages of, 900–901
William's temporary clip, 258
Wolman's disease, SAH and, 1065
Wound
  closure of, after hematoma removal, 1278–1279
  infection of, after carotid ligation, 797–798
Wound hematoma, after carotid endarterectomy, 420

X and Y radiation, interaction of, 1164
X-ray, 1162–1163
  of abnormal intracranial calcification, 690
  plain skull, 686, 690
X-ray equipment, for stereotactic surgery, 901–902
Xenon, stable, and CBF, 200
Xenon-133
  CBF measurement with, 193–194
    inhalation of, 82–83, 469
    intracarotid vs. noninvasive, 194–195
    limitations of, 195
  intra-arterial, 82
Xenon-133 emission tomography, CBF measurment with, 84

Zeiss OPMI microscope, 262–264
Zoom microscope, 239
Zoster ophthalmicus, 586–587